# New Paradigms in Caregiving and Home Care

# New Paradigms in Caregiving and Home Care

Editor: Elizabeth Stephenson

MURPHY & MOORE
www.murphy-moorepublishing.com

www.murphy-moorepublishing.com

MURPHY & MOORE

**Cataloging-in-Publication Data**

New paradigms in caregiving and home care / edited by Elizabeth Stephenson.
p. cm.
Includes bibliographical references and index.
ISBN 978-1-63987-394-4
1. Home nursing. 2. Home care services. 3. Home health aides. 4. Medical care. 5. Care of the sick. I. Stephenson, Elizabeth.
RT120.H65 N49 2022
362.14--dc23



Murphy & Moore Publishing,
1 Rockefeller Plaza,
New York City, NY 10020, USA

ISBN 978-1-63987-394-4 (Hardback)

# Contents

# Preface

Caregiving involves providing emotional, physical and practical care to people who are unable to take care of themselves. Some of the responsibilities which fall under caregiving are managing the medications, interacting with nurses and doctors, performing household chores and documenting health. The professional care which is provided to a patient within the home is termed as home care. It involves communicating effectively with the person receiving care, managing the hygiene of the patient and the surroundings, and assisting the person in eating a healthy diet. Patients with diverse types of impairment might require caregiving. These impairments can be connected to a disease, advanced age, disability or a mental disorder. This book elucidates the concepts and innovative models around prospective developments with respect to caregiving and home care. It explores all the important aspects of this field in the present day scenario. This book will help the readers in keeping pace with the rapid changes in this field.

This book is a result of research of several months to collate the most relevant data in the field.

When I was approached with the idea of this book and the proposal to edit it, I was overwhelmed. It gave me an opportunity to reach out to all those who share a common interest with me in this field. I had 3 main parameters for editing this text:

1. Accuracy - The data and information provided in this book should be up-to-date and valuable to the readers.
2. Structure - The data must be presented in a structured format for easy understanding and better grasping of the readers.
3. Universal Approach - This book not only targets students but also experts and innovators in the field, thus my aim was to present topics which are of use to all.

Thus, it took me a couple of months to finish the editing of this book.

I would like to make a special mention of my publisher who considered me worthy of this opportunity and also supported me throughout the editing process. I would also like to thank the editing team at the back-end who extended their help whenever required.

**Editor**

# 1

# Caring for Individuals with Dementia on a Continuum: An Interdisciplinary Approach Between Music Therapy and Nursing

Kendra Ray, Ayelet Dassa, Jan Maier,
Renita Davis and Olayinka Ogunlade

**Abstract**

**Background:** Music has long been used to ease symptoms of dementia. Several studies have shown the therapeutic benefits of music therapy to decrease symptoms of agitation in people with dementia (PWD). Other research has demonstrated that the use of music during caregiving can ease agitated behaviors. However, few studies have shown the clinical benefits of using translational research in practice between music therapists and certified nursing assistants.

**Introduction:** We recruited 28 nursing home residents who were diagnosed with moderate to severe dementia to determine the effects of music therapy and music in aid of caregiving on symptoms of agitation.

**Methods:** Participants were evaluated for agitation, then baseline assessments were completed 2 weeks apart. After the 2-week music therapy intervention, participants were evaluated immediately, 2 weeks post music therapy, and immediately following music in aid of caregiving.

**Results:** A repeated measures analysis of variance (ANOVA) found that after 2 weeks of music therapy, agitation was significantly reduced and symptoms continued to decline following music in aid of caregiving.

**Conclusion:** Results suggest that consideration for interdisciplinary use of music therapy and music in aid of caregiving should be considered to reduce and sustain symptoms of agitation in nursing home residents with dementia.

**Keywords:** dementia, caregiving, Alzheimer's disease, nursing, nonpharmacological, music therapy, interdisciplinary, agitation, music, brain, neuroscience

# 1. Introduction

Caring for people with dementia (PWD) has become a focal point of policy makers, researchers, and healthcare providers. With over 30 million people globally and five million people in the USA diagnosed with Alzheimer's disease and other types of dementia, the need for capable and effective caregiving is necessary [1]. Music therapy has been shown to decrease neuropsychiatric symptoms of dementia [2]. It is well known that music serves as a positive nonpharmacological intervention, and when used therapeutically has the effect to reduce agitation in people who are diagnosed with dementia [3].

Caregiver burden in nursing professionals who work in long-term care facilities is often associated with compassion fatigue, burnout, moral, and psychological distress [4–6]. Music therapists are equipped with therapeutic tools that may assist in making caregiving tasks easier. Research has shown that both music therapy and caregiver-initiated music-based interventions can reduce agitation in people with dementia [7–10]. Singing and rhythm-based interventions are two examples of therapeutic techniques that may be initiated to aid in triggering a memory, changing a mood, or moving toward a desired behavior. Paid caregivers, such as nursing professionals, may be able to assist people with dementia even without any musical skills or background.

The aims of this chapter are to provide evidence of the effectiveness of a music therapy intervention used to lower agitation symptoms in nursing home residents with moderate to severe dementia. We give examples of music in aid of caregiving that may help sustain or further reduce symptoms of agitation. We hope that this chapter may be used as a resource for practitioners and paid caregivers to broaden the scope of how music may be used collaboratively in institutional settings such as nursing homes, hospitals, and hospices.

# 2. Literature review

## 2.1. Music therapy and neurological disorders

The use of music therapy in treating mental and neurological disorders is on the rise. Over the past 60 years, music therapy has developed as a clinically applied treatment in various healthcare settings administered by trained professionals who have completed an approved music therapy program.

Bonde et al. [11] explained that the process of defining music therapy both as a profession and as a discipline can vary depending on the orientation and perspective of a particular group of practitioners, or different cultures. However, the process of defining music therapy can be reflected in the way the profession itself has emerged in different countries and through various traditions. In this way, one has to take into consideration three main factors: professional background of practitioners, needs of the clients, and approach used in treatment. Music therapy can be defined as a three-dimensional therapeutic interaction between a trained music therapist, the music, and a patient who meet to reach defined goals and objectives.

Alzheimer's disease and other types of dementia are among the disorders most commonly treated with music therapy [12]. Music therapy for individuals with dementia focuses on improved communication, memory, behavioral management, and facilitating interactive relationships with therapists and carers. Music is seen as a tool to achieve those goals, and the outcomes of music sessions are measured either quantitatively [13, 14] or qualitatively [15, 16]. Hence, in both the neuroscience and music therapy models, music is used instrumentally as an isolated material for impacting change.

The research on music therapy with PWD focuses on two main topics. One examines the effect of music therapy on an increase in desirable behaviors such as concentration span and degree of participation in an activity, and the other examines how music therapy affects the reduction of unwanted behaviors such as restlessness, anxiety, and depression [17].

Music has the power to unlock memories, to be a safe place, and offer solace for people with dementia [18]. The greatest challenge, arguably, in unraveling the myriad effects of music on the brain is the sheer complexity and interactivity of neural network stimulation observed in response to music. As early as 1984, case studies and anecdotal reports described people with dementia with severe cognitive deficits who could still play and/or sing with surprising skill [13, 19–21]. This led to the development of the preservation theory—that areas of the brain involved in the recall of music memories may be preserved from the progression of the disease. Using functional magnetic resonance imagings (fMRIs) in 2009, Janata [22] suggested a role of the dorsal medial prefrontal cortex, which is slower to atrophy in Alzheimer's disease, in connection with emotionally salient long-term memories. In a more recent study, researchers used fMRIs to identify specific brain regions where musical long-term memories seemed to be stored (in the caudal anterior cingulate and the ventral pre-supplemental motor area) in healthy adults. They then contrasted scans of these same regions of healthy older adult controls with people with mild-moderate Alzheimer's disease. The results strongly support the preservation of these regions in people with Alzheimer's disease [23]. This access allows music therapists to connect with PWD where other potential treatments may fail.

### 2.2. Using music therapy to address agitation with PWD

Neuropsychiatric symptoms, such as agitation, in dementia have been estimated to be between 80 and 90%, and more than 80% of these symptoms persist for at least 18 months [24]. In nursing homes, agitation may be prevalent in up to 20% of individuals diagnosed with dementia [25]. Agitation may interfere with the nursing staff's ability to provide care as it is one of the most difficult symptoms to manage [26].

Many studies have shown that music therapy should be considered as treatment for individuals with dementia who exhibit signs and symptoms of agitation [10, 27–29]. In a systematic review, Livingston et al. (2014) analyzed 33 randomized controlled trials and found that music therapy along with other types of nonpharmacological interventions decreases overall agitation [30]. In their randomized controlled trial, Ridder et al.'s [31] results showed that after 6 weeks of music therapy, agitation in individuals with dementia was significantly reduced, while in the control group agitation increased. Other authors [32] found similar results for nursing home residents with dementia who received music therapy for 6 weeks. In comparison with the control group, agitation was significantly reduced following music therapy and results were sustained for 1 month after the music therapy intervention.

### 2.3. Daily care for PWD

With the rising number of individuals diagnosed with dementia accompanied by neuropsychiatric symptoms such as agitation, the need for capable care staff is imminent. Nursing professionals are challenged with the difficulty of tasks associated with caregiving and the behaviors that often accompany a diagnosis of dementia. PWD experience problems with activities of daily living including bathing, dressing, and eventually decision making, which for over 60% of people with dementia leads to institutionalization for assistance with care [33].

Caregiver burden in nursing home staff who work in long-term care facilities is often associated with compassion fatigue, burnout, moral, and psychological distress. These caregivers may be at risk of burnout between 5 and 37% of the time. Outcomes from a focus group performed concluded that nurses who care for people with dementia want to alleviate their suffering and improve their quality of life and may feel strained due to inadequate resources for caregiving [34]. Two other studies indicated an increasing prevalence in psychological distress in care staff who work in nursing homes for people with dementia [5, 6].

### 2.4. The use of music by care staff

Music medicine involves passive listening of music (usually recorded) that is provided by a medical practitioner or a paid caregiver. The music used during the interaction may or may not be selected based either on the subject's musical preference. Music medicine or music in aid of caregiving (as referred to in this chapter) is different from music therapy in that there is no attempt to develop a therapeutic relationship and the interaction does not involve psychological processes [35].

A review of nonpharmacological interventions among PWD over the past two decades found that music can decrease resistance to treatment and care [3, 29]. Music helps to reduce symptoms of anxiety during activities that pose difficulties. Several studies have documented the effectiveness of the use of music by care staff for people with dementia. One study found that nursing personnel who used singing had a positive effect on the individuals with dementia, including improved posture, increased awareness of self and surroundings, motivation, and skills to perform daily tasks. The care staff who sang with residents benefited by developing mutuality and increased interactions more than those who only played background music [36, 37]. PWD showed better cooperation and fewer behaviors exhibiting resistance to care when singing and recorded music were used, compared to these activities without the use of music [36]. Other benefits that caregiver singing appeared to influence was communication, decreased levels of aggression, and disruptive screaming [36]. Gerdner [38] has created evidence-based guidelines for paid caregivers to use individualized music for people with dementia. Her techniques are often used by professional caregivers to lessen symptoms of agitation in people with dementia. Hammar et al. (2011) performed a study using a technique called Music Therapeutic Caregiving (MTC). The author compared patterns of behavior in participants whose caregiver used the MTC with patterns of behavior of participants whose caregiver performed care as usual [39]. She found that the caregivers who did not use the MTC experienced more episodes of aggression and resistance from their care recipients than those who did not. In other studies using MTC, this author reported that caregivers described a feeling of well-being, happy, and positive interactions with the person who they were caring for. The individuals with dementia demonstrated increased positive emotions and expressed pleasure and appeared more alert due to the MTC [39].

Nursing professionals who sing and play background music can have positive effects on people with dementia. Results from a randomized controlled trial found that regularly listening to music and singing familiar songs can benefit people with dementia cognitively, emotionally, and socially. In this study, researchers found that these musical activities led by the nurses, family caregivers, choral leaders, and music therapists helped to reduce psychological burden and that singing and listening to music can have positive effects for up to 6 months for people with early dementia [40].

Other researchers have described qualitatively and quantitatively how music can help to reduce agitation during caregiving [37, 41–43]. A review article found that carers for people with dementia played a significant role in decreasing agitation and in the work of music therapy for elders with dementia in nursing homes [44]. Choi et al. [45] found that music therapy was useful in not only reducing agitation in residents with dementia but also reducing irritability, distress, and anxiety in their caregivers. Numerous studies reported that caregivers who used a tape player or a CD player were effective in reducing agitation in clients diagnosed with dementia [46–48]. Using music during caregiving taps into memories, stimulates emotions, inspires, rewards engagement, and has an effect on individuals with dementia like no other treatment [49].

#### *2.4.1. Training program for care staff: utilizing music in daily care*

Since music is an accessible tool that is a part of most people's day-to-day life, main elements (recorded music, singing, and rhythm) can be used by music therapists to instruct and make it possible for care staff, even those without any musical experience, to employ it in their work with PWD. Minimizing restlessness is significant and contributes to the person with dementia's quality of life, and also improves the caregiver's ability to give optimal and safe care. Music's positive effect renders it useful for relaxation and for softening resistance, and thus alleviating the day-to-day life of the caregiver and the person with dementia.

### 2.5. Elements of music: Background music, singing, and rhythm

The various musical activities that can be used in a training program for caregivers serve as a therapeutic tool with an optimum impact. Following is a review of the literature addressing each of these musical tools in working with people with dementia.

### 2.5.1. *The effect of background music*

Studies examining musical interventions among PWD indicate that individually or culturally matched music significantly increases the music's positive effect on the person. Individually matched music was found to be the best and most effective way to reduce restlessness among Alzheimer's patients [48, 50]. The effect of culturally matched background music on the degree of the patients' restlessness was examined among the residents of a retirement home [51]. While listening to music, a marked reduction in restlessness characteristics was observed, such as less shouting, repetitive requests for attention, and so forth. Also, positive behaviors such as singing, drumming/tapping to the rhythm of the music, smiling, and others were observed. On the other hand, when music was not heard, the number of problematic behaviors increased and the number of positive behaviors decreased [51].

### 2.5.2. *The effect of singing*

Singing has a central place in music therapy with PWD. The literature shows that despite their memory loss, these patients continue to sing old songs, which remain intact in their memory for longer than songs learned at a later stage in their lives. Episodic/explicit memory for songs is not only for the melody and lyrics but also for the world of associations and personal memories that the songs evoke. In practice, the songs work like a stimulus to evoke multitude memories associated with the song [22, 52–54]. The songs stimulate and encourage conversation associated with the topic of the song. Music therapy groups that focus on singing have led to an improvement in the patients' conversational capabilities and to a lively discussion about the experience of singing in the group [55]. Singing thus provides PWD with a feeling of social belonging. Singing is comforting in that it is a familiar activity, whereas cognitive activity arouses difficulty and frustration. Singing provides respites of stimulation, awareness, a pleasant feeling, and an experience of success [52]. The feeling of success is important among PWD encountering difficulty and poor functioning, which generally lead to a damaged sense of self-worth and depression. A music therapy group that focuses on singing and evoking memories can alleviate the symptoms of depression among PWD [56]. Singing can also reduce the degree of restlessness among PWD. A decrease in problematic behavior stemming from restlessness is evident during participation in a singing-focused music therapy group [57].

### 2.5.3. *The effect of rhythm*

Rhythm has an effect on the movement system. The body reacts automatically to rhythmic musical stimulus. Even when the listener is not moving, rhythm stimulates activity in the premotor cortex as if priming the body for movement [2, 58–60]. Movement to music is a common phenomenon across cultures, and moving in time with the beat (entrainment) appears to be pleasurable [61–64]. Toe tapping, head nodding, and dance involve perception of rhythm and the beat, which can enable synchrony among individuals, whether playing, singing, or moving.

Music helps to boost physical activity and it also has a calming effect. A group of 18 participants with dementia who took part in exercise sessions with background music showed a reduction in restlessness signs after 4 weeks of activity (twice a week), compared to a group of 18 patients who did not receive the intervention, but only "regular treatment"[50].

Even though many studies have investigated the effectiveness of using music therapy and music-based activities for people with dementia, there lacks evidence of a study that describes collaborative efforts between music therapy and nursing for nursing home residents with dementia. This study was intended to examine whether music therapy could reduce agitation in nursing home residents with moderate to severe dementia and if the reduction in agitation could be sustained or further reduced through the facilitation of music to aid in caregiving by Certified Nursing Assistants (CNAs).

## 3. Methods

### 3.1. Participants

#### *3.1.1. Certified nursing assistants (CNAs)*

At MJHS, certified nursing assistants (CNAs) are responsible for providing direct care to nursing home residents. Their duties include but are not limited to dressing, feeding, toileting, bathing, and other activities of daily living. CNAs have the most frequent and most intimate contact with nursing home residents. They report directly to unit nurse supervisors and the director of nursing who oversee their assignments and duties. At the time of the study, two CNAs reported singing with residents but for pleasure instead of with the desire to decrease or alleviate agitation. Only one of the CNAs had a history of formal musical training prior to this study. Previously, she was employed as a school teacher, but had not used music during her caregiving. For this study, there were eight CNAs recruited at the Menorah Center for Nursing and Rehabilitation, six at Metropolitan Jewish Geriatric Center, and 10 at Shorefront Center for Nursing and Rehabilitation. The majority of the CNAs were Black Caribbean American, followed by Latino and Russian. All were female, aged between 35 and 60 and reported to have five or more years of experience working with nursing home residents diagnosed with dementia.

#### *3.1.2. CNA training*

The CNAs participated in a 3-day intensive training course. The purpose of the training was to educate CNAs to facilitate music in aid of caregiving activities appropriate for the participants that they provided care. Topics in the training included foundations of music, recognizing and identifying agitation, working with an iPod for music in aid of caregiving, selecting person-preferred music and music that may influence participant behavior, and preventing agitation through the use of recorded music with six protocols that are described below. CNAs were tested on music in aid of caregiving facilitation and on their ability to use an iPod in a mock-group setting at the end of the training. Video recordings of the CNAs' use of music in aid of caregiving with participants were used for training purposes as a reflective process with the music therapist and to determine if additional education was needed.

CNAs were assigned an iPod mini that was attached to their uniform. The iPod was loaded with personalized playlists created by the research music therapist. The CNAs were also given portable speakers that could be easily stored in their pockets until ready for use. Selections for each song in the playlists were created based on individualized preference and the success of observed reductions of agitation during music therapy groups. The music therapists created other general playlists that were loaded onto the iPod. These were meant to stimulate, relax, or prompt caregiving activities depending on the need of the resident. Some examples of the types of playlists included the following: sing-a-long, Russian classical, music-assisted bathing, energizing, Caribbean, etc., **Figure 1**. As needed, the music therapists created playlists for CNAs to use with residents when they were engaged in activities that triggered agitation such as bath/shower time [42].

| Sing-a-long Playlist (24 minutes)<br>Song-Artist | Album |
|---|---|
| Side by Side<br>Kate Smith | I'll Be Seeing You |
| You Are My Sunshine<br>Rosemary Clooney | Learnin' the Blues |
| Hava Nagilah<br>The Moshe Silberstein Ensemble and Chorus | The Music of Israel |
| Tumbalalaika<br>Theodore Bikel | Yiddish Folk and Theatre |
| Quizas, Quizas, Quizas<br>Celia Cruz | Cuba Bella |
| Michael Row the Boat Ashore<br>Peter, Paul and Mary | Sing Along |
| Red River Valley<br>Frank Corrales and Cisco Trio | Sing Along |
| Tzenah Tzenah<br>The Neshoma Orchestra | Jewish Play Along |
| God Bless America<br>Kate Smith | The Best of Kate Smith |

**Figure 1.** Sample sing-a-long playlist. Source: Kendra Ray, Michael McGaughy, Scott Stuart, *Music Therapy: Keys to dementia care* (New York, MJHS) 34. Print [65].

There were six music in aid of caregiving protocols written by the research music therapists and used by the CNAs in this study. A detailed description of each of these protocols can be found online at https://issuu.com/mjhs/docs/2013_dementia_workbook_lr_fnl_upt. All protocols used participants' individually preferred music based on a music therapy assessment and were created specifically for the nursing home residents who participated in this study. The developed protocols were singing, music and movement, music-assisted bath/shower, music-assisted wound care, music-assisted range of motion, and tonal protocol. A variety were created in order for the CNA to have a selection to choose from that would fit most appropriately when addressing agitation. Each protocol lists the following criteria to be considered before use: staff requirements, objectives, entrance and exit criteria, duration, safety considerations, facility/equipment required, and methods for facilitation.

Singing protocol uses live and/or recorded background music to facilitate a meaningful opportunity and to prevent or reduce verbal and/or physical agitation during activities of daily living. Music playlists or CNA lead singing should be used while providing care. Communication and singing are emphasized in this protocol.

Music and movement uses background music to engage residents to decrease symptoms of agitation, such as unexplained motor activity or verbalizations, until they decrease or are diminished. For this protocol, CNAs are asked to lead movements using sensory-stimulating items such as scarves or ribbons. Pre-recorded playlists were provided that stimulate slow to moderate movement.

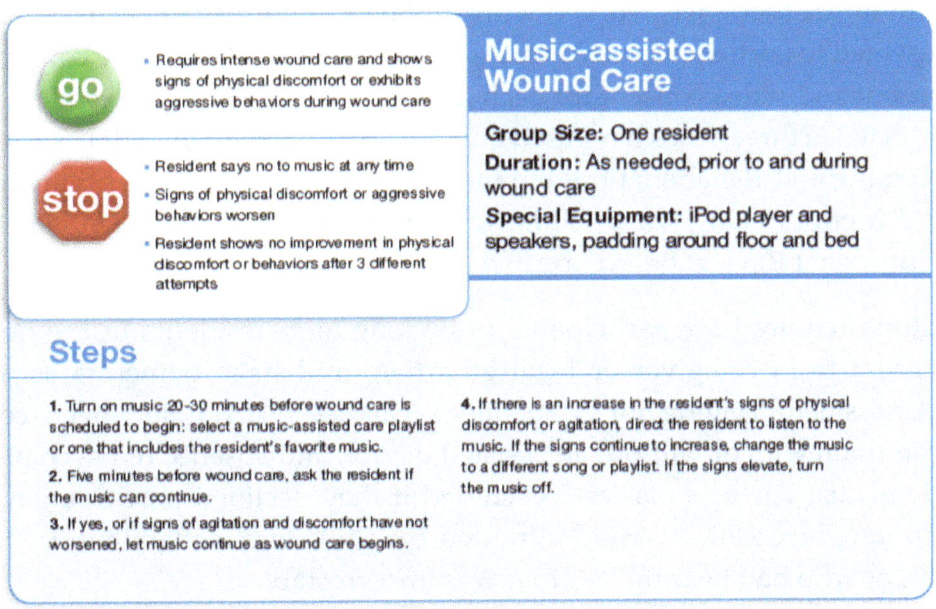


**Figure 2.** Abbreviated version of music-assisted wound care provided for CNAs and nursing staff. Source: Kendra Ray, Michael McGaughy, Scott Stuart, *Music Therapy: Keys to dementia care* (New York, MJHS) 70. Print [65].

Music-assisted bath/shower uses background music designed to decrease physical tension and aggressive behaviors often associated with bath time for nursing home residents with dementia. CNAs are encouraged to begin music during preparation of the bath/shower to reduce agitation and distract from anticipated stress. The selected music was customized with songs that have historically relaxed the resident. Communication, listening, and awareness of sensitivity to noise and temperature and other residents' preferences are emphasized.

For music-assisted wound care, staff are encouraged to play background music during preparation of wound care to distract the resident from anticipated stress or agitated behaviors. The music should continue to be played during and following the procedure to reach desired objectives that may include decreased discomfort, fewer or no aggressive behaviors toward nursing staff and less resistance to wound care. Instructions are demonstrated subsequently (**Figure 2**).

Music-assisted range of motion uses background music to motivate residents' involvement in motion exercises. The objectives are to decrease resistance to movement, and reduce episodes of agitation. CNAs are provided with songs of measured tempos that begin slowly and gradually increase in beats per minute as the playlist develops. Rhythm and movement are emphasized in this activity.

The tonal protocol is a music-based activity with an objective of reducing agitation and increasing socialization. Residents are encouraged to sing familiar songs and play tone bars as led by the CNA. Rhythm and movement are emphasized in this activity.

### *3.1.3. Residents*

The CNAs and music therapists worked with a total of 28 adults between the ages of 59 and 101 whom assented to participate in this study. Legal representatives were contacted to obtain informed consent and video consent for each individual. This was part of a larger study [10] that was conducted in three Brooklyn-based nursing homes, part of the MJHS system, Menorah Center for Nursing and Rehabilitation, the former Shorefront Center for Nursing and Rehabilitation, and Metropolitan Jewish Geriatric Center. The New York University School of Medicine Institutional Review Board approved the protocol for this study.

Inclusion criteria required for participants to be long-term residents in the nursing home, informed consent from caregiver or legal guardian, mid-stage dementia as measured by Functional Assessment Staging for Alzheimer's Disease (FAST), stabilized comorbidities, auditory recognition with or without an assisted device, and absence of psychiatric disorders other than dementia. Participants were excluded if they declined participation, were being introduced to new medications, were admitted for short-term rehabilitation, had unstable comorbidities, or who had hearing loss that was uncorrectable.

Consented participants were mostly female ($n$ = 26, 92.9%). The majority of participants were Caucasian ($n$ = 22, 78.6%) followed by African American ($n$ = 4, 14.3%). Their country of origins varied, but most were born in America ($n$ = 14, 50%). Many of the participants were taking anti-anxiety ($n$ = 4, 14.3%), antipsychotic ($n$ = 6, 21.4%) medications, but the majority was not taking any psychotropic medications ($n$ = 15, 53.6%). Participants had a documented diagnosis of dementia in their medical chart with varying types: mixed ($n$ = 12, 42.9%), Alzheimer's disease ($n$ = 7, 25%), unspecified/other ($n$ = 8, 28.5%).

### 3.4. Study design

Convenience sampling was used for recruitment. Along with chart review, we received referrals for study participation from therapeutic recreation, social work and nursing departments.

#### *3.4.1. Assessment*

The Functional Assessment Staging for Alzheimer's Disease (FAST) was used to measure staging for dementia during screening process [66]. Participants who scored between 5 and 6 on the FAST were considered eligible for participation in this study. To the validity of this study, the tester did not contribute to the intervention and had no prior relationship with study participants.

#### *3.4.2. Outcome measure*

The outcome measure of the study was the Cohen-Mansfield Agitation Inventory [67]. This tool consists of 29 agitated behaviors and the score can range from 34 to 128. The Cohen-Mansfield Agitation Inventory has high inter-rater agreement rates for each behavior for nursing home residents [67]. Other researchers found that the test/retest reliability for this tool was moderate to good in nursing home residents ($n$ = 105) who were evaluated for agitation [68].

#### *3.4.3. Music therapy intervention*

Participants in this study took part in music therapy three times a week for 2 weeks. The intervention was facilitated by two nationally board-certified music therapists who conducted music therapy assessments prior to the intervention to obtain historical, musical preferences. This information was gathered from the nursing home resident, his/her family member, recreation, or nursing staff members. Music selections for the music therapy sessions were tailored according to participants' individual preferences.

Music therapy was conducted in small groups of four to six participants in a private lounge in the nursing home where the participant lived. Each session lasted from 15 min to an hour depending on the tolerance of the participant. Musical expression was demonstrated through singing, music and movement, and tonal activities. The music therapists encouraged the residents to play a variety of rhythm instruments, djembe drums, and ocean drums. Movement was encouraged through the use of colorful scarves and ribbons. The music therapists used live music for the sessions and were self-accompanied by guitar and electronic keyboard. An in-depth description of the music therapy intervention including the songs chosen and common themes that occurred is described in our previous publication [10].

#### *3.4.4. CNA music programming*

Following the music therapy intervention, the music therapists trained CNAs to integrate music in aid of caregiving during their daily routine. The transformation design model was used to guide the training created for the CNAs [69]. The transformation design model is a framework specifically for music therapy treatment. The treatment design was created to make available scientific outcomes in clinical practice immediately [69]. The treatment design is directed by nonmusical outcomes with consideration for the nursing home residents' music and music activity preference. Steps to this model are illustrated in the following example:

1. *Gather information on nonmusical behavior*

    CNA reports that resident gets agitated especially during morning care. The CNA informs the music therapist that the resident becomes agitated as soon as it is time to get dressed. The resident kicks and screams as the CNA attempts to dress her. The resident has been checked for signs and symptoms of pain or distress.

2. *Develop treatment goals and objectives*

    Goal: Decrease agitation during morning care

    Objectives: Decrease kicking and screaming.

3. *Design functional nonmusical activities*

    Set a relaxing, musical environment for morning care activities.

4. *Design music activities*

    Music therapist visits resident's room prior to morning care and sings resident's favorite songs with her. CNA joins in singing and initiates morning care and dressing resident. Music therapist exits when appropriate.

5. *Transfer outcomes to everyday setting*

    Therapist creates a protocol for CNA to use that includes playing familiar music and singing lyrics of resident's favorite songs while dressing during morning care. Music therapist creates playlist on an iPod or a CD player of resident's preferred music based on positive outcomes observed during music therapy. Music therapist instructs CNA with resident's musical preferences to use with resident during morning care [69].

#### *3.4.5. Analysis*

IBM Statistical Package for Social Science (SPSS) Statistics software (version 21) was used to obtain frequencies, percentages, means and standard error, and confidence intervals for demographic information and repeated measures ANOVA analysis related to study participants.

A repeated measures ANOVA was conducted to analyze changes in Cohen-Mansfield Agitation Inventory scores for multiple data points. IBM SPSS Statistics software was used to perform the analysis. This method of analysis was chosen since each participant served as her/his own control and it enabled us to compare changes in agitation between multiple data points over time including the following: baseline 1 and baseline 2; baseline 1 and immediately following music therapy; after music therapy and 2 weeks post music therapy; immediately following music therapy and CNA facilitated music in aid of caregiving. This procedure helped to determine any changes in agitation that occurred during care as usual (between baseline 1 and baseline 2), following the music therapy intervention and following the CNA-initiated music activities.

## 4. Results

The goal of this study was to determine if music therapy could reduce agitation symptoms and if these changes could be sustained by music in aid of caregiving. A repeated measures ANOVA found that Cohen-Mansfield Agitation Inventory scores differed significantly between the various time points. The assumption of sphericity was met according to Mauchly's test of sphericity, $x^2$ (9) = 14.81, $p = 0.097$. Mauchly's test of sphericity demonstrated that the average agitation scores were significantly different between time frames $F$ (4, 92) = 7.03, $p < 0.001$, and that these changes can be seen visibly on a graph, **Table 1**, **Figure 3**.

| Comparisons | Mean score difference | Standard error | 95% CI | |
|---|---|---|---|---|
| | | | Lower bound | Upper bound |
| Baseline 1 vs Baseline 2 | −3.33 | 3.77 | −15.04 | 8.37 |
| Post music therapy vs Baseline 1 | −11.42* | 2.86 | −20.28 | −2.55 |
| 2 weeks post music therapy vs post music therapy | 1.71 | 2.70 | −6.67 | 10.09 |
| CNA MAC vs Baseline 1 | −16.67* | 4.03 | −29.18 | −4.15 |
| CNA MAC vs post music therapy | −5.25 | 4.49 | −19.19 | 8.69 |

*$p < 0.05$

**Table 1.** Bonferroni comparison of agitation scores at various time points.

Post hoc tests were performed using the Bonferroni adjustment for multiple comparisons. The results revealed that between first and second baseline, when participants were receiving care as usual, there were no significant differences in agitation scores (60.87 ± 23.00 vs 57.54 ± 24.17, $p$ = 1.0). When post-music therapy scores were compared to baseline 1 scores, there was a significant difference in agitation (60.87 ± 23.00 vs 49.46 ± 21.92, $p$ = 0.006) indicating that music therapy significantly contributed to reduced agitation. We measured agitation scores again 2 weeks post music therapy and found that there was a slight, but insignificant increase in agitation (49.46 ± 21.92 vs 51.17 ± 16.33, $p$ = 0.189). The agitation scores declined again following CNA-initiated music in aid of caregiving activities (49.46 ± 15.25 vs 44.21 ± 15.25, $p$ = 0.605), although these changes were not significant. The participants' agitation after music in aid of caregiving was significantly lower than the initial baseline scores (44.21 ± 15.25 vs 60.87 ± 23.00,

$p = 0.004$). These results suggest that routine care did not significantly affect agitation, but music therapy significantly decreased agitation symptoms. The effects of the music therapy intervention were not sustainable for 2 weeks post music therapy, but agitation declined again after music in aid of caregiving.

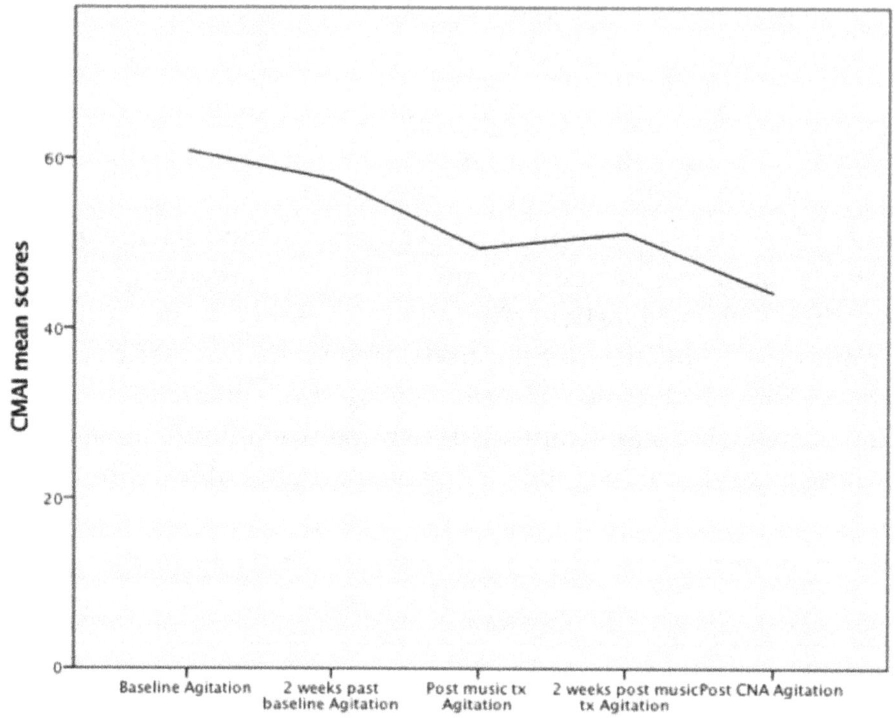


**Figure 3.** Changes in Cohen-Mansfield agitation scores over time.

## 5. Discussion and conclusion

Music therapy has been recommended as a nonpharmacological intervention to reduce behavioral symptoms related to dementia such as agitation [3, 29], though there is little research documenting the use of music as an interdisciplinary method between music therapists and nursing professionals. In the current study, we hypothesized that music therapy would reduce symptoms of agitation and that music in aid of caregiving facilitated by educated CNAs would sustain those results. We found that when compared to usual care, music therapy reduced agitation significantly, but following music therapy symptoms began to rise again slightly. When nursing home residents were introduced to music in aid of caregiving by the CNAs, agitation began to decline again. This evidence supports the initiative of researchers that nonpharmacological treatments such as music should be used to manage symptoms of agitation in PWD [70]. Because the majority of residents were taking medications to cope with agitation symptoms, our outcomes also suggest that music therapy followed by music in aid of caregiving should be considered as an interdisciplinary, yet complimentary treatment alongside pharmaceutical therapy.

Prior to the intervention, we observed that many of our residents exhibited symptoms of agitation that included spitting on staff members, cursing, and yelling. These behaviors led to CNAs spending much of their time trying to redirect and console residents using techniques that were often ineffective. The reduction of agitation scores that occurred following the music in aid of caregiving indicates that the education for the CNAs and provision of music-based tools were sufficient.

Our study followed the transformational design which presents the theory that nonmusical behaviors can be changed through the introduction of a music therapy treatment plan [69]. For this study, music therapy followed by CNA education and facilitation of music in aid of caregiving activities led to a decrease in agitation for most of our participants. The plan began with specific goals set by the music therapy researchers who used therapeutic techniques to reduce agitation. Next, music in aid of caregiving or "pleasant (musical) diversions from daily routines or struggles" [52] were used to assist in sustaining the goals set by the music therapists. These protocols (e.g., singing and music-assisted bathing) allowed for CNAs to practice skills that may have been effective during music therapy sessions [52]. From our observations, the results positively affected not only the PWD as evidenced by fewer symptoms but also the CNA who was providing care.

### 5.1. Conclusion

The tremendous need for nonpharmacological treatment in patients with dementia particularly highlights the importance of making music accessible as a simple and everyday tool that can help in these patients' care. The authors believe that music therapists should challenge this need and that specific training for caregivers at home or in institutions will help ease the burden of care and promote the well-being of both caregivers and people with dementia. Music therapists who work with people with dementia should expand their knowledge and expertise beyond the boundaries of the music therapy room. For that, we must differentiate between music therapy, which is performed by a professional and certified person and the use of music in aid of caregiving done by anyone who cares for people with dementia without the need for any musical background or skill. By promoting training programs in institution settings and at home, we can provide better care for those who need it.

A larger study is needed to test the effects of our intervention and provide evidence of its usefulness. We would like to propose that music in aid of caregiving is not only useful in nursing situations with CNAs but also may be beneficial for all nursing professionals to use to reduce resistance to care while giving medication and for wound care.

Because of the brain's ability to process music even in late stages of dementia [23], it may be beneficial for other healthcare practitioners besides nurses to consider adding music as a tool to aid them in their treatment. Presently, the protocols in this study have been adapted for work with home health aides, family caregivers, occupational and physical therapists, and social workers in multiple types of settings. It is currently being used in the United States, Israel, and Spain. Our future research includes work with a physiotherapist using music to aid with walking. This work will be based on a music therapy technique for patients with neurological problems that make use of rhythm to organize locomotion. Based on previous research with patients with Alzheimer's in which individuals required assistance with walking and inertia, we will test the rhythmic stimulus that may have a physiological effect and help to organize control over walking. This intervention may also reduce the need for multiple caregivers who assist the patient with walking [71].

In conclusion, the limits for the use of music in aid of caregiving are inexhaustible, but larger samples with more stringent designs are needed to confirm its worthiness. Since music is an accessible tool that is part of most people's day-to-day life, it is possible for even those without musical experience, to employ it in their work with a PWD. Minimizing restlessness is significant and contributes to the person with dementia's quality of life, and also improves caregiver's ability to give optimal and safe care. Music's positive effect renders it useful for relaxation and for softening resistance, and thus alleviating the day-to-day life of the caregiver and the person with dementia.

## Author details

Kendra Ray[1,2*], Ayelet Dassa[3,4], Jan Maier[5], Renita Davis[6] and Olayinka Ogunlade[7]

*Address all correspondence to: kray@mjhs.org

1 MJHS, Menorah Center for Nursing and Rehabilitation, Brooklyn, NY, USA

2 Drexel University, Philadelphia, PA, USA

3 Bar-llan University, Ramat Gan, Israel

4 Alzheimer's Medical Center, Ramat Gan, Israel

5 Jemsong, LLC, Waltham, MA, USA

6 Troy University at Phenix City, AL, USA

7 Gemma Regis Center for Music Therapy, Lagos, Nigeria

## References

[1] Prince M, Bryce R, Albanese E, Wimo A, Ribeiro W, Ferri CP. The global prevalence of dementia: a systematic review and metaanalysis. Alzheimer's & Dementia: The Journal of the Alzheimer's Association. 2013;9(1):63–75.e2.

[2] Patel AD, Iversen JR. The evolutionary neuroscience of musical beat perception: the action simulation for auditory prediction (ASAP) hypothesis. Frontiers in Systems Neuroscience. 2014;8:57.

[3] Ueda T, Suzukamo Y, Sato M, Izumi S. Effects of music therapy on behavioral and psychological symptoms of dementia: a systematic review and meta-analysis. Ageing Research Reviews. 2013;12(2):628–41.

[4] Albers G, Van den Block L, Stichele RV. The burden of caring for people with dementia at the end of life in nursing homes: a postdeath study among nursing staff. International Journal of Older People Nursing. 2014;9:106–17.

[5] Astrom S, Nilsson M, Norberg A, Winbald B. Empathy, experience of burnout and attitudes towards demented patients amoung nursing staff in geriatric care. Journal of Advanced Nursing. 1990;15:1236–44.

[6] Kuremyr D, Kihlgren M, Norberg A, Astrom S, Karlsson I. Emotional experiences, empathy and burnour among staff carring for demented patients at a collective living unit and a nursing home. Journal of Advanced Nursing. 1994;19:670–9.

[7] Garland K, Beer E, Eppingstall B, O'Connor DW. A comparison of two treatments of agitated behavior in nursing home residents with dementia: simulated family presence and preferred music. The American Journal of Geriatric Psychiatry: Official Journal of the American Association for Geriatric Psychiatry. 2007;15(6):514–21.

[8] Guetin S, Portet F, Picot MC, Pommie C, Messaoudi M, Djabelkir L, et al. Effect of music therapy on anxiety and depression in patients with Alzheimer's type dementia: randomised, controlled study. Dementia and Geriatric Cognitive Disorders. 2009;28(1): 36–46.

[9] Raglio A, Bellelli G, Traficante D, Gianotti M, Ubezio MC, Villani D, et al. Efficacy of music therapy in the treatment of behavioral and psychiatric symptoms of dementia. Alzheimer Disease and Associated Disorders. 2008;22(2):158–62.

[10] Ray KD, Mittelman MS. Music therapy: A nonpharmacological approach to the care of agitation and depressive symptoms for nursing home residents with dementia. Dementia. 2015.

[11] Wigram T, Pedersen N, Bonde LO. A Comprehensive Guide to Music Therapy: Theory, Clinical Practice and Training. London: Jessica Kingsley Publishers, Ltd; 29–35, 2002.

[12] Hara M. Music in dementia care: increased understanding through mixed research methods. Music and Arts in Action. 2011;3(2):34–58.

[13] Cuddy L, Duffin J. Music, memory, and Alzheimer's disease; Is music recognition spared in dementia, and how can it be assessed? Medical Hypotheses. 2005;64(2):229–35.

[14] Vink AC, Bruinsma MS, Scholter RJPM. Music therapy for people with dementia. The Cochrane Collaboration. 2011(4):1–50.

[15] Clair AA. The effect of singing on alert responses in persons with late stage dementia. Journal of Music Therapy. 1996;33:234–47.

[16] Simpson F. Creative music therapy: Last resort? In: Aldridge D, editor. Music Therapy for People with Dementia. London: Jessica Kingsley Publishers; 2000. p. 166–83.

[17] Music therapy in dementia treatment. Presentatoin to the 19th International Symposium on Research in Music Behavior; 2011; Barcelona, Spain.

[18] Clark CN, Warren JD. Music, memory and mechanisms in Alzheimer's disease. Brain: A Journal of Neurology. 2015;138(Pt 8):2122–5.

[19] Beatty WW, Winn P, Adams EW, Wilson DA, Prince JR, et al. Preserved cognitive skills in dementia of the Alzheimer's type. Archives of Neurology. 1994;51:1040–6.

[20] Beatty WW, Zavadil KD, Bailly R, Rixen G, et al. Preserved musical skill in a severely demented patient. International Journal of Clinical Neuropsychology. 1988;10(4):158–64.

[21] Sacks OW. Musicophillia. New York: Alfred A. Knopf; 2007.

[22] Janata P. The neural architecture of music-evoked autobiographical memories. Cerebral cortex (New York, NY: 1991). 2009;19(11):2579–94.

[23] Jacobsen JH, Stelzer J, Fritz TH, Chetelat G, La Joie R, Turner R. Why musical memory can be preserved in advanced Alzheimer's disease. Brain: A Journal of Neurology. 2015;138(Pt 8):2438–50.

[24] Steinberg M, Tschanz JT, Corcoran C, Steffens DC, Norton MC, Lyketsos CG, et al. The persistence of neuropsychiatric symptoms in dementia: the Cache County Study. International Journal of Geriatric Psychiatry. 2004;19(1):19–26.

[25] Morley JE. Dementia-related agitation. Journal of the American Medical Directors Association. 2011;12(9):611–2.e2.

[26] Faull C, Carter YH, Daniels L. Handbook of Palliative Care. MA: Blackwell Publishing; 2005.

[27] Cox E, Nowak M, Buettner P. Managing agitated behavior in people with Alzheimer's disease: the role of live music. The British Journal of Occupational Therapy. 2011;11:517–24.

[28] Raglio A, Bellelli G, Traficante D, Gianotti M, Ubezio MC, Gentile S, et al. Efficacy of music therapy treatment based on cycles of sessions: a randomised controlled trial. Aging & Mental Health. 2010;14(8):900–4.

[29] Patel B, Perera M, Pendleton J, Richman A, Majumdar B. Psychosocial interventions for dementia: from evidence to practice. Advances in Psychiatric Treatment. 2014;20:340–9.

[30] Livingston G, Kelly L, Lewis-Holmes E, Baio G, Morris S, Patel N, et al. Non-pharmacological interventions for agitation in dementia: systematic review of randomised

controlled trials. The British Journal of Psychiatry: The Journal of Mental Science. 2014;205(6):436–42.

[31] Ridder HM, Stige B, Qvale LG, Gold C. Individual music therapy for agitation in dementia: an exploratory randomized controlled trial. Aging & Mental Health. 2013;17(6):667–78.

[32] Lin Y, Chu H, Yang CY, Chen CH, Chen SG, Chang HJ, et al. Effectiveness of group music intervention against agitated behavior in elderly persons with dementia. International Journal of Geriatric Psychiatry. 2011;26(7):670–8.

[33] Rabins PV, Blass DM. In the Clinic. Dementia. Annals of Internal Medicine. 2014;161(3):ITC1; quiz ITC16.

[34] Edberg AK, Bird M, Richards DA, Woods R, Keeley P, Davis-Quarrell V. Strain in nursing care of people with dementia: nurses' experience in Australia, Sweden and United Kingdom. Aging & Mental Health. 2008;12(2):236–43.

[35] Dileo C. Effects of music and music therapy on medical patients: a meta-analysis of the research and implications for the future. Journal of the Society for Integrative Oncology. 2006;4(2):67–70.

[36] Gotell E, Brown S, Ekman SL. Influence of caregiver singing and background music on posture, movement, and sensory awareness in dementia care. International Psychogeriatrics/IPA. 2003;15(4):411–30.

[37] Gotell E, Brown S, Ekman SL. Caregiver singing and background music in dementia care. Western Journal of Nursing Research. 2002;24(2):195–216.

[38] Gerdner LA. Consumer version of evidence-based guidelines: Individualized music for elders with dementia. In: Titler M, editor. Series on Evidence-Based Practice for Older Adults. Iowa City, IA: The University of Iowa College of Nursing Gerontological Nursing Interventions Research Center; Research Dissemination Core; 2007.

[39] Hammar LM. Caregivers' Singing Facilitates Mutual Encounter: Implementation and Evaluation of Music Therapeutic Caregiving in Complex Dementia Care Situations. Karolinska Institute. Stockholm, Sweden; 2011.

[40] Sarkamo T, Tervaniemi M, Laitinen S, Numminen A, Kurki M, Johnson JK, et al. Cognitive, emotional, and social benefits of regular musical activities in early dementia: randomized controlled study. The Gerontologist. 2014;54(4):634-50 doi:10.1093/geront/gnt100.

[41] Hoeffer B, Talerico KA, Rasin J, Mitchell CM, Stewart BJ, McKenzie D, et al. Assisting cognitively impaired nursing home residents with bathing: effects of two bathing interventions on caregiving. The Gerontologist. 2006;46(4):524–32.

[42] Ray KD, Fitzsimmons S. Music-assisted bathing: making shower time easier for people with dementia. Journal of Gerontological Nursing. 2014;40(2):9–13.

[43] Thomas D, Heltman R, Alexander T. The effects of music on bathing cooperation for residents with dementia. Journal of Music Therapy. 1997;34(4):246–59.

[44] Wall M, Duffy A. The effects of music therapy for older people with dementia. British Journal of Nursing 2010;19(2):108–13.

[45] Choi AN, Lee MS, Cheong KJ, Lee JS. Effects of group music intervention on behavioral and psychological symptoms in patients with dementia: a pilot-controlled trial. The International Journal of Neuroscience. 2009;119(4):471–81.

[46] Cohen-Mansfield J, Werner P. Management of verbally disruptive behaviors in nursing home residents. The Journals of Gerontology Series A, Biological Sciences and Medical Sciences. 1997;52(6):M369–77.

[47] Gerdner LA, Swanson EA. Effects of individualized music on confused and agitated elderly patients. Archives of Psychiatric Nursing. 1993;7(5):284–91.

[48] Gerdner LA. Effects of individualized versus classical "relaxation" music on the frequency of agitation in elderly persons with Alzheimer's disease and related disorders. International Psychogeriatrics/IPA. 2000;12(1):49–65.

[49] Weeks S. Connecting through music with people with dementia: A guide for caregivers. Journal of Mental Health. 2011;20:503.

[50] Sung HC, Chang AM, Lee WL. A preferred music listening intervention to reduce anxiety in older adults with dementia in nursing homes. Journal of Clincal Nursing. 2010;19(7–8):1056–64.

[51] Ziv N, Granot A, Hai S, Dassa A, Haimov I. The effect of background stimulative music on behavior in Alzheimer's patients. Journal of Music Therapy. 2007;44(4):329–43.

[52] Clair AA, Memmott J. Therapeutic Uses of Music with Older Adults. Silver Spring, MD: American Music Therapy Association; 2008.

[53] Tomaino C. The role of music in the rehabilitation of persons with neurologic diseases. Music Therapy Today (online). 2002.

[54] Koelsch S. Music-evoked emotions: principles, brain correlates, and implications for therapy. Annals of the New York Academy of Science 2015;1337:193–201.

[55] Dassa A, Amir D. The role of singing familiar songs in encouraging conversation among people with middle to late stage Alzheimer's disease. Journal of Music Therapy. 2014;51(2):131–53.

[56] Ashida S. The effect of reminiscence music therapy sessions on changes in depressive symptoms in elderly persons with dementia. Journal of Music Therapy. 2000;37(3):170.

[57] Svansdottir HB, Snaedal J. Music therapy in moderate and severe dementia of Alzheimer's type: a case–control study. International Psychogeriatrics/IPA. 2006;18(4): 613–21.

[58] Kung SJ, Chen JL, Zatorre RJ, Penhune VB. Interacting cortical and basal ganglia networks underlying finding and tapping to the musical beat. Journal of Cognitive Neuroscience. 2013;25(3):401–20.

[59] Grahn JA, Brett M. Rhythm and beat perception in motor areas of the brain. Journal of Cognitive Neuroscience. 2007;19(5):893–906.

[60] Grahn JA, Rowe JB. Feeling the beat: premotor and striatal interactions in musicians and nonmusicians during beat perception. The Journal of Neuroscience: The Official Journal of the Society for Neuroscience. 2009;29(23):7540–8.

[61] Drake C, Penel A, Bigand E. Tapping in time with mechanically and expressively performed music. Music Perception. 2000;18:1–24.

[62] Nettl B. An ethnomusicologist contemplates universals in musical sound and musical culture. In: Wallin NL, Merker B, Brown S, editors. The Origins of Music. Cambridge, MA: MIT Press; 2000. p. 463–72.

[63] Brown S, Jordania J. Universals in the world's musics. Psychology of Music. 2013;41:229–48.

[64] Zatorre RJ, Salimpoor VN. From perception to pleasure: music and its neural substrates. Proceedings of the National Academy of Sciences of the United States of America. 2013;110(Suppl 2):10430–7.

[65] Ray KD, McGaughy M, Stuart S. Music Therapy: Keys to Dementia Care. New York, NY: MJHS; 2013.

[66] Sclan SG, Reisberg B. Functional assessment staging (FAST) in Alzheimer's disease: reliability, validity, and ordinality. International Psychogeriatrics/IPA. 1992;4(Suppl 1): 55–69.

[67] Cohen-Mansfield J, Marx MS, Rosenthal AS. A description of agitation in a nursing home. Journal of Gerontology: Medical Sciences. 1989;44(3):M77–M84.

[68] Zuidema SU, Buursema AL, Gerritsen MG, Oosterwal KC, Smits MM, Koopmans RT, et al. Assessing neuropsychiatric symptoms in nursing home patients with dementia: reliability and Reliable Change Index of the Neuropsychiatric Inventory and the Cohen-Mansfield Agitation Inventory. International Journal of Geriatric Psychiatry. 2011;26(2):127–34.

[69] Thaut M. Rhythm, Music, And the Brain: Scientific Foundations and Clinical Applications. New York, NY: Taylor & Francis; 2008.

[70] Herrman N, Gauthier S. Diagnosis and treatment of dementia: Management of severe Alzheimer's disease. Canadian Medical Association Journal. 2008;179(12):1279–87.

[71] Clair AA, O'Konski M. The effect of rhythmic audotiry stimulation (RAS) on gait characteristics of cadence, velocity, and stride length in persons with late stage dementia. Journal of Music Therapy. 2006;43(2):154–63.

# 2

# Influence of Caregiver Practices Child Undernourishment and Development

Assol Cortés-Moreno

**Abstract**

Children living in poverty are at risk of malnutrition and developmental delays. In addition to environmental constraints, caregiver practices can exacerbate or mitigate effects of economic scarcity on these issues. This study explores the influence of rearing practices and socioemotional caregiver factors on the nutritional status and psychological development in a sample of Mexican children; also, the participation of some sociodemographic variables is analyzed. Sixteen children (9–19 months old) at risk of malnutrition or malnourished and their main caregivers participated. In addition to the nutritional status, infant development was assessed using the Bayley Child Development Scales. The caregiver answered questionnaires on demographics, parenting practice (RPS Questionnaire), and parenting stress (Parenting Stress Index). According to expectations, positive relations between responsive-rearing practices and children-favorable condition were found, and negative associations between parental stress and child indicators of optimal nourishment and development were also found. Some demographic factors were associated with the caregiver and the child variables. Results found have limitations imposed by the sample size to conclude on the direction of the effects in the relationships obtained. Despite this, the results show the relevance of the caregiver's characteristics and practices.

**Keywords:** caregiving, stunting, child development, poverty, parenting stress

## 1. Introduction

### 1.1. Background

As developing countries improve their economies, they increase the availability of food and, theoretically, can meet the food needs of their population. However, the current situation of the problem shows that the phenomenon of food consumption is intricate; a direct relationship between a country's economic growth and reducing the risk of malnutrition is not always observed [1].

In addition to the macroeconomic factors, other variables of the physical and social context affect the availability of food. The physical approachability is determined by characteristics of a geographical area, such temperature, altitude, and humidity. In the same way, social factors such as population growth, change in the role of women in work and family life, and changes in the perception of the relations between diet and health also define access to food [2, 3]. Moreover, culture as a belief system and customs derived from it influences habits of people, which are concretized in the selection, conservation, and preparation of foods, resulting in the use or waste of food resources. According to Bourges [4], the availability and cultural access to food refer to the way in which customs and traditions delimit the acceptance or rejection of some products or the way in which they should be prepared and consumed.

Eating habits developed from these factors and others of an individual nature act, in a beneficial or harmful way, on the health condition and the people's quality of life. Inadequate habits result in a risk powerfully associated with various conditions of infectious origin and conditions related to nutrient deficiencies and non-hereditary chronic-degenerative diseases (NHCDs). Conversely, when eating habits are correct, they become a protective factor for such problems. The imbalance between food intake and energy expenditure leads to a condition of malnutrition. When this is the result of excessive feeding, overweight or obesity is present, these conditions constitute risk factors for several NHCDs; on the other hand, poor nutrition derived from food sub-consumption is generically known as undernourishment [5].

### 1.2. Undernourishment sequels

Undernourishment or malnutrition is the result of reduced food intake and repeated occurrence of infectious illness [6]. A low height-for-age or stunting represents a chronic malnutrition, a little weight-for-height or wasting denotes a recent loss, and low weight-for-age is a mixed index influenced by both stunting and wasting. Micronutrient deficiencies, such as iron, iodine, or zinc, may also occur [7].

Undernourishment can have grave consequences on the physiological and psychological development. The magnitude of the sequelae is determined, in part, by the severity, duration, and temporality of specific or generalized gaps. The most sensitive stages to sub-nutrition are gestational age and the first year of life because damage at this period reduces neuronal proliferation, which cannot be compensated later. Likewise, other developmental processes of the central nervous system (CNS), such as myelination, continue during childhood, so the occurrence of a severe nutritional deficit has the potential to modify the rate of integration of neural structures, related to the emergence of different cognitive and behavioral skills [8, 9]. Critical moments in the development of CNS structures are as follows:

1. Myelination begins slowly at 16 weeks in the spinal cord and nerve roots of the brain and continues during infancy and childhood.
2. The vestibuloacoustic system (balance), the parietal cortex (integration of motor responses), and the hippocampus, already myelinated, mature at 12 months of age.

3. The language area of the left temporal lobe is myelinated at approximately 18 months of age.
4. Other structures are more slowly myelinated through infancy and childhood: (a) the structures involved in focusing and maintaining attention (reticular formation, a portion of the nucleus, the superior colliculus, and the lateral part of the thalamus) begin myelination at 10 months, and the process continues during childhood, adolescence, and adulthood.
5. The periods of accelerated development of the frontal lobe (which has a circuit integration function necessary for the higher processes) occur from birth to 2 years, from 7 to 9 years, and in the middle adolescence.

However, when nutrient deficiencies occur at a late stage, the effects may be attenuated as the process of structural development of the CNS is more advanced and it is highly likely that the child already has basic behavioral repertoires, necessary for the acquisition of more complex psychological processes. At that time, the social context surrounding the child can play a crucial role. If the child is given the necessary stimulation and care, the effects of malnutrition can be compensated [10] .

In the behavioral dimension, there is apathy and lack of initiative, emotional monotony, poor social interaction, lack of curiosity and exploration of the environment, and physical closeness to the mother. These forms of response condition malnourished children to perform developmental test unwell when compared to children in optimal nutritional status [9, 11–13]. They also limit the forms of interaction with others, which facilitates that the adverse effects remain for years [14].

### 1.3. The caregiver role on undernourishment: isolation hypothesis

Poverty and a disorganized psychosocial environment increase exposure to biological and social risks that affect development through changes in the structure and function of the CNS, as well as through the establishment and consolidation of deficient patterns of interaction between the child and his/her physical and social environment [3, 15, 16]. In this way, different variables of both levels act synchronously, and the scope of each of them will vary according to the characteristics of the individual, the social circumstances, and the moment of the child development. The first factor, the type of lack, can determine the nature of the consequences associated with undernourishment, because each nutrient has different functions in the organism according to its composition. The second factor, the social environment, is equally critical to understanding the problem, since an unfavorable social surrounding alone can constitute a risk factor for the child development, especially when this is conjugated with a nutritional status deteriorated.

Findings reported in the last two decades of the twentieth century that included the observation of the child's reactions in interaction with other people led to revalue the *functional isolation* hypothesis as a conceptual element explaining the processes involved to perpetuate the effects of underconsumption of food. This was formulated by Levitsky and Barnes [17] when they restricted food to newborn rodents during the first 7 weeks of life and underwent a 10-week recovery period where they observed that the adverse effects of malnutrition on performance in several tests were mediated by the decrease in the animal activity level. The additional environmental stimulation provided in the recovery period improved the performance in the tests used.

The *functional isolation* hypothesis applied to human undernourishment suggests the mechanism by which the performance of malnourished children is affected in psychological tests [18]. Equally, it contributes to explain how these effects last: when there is scarce food intake, physical growth is limited and activity is diminished when compared to that of well-nourished children; this appearance means that the contacts of the caregivers are few and that their behavior is the one shown for younger children; the child is less likely to explore their environment and therefore motor, social, and learning abilities do not reach the levels that characterize development under optimum conditions. When these patterns occur recurrently, the effects are cumulative and the child does not acquire the competencies to cope with the demands of the environment (**Figure 1**).

Studies show that attention, emotion, and affection are the behavioral traits that can be recognized as mediators of learning processes and in turn are most affected by malnutrition [18–20]. Changes in these dimensions reduce reactivity and/or motivation and interfere with processes of selective attention, motor exploration, and also alter the response styles in problem-solving tasks [21], or on the other hand, this changes can be attended to the work but their answers are slower in comparison to a eutrophic child. When the analysis of infant behavior was performed using finer observational categories than in previous studies, it was found that the differences between anemic and non-anemic children were mainly in the orientation toward the mother and in the rapidity of reactions: children with low iron levels tended to be less oriented toward the mother when there was a novel stimulus and their answers were more durable than those exhibited by children with normal iron levels [20]. Similarly, social behaviors such as smiling or approaching the mother used to last longer.

Such forms of response affect the synchrony of interactions between the child and his or her primary caregiver by promoting ineffective behavioral patterns to stimulate child development.

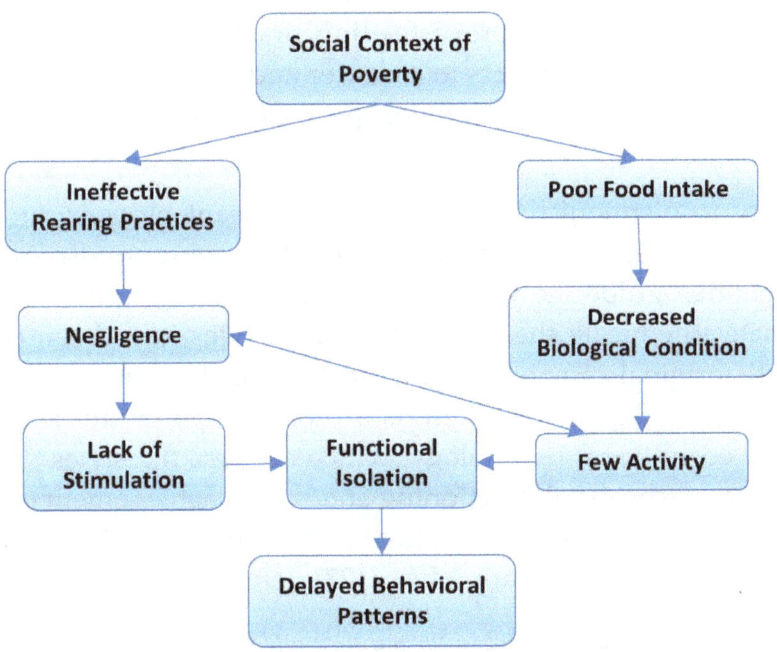
Social Context of Poverty
Ineffective Rearing Practices
Poor Food Intake
Negligence
Decreased Biological Condition
Lack of Stimulation
Functional Isolation
Few Activity
Delayed Behavioral Patterns

**Figure 1.** Representation of functional isolation hypothesis.

Stanfield [22] points out how the dynamics of the mother or caregiver can be altered by interacting with a child who shows less attention and/or little activity and affective monotony: on the one hand, the mother can accept the loss of the interrelation between her and the child or perceive it as a child that does not cause problems, thus developing a neglectful style and an additional form of environmental deprivation; or on the other hand, it may show concern and increase interest in the child by increasing the time of contact with him/her and making him/her more dependent and with less initiative for exploration.

Sensitive, reciprocal, and development-conducive maternal behaviors depend in part on the signals the child emits and on the reactions he or she exhibits to adult attempts to establish an exchange; a hyporeactive child makes it difficult to establish synchrony in caregiver-child interactions, since the adult does not have the necessary keys to adapt his/her behavior and thus satisfies the child's needs [23, 24]. The functional isolation in conditions of poverty or social disorganization can be interpreted as a double-risk model for optimal child development: the biological risk (undernourishment) that restricts the child's response team, necessary to meet the demands provided by the child environment, and social risk, determined by the alteration of the patterns of interaction between the child and the caregivers.

The modification of risk factors to protective factors conducive to a healthy and adequate environment to stimulate child growth and development must necessarily require an understanding of the problem of malnutrition from a broader and more inclusive perspective, multiple dimensions of this health issue highlighting the role of the caregiver as one of the most relevant explanatory variables.

### 1.4. Rearing practices

The parenting practices used by the primary caregiver determine to a large extent the quantity, quality, and manner in which children receive food. Developing skills to interpret and respond to the child's needs can improve feeding practices even in marginal populations [25]. Therefore, it is necessary to address in a clearer and the more precise way the ecological conditions in which the child develops and the specific demands of the social environment in which he/she participates.

Here, it is necessary to distinguish between what is meant by *parenting styles* and *parenting practices* or *rearing practices*. The first term refers to a compound of relatively invariable attitudes and beliefs that guide the way of communicating with the child and establishing an emotional climate to educate the child. Parenting styles have been extensively studied through Baumrind's original categorization that includes four styles: authoritarian, democratic, permissive, and negligent [26]; there is a broad range of studies, mainly within the areas of clinical and educational psychology, which address the styles of parenting relating them to results on the psychosocial functioning and school achievement of the child and adolescent. By contrast, the term parenting practice has been used to refer to concrete actions that meet parents in education and childcare. Myers [27] defines them as

> *Generally accepted activities that respond to the survival and development needs of children in their first months and years of life, so as to ensure the survival and maintenance (and sometimes development) of the group or culture as well as of the child (p. 431).*

These activities include food, hygiene care, and health preservation, as well as those focused on adjusting social and educational demands. It highlights three characteristics that must be addressed when describing and/or analyzing a practice: action (what it does), the person who performs it (who does it), and how to carry it to term (how it does it). The level of responsiveness or sensitivity to detect signs that account for the needs of the infant is an essential feature of the rearing practice that maintains the correct child nutritional status and favors a better psychological development.

Both the physical and social conditions of a family and the prevailing customs and beliefs in their culture define the set of practices designated for the care of children. The practices used to feed the child are then determined by a number of factors, including the ethnic group of belonging, beliefs about food [28], the educational level of the caregiver, family income, physical housing conditions [29–31], and how the adult perceives the child's health status and the child's ability to perform different activities [15].

Also, there are many factors that can significantly deteriorate child-care patterns related to food, health preservation, and development, such as the family environment characterized by apathy and disorganization [32], and emotional disturbances such as depression and parental stress [33, 34]. Addressing these factors is critical as, as a child health regulatory axis, parenting practices will determine the degrees of exposure to factors that protect or impair health. On the contrary, it is very likely that appropriate raising conditions will operate as a development-promoting element and thereby compensate for the lack of economic resources in the family or the existence of unfavorable environmental factors. Through sensitive practices and quality care, one can ensure proper child feeding to prevent undernourishment, and in the case of having suffered, one can reverse or minimize the adverse impact on psychological development.

From the above, it is evident that the practices of aging should be incorporated in a more systematic way to the analysis of the relationship between the psychosocial conditions of children at risk of malnutrition and the scope in terms of psychological development. Focusing on behavior and socio-emotional conditions of caregivers can provide valuable information to be incorporated into undernourishment prevention strategies and intervention programs aimed at reversing or minimizing their impact on child development.

## 1.5. Objective and hypothesis

### *1.5.1. General objective*

The present work addresses this problem, from the point of view of Health Psychology, and aims at exploring the influence of rearing practices and socioemotional caregiver factors on the nutritional status and psychological development in a sample of Mexican children. Additionally, some sociodemographic variables involved will be analyzed.

### *1.5.2. Particular objectives*

**a.** Analyzing if relations between nutritional status and development in children are present.

**b.** Examine the relations between the variables of the caregiver, child nutrition, and child performance of mental and psychomotor development test.

c. To explore if in the studied sample some demographic variables are involved in the parenting, children nutritional condition, and their development.

*1.5.3. Hypothesis*

It expects to find:

Hypothesis 1: The more obvious undernourishment is, the lower scores on developmental tests.

Hypothesis 2: Levels of parental stress and anxiety in caregiver will be negatively related to indicators of nutritional status and child development.

Hypothesis 3: Scores on the responsive parenting will relate positively to the infant's nutritional status and development.

## 2. Method

### 2.1. Participants

Non-random sampling was used. The sample is part of a longer study whose objective is to assess an intervention strategy, based on the responsive parenting, to reverse child undernourishment and its effects on motor and cognitive development. Participants were invited through outpatient clinics of the State of Mexico Health Institute (ISEM) located in marginalized areas at the municipality of Tlalnepantla. Thirty-three caregiver-child dyads were involved in this research, but only 16 of them completed all measures. Children were 9–19 months old ($M$ = 10.9): 68.7% ($n$ = 11) girls and 31.3% ($n$ = 5) boys, and they were at risk of undernutrition ($n$ = 10) or were moderately undernourished ($n$ = 4). Fourteen of caregivers were child's mothers ($M$ = 23.9 years old), and two more were their grandmothers ($M$ = 48 years old). All participants came from economically deprived families: three were income vulnerable, nine had moderate multidimensional poverty, and four extreme multidimensional poverty. In two households, the father was absent.

### 2.2. Measures and instruments

*2.2.1. Sociodemographics and health history*

An interview questionnaire was applied to obtain information about schooling and age of the mother, father and the main caregiver—when not the mother—type of work, and family structure. There are also questions on child and family health status, and child appetite perceived by the caregiver. In addition, the *National Council for the Evaluation of Social Development Policy (CONEVAL) Instrumen*t was used to obtain the Wellness Index. CONEVAL [35] proposes a set of indicators complementary to those used in the Multidimensional Measurement of Poverty Methodology, which aim to determine if a family's income is insufficient to meet their needs and if there are scarcities in each of the six indicators in order to identify the population in a situation of multidimensional poverty. The Wellness Index show five levels: extreme multidimensional poverty, moderate multidimensional poverty, vulnerable by social scarcity, vulnerable by income, and nonvulnerable.

### 2.2.2. *Anthropometrics*

Once the child measures of weight and supine length were obtained, according to the technique suggested by the World Health Organization (WHO) [36], *z*-scores were calculated for body mass index (BMI), body weight (BW), and body height (BH), using the tables included in the ANTHRO 2005 software as a reference measure [37]. All children whose measurements fell between ≤1 and 2 standard deviations below the median in any of the parameters, BMI, BW, or BH, were considered at risk of malnutrition (wasting, underweight, and stunting, respectively). Children whose measurements were 2 standard deviations below the median in any of the three parameters were considered cases of undernourishment.

### 2.2.3. *Child development*

*Bayley Scales of Infant Development* (BSID) Spanish-language version of these scales was used, designed to assess developmental status in children aged 1–40 months [38]. This instrument provides the child's assessment base through two components: (1) The Mental Development Scale that assesses sensory-perceptual acuity, discrimination, and responsiveness to stimuli; memory and solution; early vocalizations, as well as first classification and generalization. The results of this scale are expressed in standardized scores or Mental Development Index (MDI) and (2) the Psychomotor Scale provides information on the degree of body control, coordination of large muscles, and fine coordination of hands and fingers. The results of this scale are expressed in standardized scores or Psychomotor Development Indexes (PDI).

### 2.2.4. *Parenting Stress Index (PSI)*

This instrument provides a measure of maternal discomfort related to child-rearing work: higher scores, greater worry, and inadequate parenting to promote child development [39]. It comprises three dimensions: child characteristics, parent characteristics, and life stressors. The first two are constructed as a Likert scale and composed of the following subscales: (1) child characteristics: Adaptability, Acceptability, Demandingness, Mood, Distractibility/Hyperactivity and Reinforcement of Parents and (2) parent characteristics: Depression, Attachment, Role Restriction, Sense of Competence, Social isolation, Relationship with the Spouse, and Parental Health. A version adapted for children from northern Mexico [40] was used, with 38 items for child dimension, 35 for parent dimension, and 21 of stressors related to vital events. In this study, some lexical changes were made to suit the population of central Mexico. The internal consistency showed the following values of Cronbach's $\alpha$: $r = 0.75$ for child subscales, $r = 0.78$ for parent subscales, and $r = 0.84$ for the whole instrument.

### 2.2.5. *Anxiety*

Trait-State Anxiety Inventory (IDARE). The Spielberger and Díaz Guerrero [41], Anxiety Inventory: Status—Index (IDARE) consists of two separate self-assessment scales used to measure two different dimensions of anxiety: (1) Anxiety-Trait (A-Trait) and (2) Anxiety-State (A-State). The self-assessment inventory, IDARE, ranges from a minimum score of 20 to a maximum score of 80, on both the A-State scale and the A-Trait scale. The interpretation of both scales is according to the following scores: <30 low anxiety, 30–44 moderate, and >45 high.

#### *2.2.6. Rearing practices*

This aspect was assessed using the *Responsive Practice and Stimulation Questionnaire* (RPS-Q); this instrument allows to detect the sensitivity and effectiveness of the caregiver to meet the basic physical and psychological child needs, and care patterns adopted by adults in daily situations to meet the needs of children at complementary feeding age. It is made up of 23 Likert items, ranging from 1 for the "never" answer to 5 for the "always" option. The items are grouped into four factors: Stimulation from Play, Responsive Practice, Skills Promotion, Planned Attention, and Willingness to childcare. The internal consistency of the instrument yields Cronbach's alpha of 0.83 and correlations with the total score between 0.26 and 0.61 [42].

### 2.3. Procedure

All persons with a child younger than 24 months in outpatient clinics, who attended the child's vaccination, were invited to participate in talks on health, nutrition, and child development. At conferences, the child's primary caregivers were called to take part in the research. Once the caregivers were informed about the purpose of the study and the type of participation that they and their children would have, then each couple was evaluated by two psychology interns previously trained in the use of the instruments. In the first instance, the child's weight and height measurements were taken; then both observers applied the development scales with caregiver collaboration. It was preferred first to use the Psychomotor Scale since this order facilitates the child's responses on the Mental Scale; an evaluator presented the tests and another noted the answers. In case the child showed signs of fatigue or distress, a new appointment was arranged to continue with the application of the scales. The evaluation of child development was videotaped for later review by those responsible for the research. The RPS Questionnaire was applied as an interview at the health center after evaluating the child. Subsequently, a home visit of the participants was carried out for the application of the Demographic data questionnaires, corroborating the conditions of family life. It also applied the instruments that evaluate parental stress and anxiety. After qualifying the instruments, the report was given to the caregiver and an appointment was made to be involved in an intervention program, not reported in this work and which is in progress.

### 2.4. Data analysis

Descriptive statistics were obtained for sociodemographic, nutritional and child development, and parental variables. Non-parametric Mann-Whitney *U*-tests were used to observe the effects of nominal dichotomous variables and Kruskal-Wallis for nominal variables with more than two values. The relationship between parental variables, anxiety and parenting stress with effective parenting practices, as well as between parenting and child variables, was evaluated using a Spearman Rho correlation test. All analyses were performed using the statistical software SPSS, version 20 [43].

## 3. Results

Sociodemographic characteristics of the sample are presented first. Subsequently, based on the nutritional state and the level of mental and psychomotor development, the characterization of the child variables and the demographic variables related to the variability of these measures.

Descriptive statistics corresponding to the RPS-Q and the variables of the socio-affective adjustments (Parenting Stress Index (PSI) and IDARE) are shown, as well as the demographic variables that are related to these variables are addressed. At the last point of the data presentation, the relationships between the caregiver's variables, the effective parenting practices, as well as the socio-affective variables with the child's nutritional status and scores obtained on the Bayley Infant Development Scales are presented.

### 3.1. Sociodemographics and general health

Although all the families of the participants had some degree of lack, from being vulnerable by income to having extreme multidimensional poverty, there were no differences attributable to this variable in terms of family structure, the degree of mother or father studies, father absence, or the child's usual health. In the same way, children gender was not associated with the child's health, nor the perceived appetite. The results of child health and disease management by the caregiver indicated that 18.8% of the children had suffered diarrhea in the last 2 weeks, 62.5% of caregivers approached management of the disease adequately, and 37.5% inadequately; while 50% of children had respiratory disease in the previous 2 weeks, 81.2% with adequate management and 18.8% with poor management, 56.3% of caregivers reported using home remedies to treat children's illnesses.

### 3.2. Child variables

A criterion for inclusion in the study was that the children were at risk of malnutrition or already present. In **Table 1**, it can be seen that the parameter most affected is body height, which indicates a history of nutrient deficiencies. However, in all three parameters there were cases of moderate malnutrition: one was wasting, one was underweight, and nine were stunting. None of the participating children were severely malnourished.

Regarding the developmental scales, it was found that the average of the children is with the expected values for a healthy child on both the psychomotor scale and the mental scale. However, it can be observed in minimum values that there were cases in which the execution

| Measures | Min | Max | *M* | *SD* |
|---|---|---|---|---|
| **Anthropometrics** | | | | |
| Body Mass Index | **−2.23** | 1.93 | −0.45 | 1.14 |
| Body Weight | **−2.53** | 0.85 | **−1.01** | 0.69 |
| Body Height | **−2.82** | 1.81 | **−1.25** | 1.33 |
| **BSID** | | | | |
| Mental | **81** | 119 | 101.81 | 12.96 |
| Psychomotor | **75** | 119 | 102.13 | 14.29 |

Note: Out-of-range values are shown in bold.

**Table 1.** Descriptive values of ant and child anthropometrics and Bayley Scales of Infant Development scores.

of the infants was lower than expected: three children showed a slight psychomotor retardation and three others low score on the mental scale.

When calculating the correlation between the nutritional status scores and results on the developmental scales, a statistically significant positive correlation was found between the psychomotor development index and the body mass index ($r = 0.52$, $p < 0.05$), and negative with the body height parameter ($r = 0.46$, $p < 0.05$).

The non-parametric analysis based on different demographic variables did not reveal any difference in the child's nutritional status associated with demographic variables like child's gender, family or caregiver type, birth order, age or schooling of both parents, but a statistically significant correlation was found between the age of the child and the BW parameter ($r = -0.56$, $p < 0.05$), the older the child, the less weight gain was observed.

Concerning the developmental tests, the PDI scores showed a positive correlation with the Wellness Index ($r = 0.502$, $p < 0.05$) and with the BW, showing better scores as this parameter approaches typical values ($r = 520$, $p < 0.05$), while the MDI was affected by the child's gender ($U = 7.5$, $p < 0.05$), with girls showing higher scores ($M = 108.81$) compared to boys ($M = 90.80$). No other sociodemographic variables showed an effect.

### 3.3. Caregiver variables

**Table 2** shows the descriptive statistics of the variables related to parenting. It can be seen that the means of the total RPS-Q score and the scores of the five factors that make up the instrument were within the range of an adequate rearing practice. However, in each factor there are cases within the values of less effective practices: two cases related to Stimulation from Play, Responsive Practice, and Skills Promotion; three corresponded to the Willingness to attend the child and four to Planned Attention. In the total score, two caregivers are observed with values of little effective practice and one that corresponds to inadequate practices.

The variability of the values of the effective practice was affected by the Wellness Index, since to better living conditions, the scores were more favorable in Responsive Practice ($r = 0.625$, $p < 0.01$), Promotion of Skills ($r = 521$, $p < 0.05$), Willingness ($r = 0.520$, $p < 0.05$), and total score ($r = 0.515$, $p < 0.05$). Willingness correlated positively to child's age ($r = 0.503$, $p < 0.05$). A significant difference was also found in the values of the Responsive Practice according to child's gender ($U = 8$, $p < 0.05$), caregivers show higher scores with girls ($M = 4.7$) than children ($M = 4.06$). The other sociodemographic variables did not show significant effects on the RPS-Q.

Results in the PSI showed high levels of parental stress related to the child's characteristics. The subscales whose values exceeded adequate coping scores for childcare were the following: adaptability that gives information about the parent's perception of the child's ability to adjust to changes in the physical and social environment; demandingness, where high values indicate that the caregiver perceives that the child requires too much attention and care; and Reinforcement of Parents, in this subscale values higher than expected report distress generated by not finding the relationship with the child as a source of gratification. Parents characteristics dimensions show that the averages in all subscales are within a suitable range. However, it is necessary to note that in both the dimensions, child and parent, the maximum

| Measures | Min | Max | *M* | *SD* |
|---|---|---|---|---|
| **RPS-Questionnaire** | | | | |
| Stimulation from Play | **3** | 5.00 | 4.31 | 0.69 |
| Responsive Practice | **3.67** | 5.00 | 4.52 | 0.50 |
| Promoting skills | **2.33** | 5.00 | 3.96 | 0.86 |
| Planned Care | **4** | 5.00 | 4.66 | 0.44 |
| Willingness | **3** | 5.00 | 4.00 | 0.75 |
| Total score | **3.13** | 5.00 | 4.26 | 0.49 |
| **Parenting Stress Index** | | | | |
| *Child characteristics* | 92.64 | **155.50** | **116.87** | 14.69 |
| Adaptability | 19.05 | **44.45** | **32.15** | 3.91 |
| Acceptability | **7.02** | **23.40** | 13.09 | 7.89 |
| Demandingness | 13.5 | **45.00** | **22.08** | 8.39 |
| Mood | 6 | **17.00** | 11.12 | 3.75 |
| Distractibility/Hyperactivity | 20.64 | **34.83** | 26.53 | 2.75 |
| Reinforcement of parents | 9 | **14.50** | **11.90** | 1.25 |
| *Parent characteristics* | **83.50** | 133.75 | 114.15 | 14.30 |
| Depression | **10.5** | **25.50** | 18.84 | 4.38 |
| Isolation | **6** | **22.00** | 12.69 | 6.36 |
| Attachment | 8.75 | **24.50** | 14.76 | 5.90 |
| Role Restriction | **8.75** | **28.00** | 18.92 | 6.95 |
| Competence | **10** | **34.00** | 20.25 | 4.65 |
| Spouse | **8** | **29.00** | 16.50 | 4.14 |
| Health | **7.5** | **23.75** | 12.19 | 4.88 |
| Total score | 187.9 | **273.75** | 219.94 | 21.23 |
| **IDARE** | | | | |
| State Anxiety | 23 | **69.00** | **43.13** | 12.48 |
| Trait Anxiety | 21 | **55.00** | **38.25** | 9.21 |

Note: Out-of-range values are shown in bold.

**Table 2.** Caregiver descriptive values.

values found to exceed the cutoff point of the accepted stress levels in all the subscales, and in the parent dimension there are several that show shallow values.

Again, the gender of children marked differences. In this case, it was the Adaptability subscale, where caregivers present stress above the cutoff point in the parenting of the girls ($M$ = 35.21), while distress generated from care of boys is within the typical ($M$ = 25.4); this

| Measures | BMI | BW | BH | MDI | PDI |
|---|---|---|---|---|---|
| **RPS-Questionnaire** | | | | | |
| Stimulation from Play | −0.205 | −0.049 | 0.059 | 0.386 | 0.136 |
| Responsive Practice | **0.544*** | 0.188 | −0.378 | **0.487*** | **0.457*** |
| Promoting skills | 0.301 | 0.169 | −0.124 | −0.001 | **0.440*** |
| Planned Care | 0.141 | 0.048 | −0.089 | 0.198 | 0.063 |
| Willingness | −0.090 | −0.248 | −0.075 | 0.121 | **0.502*** |
| Total | 0.171 | 0.043 | −0.138 | 0.344 | 0.346 |
| **Parenting Stress Index** | | | | | |
| *Child characteristics* | −0.259 | 0.100 | 0.085 | 0.438 | 0.166 |
| Adaptability | 0.199 | 0.277 | −0.145 | 0.234 | 0.192 |
| Acceptability | 0.091 | 0.034 | 0.058 | **−0.752**** | 0.102 |
| Demandingness | **−0.438*** | −0.264 | 0.125 | −0.116 | **−0.512*** |
| Mood | 0.098 | 0.064 | −0.241 | 0.299 | 0.058 |
| Distractibility/Hyperactivity | **−0.473*** | 0.070 | **0.507*** | 0.176 | −0.257 |
| Reinforcement of Parent | 0.071 | 0.219 | 0.170 | −0.108 | −0.129 |
| *Parent characteristics* | 0.150 | 0.181 | 0.062 | 0.100 | −0.032 |
| Depression | −0.371 | −0.006 | 0.324 | **−0.445*** | **−0.538*** |
| Isolation | 0.135 | 0.376 | 0.076 | −0.051 | −0.100 |
| Attachment | −0.154 | 0.211 | 0.265 | 0.039 | −0.366 |
| Role Restriction | 0.311 | −0.034 | **−0.497*** | 0.045 | 0.327 |
| Competence | 0.284 | −0.226 | −0.331 | −0.021 | 0.194 |
| Spouse | −0.033 | 0.067 | 0.089 | −0.358 | −0.093 |
| Health | 0.274 | 0.375 | 0.139 | −0.125 | −0.213 |
| Total | 0.132 | 0.193 | −0.132 | −0.324 | −0.056 |
| **IDARE** | | | | | |
| State Anxiety | 0.056 | 0.013 | 0.004 | **−0.441*** | −0.122 |
| Trait Anxiety | −0.119 | 0.111 | 0.409 | −0.324 | 0.083 |

BMI = Body mass.*<0.05.
**<0.01.

**Table 3.** Show correlation values between child and caregiver variables.

difference was statistically significant ($U = 9, p < 0.05$). It was found that at older children, caregivers perceived that raising the child made them more problematic with the couple ($r = 529$, $p < 0.05$) and higher levels of father's schooling, the less gratification the parents felt about the relationship with the infant ($r = 0.658$, $p < 0.05$). By contrast, the Wellness Index showed a negative relation with the difficulties seen by the caregiver to capture and understand the child's needs, obtaining lower scores in the Attachment subscale ($r = -0.563$, $p < 0.05$).

Averages anxiety state and trait found at moderate levels. Six caregivers showed high anxiety-state and two anxiety-trait levels. The only sociodemographic variables associated with IDARE scores were the age of the mother ($r = -0.533$, $p < 0.05$ for anxiety-state and $r = -528$, $p < 0.05$ for anxiety-trait) and of the father ($r = -0.703$, $p < 0.05$ for anxiety-state and $r = -0.845$, $p < 0.01$ for anxiety-trait).

### 3.4. Parenting variables and child nutritional status and development

Best scores on the RPS-Q correlate with better indicators in the child. In particular, Responsive Practice is positively associated with body mass index, mental development, and psychomotor development. The PDI also correlates with the Skills Promotion and Willingness factors, as can be seen in **Table 3**.

Following the values in the same table, some negative correlations, moderate or high, can be observed between parenting stress scores and child variables. Lower values of the BMI were associated with two subscales: Demandingness denoting distress generated by the appreciation that the demands of the children are too much, and Distractibility/Hyperactivity related to discomfort because child behavior is valued as erratic and lacking attention. The parameter who can indicate chronic malnutrition (BH) finds a negative correlation with the subscale Role Restriction that shows the interpretation of its role of caregiver as a restriction to its freedom, and positive with Distractibility.

The child's mental development shows a negative correlation with the values of Acceptability—the high scores in this subscale result when children possess physical, intellectual, and/or emotional characteristics that do not harmonize with what parents expect—and Depression, as well as with IDARE scores for state anxiety. On the other hand, the psychomotor development was related, also negatively, with Demandingness and Depression.

## 4. Discussion

Fitting to the objective, this work explored the influence of rearing practices and socioemotional caregiver factors on the nutritional status and psychological development in a sample of Mexican children. At the outset, it is important to mention that relevant relationships were found between the variables under study; however, the reduced size of the sample requires assessing the findings with due caution.

All children who participated in this study lived in conditions of economic and social scarcities [35] and were at risk of undernourishment or suffer it. Because of this, the variability of the values of the different measures is not very wide. Given the relative homogeneity of the sample in the sociodemographic variables, the possible contribution of parenting in the results on nutrition and child development was highlighted.

The parameter that was most affected was BH whose low values indicate a history of malnutrition and/or diseases, although the means of the other two parameters did not reach the values corresponding to emaciation and low weight, there were cases of mild and moderate undernourishment which corresponded to emaciation and low weight. According to the first hypothesis, it was expected that if the anthropometric parameters were adversely affected, this would be reflected in levels of mental and psychomotor development. This hypothesis was partially corroborated since the prediction is supported by BMI, a needle of recent faltering, data that correlate positively with the PDI, but the same was not true for parameter BH, an indicator of chronic malnutrition because the results pointed to a negative correlation of this parameter with the PDI. That is, at more height for age a lower development score was found.

This finding does not harmonize with most of the antecedent literature that demonstrates the existence of adverse effects of nutrient deficiencies on different indicators of psychomotor development in early ages [9, 10, 18, 19, 44]. There are three possible alternative explanations for this result. The first has to do with the size of the sample and the method of non-random extraction, given with small sizes the samples can be affected by very few atypical cases; in a previous study, carried out with a similar population in the State of Mexico that included a larger sample, stunting highlighted as one of the factors with greater weight to explain development deficits [45]. The second possibility is related to the lack of information on the specific children's nutritional deficiencies, since many of the developmental deficit caused by malnutrition, mainly those that corroborate the functional isolation hypothesis, consider the deficiency of anemia [18, 19]; in this study, we did not have the possibility of having information about serum iron levels. The third possibility relates to the explanation of David Seckler, and recovered by Pollitt [46], to understand cases where there is child malnutrition and development is not affected. It is an idea where the evolutionary principles of biological adaptation are applied, which argues that food deficiencies slow the child's growth rate in order to maintain a functional physiological balance, and therefore children with mild or moderate malnutrition maintain the capacity of adaptation to adverse circumstances. Considering that the children in the sample had mild (risk) and moderate undernourishment, the assumption of biological adaptation is plausible and could help to understand why, despite the slow growth, infants present adequate levels of psychomotor development.

With respect to the second hypothesis where it was predicted that at higher levels of parenting stress and anxiety the caregiver would have worse outcomes in the child's nutrition and development, the results point to its confirmation. Except for the distractibility factor, the relationships between the parenting stress factors with BMI parameters and BH were negative. Then, we may consider the possibility that in this sample the stress concerning the child caregiving is connected with the state of nutrition, although perhaps not directly. Some studies on this aspect [47, 48] have found associations between alterations in caregiver-child interactions at the mealtime, where the refusal to eat in the infant and the negative effect in both the caregiver and the child prevail, and high levels of parenting stress [34, 49, 50]. It can be assumed here that the parenting stress is the result of insufficient caregiver practices to promote child feeding. As long as their instrumental behavior is ineffective for the childcare, it can generate the distress regarding the nurturing and thus impede its future practices. In other studies, a decrease in parenting stress or anxiety following interventions aimed at reducing problematic behavior at mealtime [51, 52] has been described. The same can happen with regard to the development of the child, since the strongest relationships between anxiety and PSI scores and delay in psychomotor and mental scales occurred with the perception of a dependent child making many demands toward his caregiver, and also with the discomfort generated by the child's failure to meet expectations in terms of physical, intellectual, or emotional characteristics.

Results concerning parenting practices, measured using the RSP-Q, showed a positive relationship between the BMI and the Responsive Practice factor, which describes the caregivers' sensitivity and her/his resources to detect and react to needs based on the signals provided by the infant. This finding is in agreement with previous research on the importance of responsive parenting on child feeding [22–24]. An even clearer relationship was observed between this variable and child development, as the results showed positive correlations between developmental test scores and Responsive Practice, in addition to the factors of skill promotion and Willingness. These results replicate what was found in other studies and support the third hypothesis of this research. The level of sensitivity to detect signals that account for the infant's needs and the ability to respond to them in a timely and fitting manner are essential features of the parenting practice, which allows the child to maintain adequate nutritional status and favor a better psychological development; otherwise negligence or little skill in childcare is a further risk for malnutrition to occur with its adverse effects on child development [18, 45, 53].

Among the sociodemographic variables, the Wellness Index stood out as an important factor, since the results showed positive relationships with the variables of the child weight for the age and the index of psychomotor development. It also had a presence on the results about caregiver characteristics, mainly on the effective parenting practices related to the skills promotion and the responsiveness to child demands [28]. Another relevant demographic factor was the child gender, as it was found that caregivers were more responsive to the needs of girls, who scored better than children on the mental scale, despite being perceived as having difficulty adapting to the demands of the environment.

The children age also appeared as an important variable, the older infants showed greater affectation to the weight gain, despite showing a positive association with the caregiver's willingness for their care. An element that could explain weight loss according to the child's age is that caregivers are facing more problems feeding the child, related to neophobias and rejection. Even though they are responsive and encourage the child to eat, but many sometimes do not use the appropriate strategies for the child to accept the food [54]. Although it found an only association with a characteristic of the caregiver, the age of both parents seems to be attenuating the levels of anxiety, which were linked with those resulting from the mental development of the children.

Although the sample of this study is small and made with Mexican population, it can be assumed that the results found here can be extended, conserving the cultural peculiarities of each region, to other populations where the problem of malnutrition is present together with precarious living conditions and where caregivers of developing children face situations of high demand. The variables explored have also been relevant in studies carried out in different latitudes, such as poverty and malnutrition [1]; a low sociocultural level associated to affective instability and malnutrition [33, 55]; likewise, relations between ineffective parenting practices and malnutrition [24, 56] or disadvantages in psychological development [18].

However, these relationships were analyzed in this research from the use of different measurement instruments, particularly the Wellness Index and the RPS-Q. Likewise, adapted and validated versions for the Spanish-speaking population of instruments of extended use were employed, such as the BSID, the IDARE, and the Parenting Stress Index. The Wellness Index is a World Bank proposal that has recently been used to measure poverty on a large scale; unlike previous ordinal measures where the greatest weight fell on family income, it is based on a cardinal measurement with different axes to determine the degree of people's economic and social deprivation, social support and rights. Thus, a multidimensional poverty index reflects incidence, intensity, and composition picture of acute poverty [57, 58]. Because this way of measuring poverty is indicated for developing countries, several of them have already developed an index adapted to their specific conditions [59]. Recovering this measure for an investigation, such as that described here, represents an advantage due to the profusion of information obtained.

Regarding the extension of the use of the RPS-Q as a rearing practice measure in different contexts, it is suggested that this methodology can be used in other country settings making cultural adaptations. Despite its reliability and validity was performed in the Mexican population, the questionnaire was built considering basic principles of the rearing process that can be generalizable to diverse populations. The underlying sensitivity and responsiveness of caregiving constructs have been described as the ability to recognize and interpret the signals which the other emits about their needs and also respond to them in an appropriate and timely mode [23, 25].

Responsive parenting has been identified in observations of caregiver-infant interactions in different countries [60, 61]. This characteristic is identified through indicators of attention to the other, the relevance and contingency of responding, as well as the amount of socioemotional support provided to the child; these dimensions are present in every care interaction. The RPS-Q made it possible to obtain one of the most important contributions of this work showing relations between affective and emotional aspects with the effective caregiver practices that, ultimately, mediate the child's feeding behavior, as well as the exposure of stimuli environmental factors that contribute to their motor and mental development.

In this study, it was possible to describe several relationships between variables that may constitute risk factors or protection for child development problems associated with malnutrition. It is necessary to confirm these relationships with a larger sample that allows, at the same time, to test models that propose the directionality of the variables of the child and the caregiver, as well as the possible role as mediators or moderators of the characteristics of the caregiver and their rearing practices, between the effects of malnutrition on the development of the child.

## Acknowledgements

This research was made possible thanks to financial support from UNAM DGPA-PAPIIT program. Granted project IN307914.

The author is grateful to authorities of the Sanitary Jurisdiction of the Institute of Health-State of Mexico (ISEM), Tlalnepantla, for facilities provided to fulfill the objectives of this study, as well as to the staff of the Health Centers ISEM, Lázaro Cárdenas II, Lázaro Cardenas III, and Benito Juárez. Also thanks to fellows participating in the project for the field work.

A special acknowledgment to all caregivers and their children for taking part in this study, as well as Addalid Sánchez Hernández for the supervision of fellows and their active participation in the research activities.

## Author details

Assol Cortés-Moreno

Address all correspondence to: assol@unam.mx

National Autonomous University of Mexico, Faculty of Higher Education Iztacala, Mexico

## References

[1] Subramanyam MA, Kawachi I, Berkman LF, et al. Is economic growth associated with reduction in child undernutrition in India? PLoS Medicine. 2011;**8**:15

[2] Schmidhuber J. The outlook for long-term changes in food consumption patterns: concerns and policy options. In: FAO Scientific Workshop on Globalization of the Food System: Impacts on Food Security and Nutrition. Rome: Food and Agriculture Organization of the United Nations; 2003

[3] Cuevas-Nasu L, Rivera-Dommarco JA, Shamah-Levy T. Inseguridad alimentaria y estado de nutrición en menores de cinco años de edad en México. Salud Pública de México. 2014;**56**:47-53

[4] Bourges H. Costumbres, prácticas y hábitos alimentarios. Cuadernos de Nutricion. 1990; **13**:17-22

[5] Rivera Dommarco J, Shamah Levy T, Villalpando Hernández S, et al. Encuesta Nacional de Nutrición 1999. 2001. Available from: http://scholar.google.com/scholar?hl=en&btnG=Search&q=intitle:Encuesta+Nacional+de+Nutrici?n+1999#0

[6] UNICEF. Annual Report. 2014. Epub ahead of print 2014. DOI: 10.1017/CBO9781107415324.004

[7] Olaiz-Fernández G, Rivera-Dommarco J, Shamma-Levy T, et al. Encuesta Nacional de Salud y Nutrición 2006. Morelos: Cuernavaca; 2006

[8] Hughes D, Bryan J. The assessment of cognitive performance in children: Considerations for detecting nutritional influences. Nutrition Reviews. 2003;**61**:413-422

[9] de Andraca I, Castillo M, Walter T. Psychomotor development and behavior in iron-deficient anemic infants. Nutrition Reviews. 1997;**55**:125-132

[10] Drewett R, Wolke D, Asefa M, et al. Malnutrition and mental development: Is there a sensitive period? A nested case-control study. Journal of Child Psychology and Psychiatry. 2001;**42**:181-187

[11] Boddy J, Skuse D, Andrews B. The developmental sequelae of nonorganic failure to thrive. Journal of Child Psychology and Psychiatry. 2000;**41**:1003-1014

[12] Sandjaja N, Poh BK, Rojroonwasinkul N, et al. Relationship between anthropometric indicators and cognitive performance in Southeast Asian school-aged children. British Journal of Nutrition. 2013;**110**(Suppl):S57-S64

[13] Corbett SS, Drewett RF. To what extent is failure to thrive in infancy associated with poorer cognitive development? A review and meta-analysis. Journal of Child Psychology and Psychiatry. 2004;**45**:641-654

[14] Flores ME, Troyo R, Haro LP, et al. La desnutrición del siglo XXI y su impacto en las emociones y afrontamientos en niños escolares. Investigación en Salud. 2005;**VII**:188-195

[15] Walker SP, Wachs TD, Gardner JM, et al. Child development: Risk factors for adverse outcomes in developing countries. Lancet. 2007;**369**:145-157

[16] Meeks JM, Grantham-McGrgor S, Chang SM, et al. Activity and behavioural development in stunted and nonstunted children and response to nutritional supplementation. Child Development 1995; **66**:1785-1797

[17] Levitsky D, Barnes R. Nutritional and environmental interactions in the Behavioral development of the rat: Long-term effects. Science. 1972;**176**:68-71

[18] Pollitt E, Golub M, Gorman K, et al. A reconceptualization of the effects of undernutrition on children's biological, psychosocial and behavioural development. Social Policy Report's Society for Research in Child Development. 1996;**10**:1-22

[19] Lozzoff B, Klein NK, Nelson EC, et al. Behavior of infants with iron-deficiency anemia. Child Development. 1998;**69**:24-36

[20] Lozoff B, Corapci F, Burden MJ, et al. Preschool-aged children with iron deficiency anemia show altered affect and behavior. The Journal of Nutrition. 2007;**137**:683-689

[21] Strupp B, Levitsky D. Enduring cognitive effects of early malnutrition: A theoretical reappraisal. The Journal of Nutrition. 1995;**125**:2221-2232

[22] Stanfield P. Some aspects of the long-term effects of malnutrition on the behaviour of children in the third world. The Proceedings of the Nutrition Society. 1993;**52**:201-210

[23] Mentro AM, Steward DK, Garvin BJ. Infant feeding responsiveness: A conceptual analysis. Journal of Advanced Nursing. 2002;**37**:208-216

[24] Bentley ME, Wasser HM, Creed-Kanashiro HM. Responsive feeding and child undernutrition in low- and middle-income countries. The Journal of Nutrition. 2011;**141**:502-507

[25] Black MM, Aboud FE. Responsive feeding is embedded in a theoretical framework of responsive parenting. The Journal of Nutrition. 2011;**141**:490-494

[26] Baumrind D, Larzelere RE, Owens EB. Effects of preschool parents' power assertive patterns and practices on adolescent development. Parenting. 2010;**10**:157-201

[27] Myers RG. Comprensión de las diferencias culturales en las distintas prácticas y creencias relativas a la crianza de los niños. In: Los doce que sobreviven: fortalecimineto de los programas de desarrollo para la primera infancia. Whasington, DC: Organización Panamericana de la Salud/Fondo de las Naciones Unidas Para la Infancia; 1993. pp. 427-460

[28] Alvarado BE, Tabares RE, Delisie H, et al. Creencias maternas, prácticas de alimentación y estado nutricional en niños Afro-Colombianos. Archivos Latinoamericanos de Nutrición. 2005;**55**:55-66

[29] Engle PL. Infant feeding styles: Barriers and opportunities for good nutrition in India. Nutrition Reviews. 2002;**60**:S109-S114

[30] Needlman R. Failure to thrive: Parental neglect or well-meaning ignorance? American Family Physician. 2001;**1**:1867-1869

[31] Pelto GH, Backstrand JR. Interrelationships between power-related and belief-related factors determine nutrition in Populations1. American Society of Nutrition Science. 2003;**133**:297S-300S

[32] Kerr MA, Black MM, Krishnakumar A. Failure-to-thrive, maltreatment and the behavior and development of 6-year-old children from low-income, urban families: A cumulative risk model. Child Abuse & Neglect. 2000;**24**:587-598

[33] Surkan PJ, Kennedy CE, Hurley KM, et al. Maternal depression and early childhood growth in developing countries: Systematic review and meta-analysis. Bulletin of the World Health Organization. 2011;**89**:608-615

[34] Ashiabi GS, O'Neal KK. Children's health status: Examining the associations among income poverty, material hardship, and parental factors. PLoS One. 2007;**2**:e940

[35] Consejo Nacional de Evaluación de la Política de Desarrollo Social [CONEVAL]. Metodología para la Medición Multidimensional de la Pobreza en México. México, DF, México: CONEVAL; 2014

[36] WHO Expert Comittee. Physical Status: The Use and Interpretation of Anthropometry. Geneva, Switzerland: WHO Expert Comittee; 1995

[37] World Health Organization. ANHRO 2005. 2006. Available from: https://www.google.com.mx/search?q=anthro+2005+software&oq=anthro+2005&aqs=chrome.2.69i57j015.6680j0j7&sourceid=chrome&ie=UTF-8

[38] Bayley N. Escalas de Desarrollo Infantil. Téccnicos Especialistas Aplicados: Madrid, España; 1977

[39] Abidin R. Parenting Stress Index. Odessa, PL: Psychological Assessment Resources, Inc.; 1995

[40] Montiel MM, Vera JÁ. Análisis de las propiedades psicométricas del índice de estrés de la crianza en una población rural del estado de Sonora. La Psicol Soc en México. 1998;**6**:86-90

[41] Spielberg C, Díaz-Guerrero R. IDARE: Inventario de ansiedad: Rasgo-Estado [IDARE: inventory of anxiety]. México, D.F, México: El Manual Moderno; 2002

[42] Cortés MA, Romero SP, Sánchez TG. Diseño y validación inicial de un instrumento para evaluar prácticas de crianza en la infancia. Universitas Psychologica. 2006;**5**:37-49

[43] IBM. IBM SPSS Statistics. Chicago, USA: IBM Corporation; 2011

[44] Subramanian SV, Mejía-Guevara I, Krishna A. Rethinking policy perspectives on childhood stunting: Time to formulate a structural and multifactorial strategy. Maternal & Child Nutrition. 2016;**12**:219-236

[45] Cortés A, Avilés AL. Factores demográficos, crianza e historia de salud: vinculación con la nutrición y el desarrollo infantil. Universitas Psychologica. 2011;**10**:789-802

[46] Pollitt E. Desnutrición energético proteica I: causas, clasificación y epidemiología. In: Consecuencias de la desnutrición en el escolar peruano. Lima, Perú: Pontificia Universidad Católica del Perú; 2002. pp. 157-171

[47] Ramsay M. Feeding skill, appetite and feeding behaviours of infants and young children and their impact on growth and psychosocial development. Early Childhood Development [online]. 2004:1-9. Available from: http://www.child-encyclopedia.com/sites/default/files/textes-experts/en/535/feeding-skill-appetite-and-feeding-behaviours-of-infants-and-young-children-and-their-impact-on-growth-and-psychosocial-development.pdf

[48] Flancbaum M, Oppenheimer CW, Abela JRZ, et al. The effects of rumination on the timing of maternal and child negative affect. Journal of Clinical Child and Adolescent Psychology. 2011;**40**:596-606

[49] Cortés-Moreno A, Méndez-Lozano SM. Estrés parental, interacciones diádicas al comer y desnutrición en el periodo de alimentación complementaria. Journal of Behavior, Health & Social Issues. 2012;**3**:113-125

[50] Surkan PJ, Kawachi I, Ryan LM, et al. Maternal depressive symptoms, parenting self-efficacy, and child growth. American Journal of Public Health. 2008;**98**:125-132

[51] Lukens CT, Silverman AH. Systematic review of psychological interventions for pediatric feeding problems. Journal of Pediatric Psychology. 2014;**39**:903-917

[52] David GG, Angélica RJ. Conducta materna en la mesa y consumo alimentario en infantes: evaluación de un programa. Universidad Nacional Autónoma de México. 2013. Available from: http://132.248.9.195/ptd2013/septiembre/0701201/Index.html

[53] Walker SP, Chang SM, Wright A, et al. Early childhood stunting is associated with lower developmental levels in the subsequent generation of children. The Journal of Nutrition. 2015;**145**:823-828

[54] Moore AC, Akhter S, Aboud FE. Responsive complementary feeding in rural Bangladesh. Social Science & Medicine. 2006;**62**:1917-1930

[55] Rahman A, Iqbal Z, Bunn J, et al. Impact of maternal depression on infant nutritional status and illness: A cohort study. Archives of General Psychiatry. 2004;**61**:946-952

[56] Wondafrash M, Amsalu T, Woldie M. Feeding styles of caregivers of children 6-23 months of age in Derashe special district, Southern Ethiopia. BMC Public Health. 2012;**12**:235

[57] Alkire S, Santos ME. Acute Multidimensional Poverty: A New Index for Developing Countries. Epub ahead of print 2010. DOI: 10.2139/ssrn.1815243.

[58] Gasper D. In: McGillivray M, editor. Human Well-being: Concepts and Conceptualizations BT – Human Well-Being: Concept and Measurement. London: Palgrave Macmillan UK; 2004. pp. 23-64

[59] Alkire S, Santos ME. Measuring acute poverty in the developing world: Robustness and scope of the multidimensional poverty index. World Development. 2014;**59**:251-274

[60] Eshel N, Daelman B, de Mello MC, et al. Responsive parenting: Interventions and outcomes. Bulletin of the World Health Organization. 2006;**84**:991-998

[61] Nahar B, Hossain MI, Hamadani JD, et al. Effects of psychosocial stimulation on improving home environment and child-rearing practices: Results from a community-based trial among severely malnourished children in Bangladesh. BMC Public Health. 2012;**12**:622

3

# Improving Quality of Life: Home Care for Chronically Ill and Elderly People

Natalia López Celani, Sergio Ponce,
Olga Lucía Quintero and Francisco Vargas-Bonilla

**Abstract**

In this chapter, we propose a system especially created for elderly or chronically ill people that are with special needs and poor familiarity with technology. The system combines home monitoring of physiological and emotional states through a set of wearable sensors, user-controlled (automated) home devices, and a central control for integration of the data, in order to provide a safe and friendly environment according to the limited capabilities of the users. The main objective is to create the easy, low-cost automation of a room or house to provide a friendly environment that enhances the psychological condition of immobilized users. In addition, the complete interaction of the components provides an overview of the physical and emotional state of the user, building a behavior pattern that can be supervised by the care giving staff. This approach allows the integration of physiological signals with the patient's environmental and social context to obtain a complete framework of the emotional states.

**Keywords:** home care, domotics, health monitoring, emotions recognition, elderly care giving

## 1. Introduction

The statistics and surveys of the World Health Organization (WHO) [1] reveal an increasing in life expectation (expecting 400 millions of population over 60 years old at 2050), longer treatments for chronic diseases as cancer, diabetes, cardiovascular conditions, and prevalence of Alzheimer's disease and dementia, which leads to an increase in health costs and a social problem for personal care and hospitalization. According to the prediction of the United Nations, 65 years and older will occupy 15.7% of the total population in 2030 [2].

A recent survey in Europe has shown the socioeconomic impact of this problem, because chronic illness and aging affect 8 out of 10 people aged over 65 in Europe and consume 70–80% of health care budgets, both by the increasing number of patients and by the focus in acute diseases that manage the resources inefficiently for this case. In this perspective, the chronicity is a major societal challenge to develop strategies to enhance quality of life and prevent unnecessary hospitalizations. Similar situation has been reported in the United States, with an older proportion of 14.9% in 2015 [3], where the population aged 80 and over is projected to more than triple between 2015 and 2050.

In the Latin-American region, the situation is not different. According to the Pan-American Health Organization's (PAHO) report on Innovative Care for Chronic Conditions [4], 76% of deaths (4 million people annually) are due to chronic conditions and only 1 of 10 people receives adequate treatment. All countries in the region show an accelerated increase in aging population, due to a better life expectative, but the adverse side is the risk of chronic diseases and the increment in the public health costs, which are already insufficient for current needs.

Besides legislative and educational support to this problem, is necessary to change the structure of health systems and the paradigm of caring for the elderly and the chronically ill, promoting home care and family support in a controlled environment. This initiative has to be accompanied for the educational, management, and budget changes that will be essentials for the next decades.

Technology will be a key instrument for a new concept of home care and continuous monitoring. New and smaller devices and communication possibilities lead to a more humanitarian model of assisted alternative to institutionalization as a great potential to reduce the burden of chronic diseases by making better use of this knowledge. A multidisciplinary approach is needed, because an integral scheme must to consider physiological, emotional, social, and environmental conditions that promote the well-being and support for the patients.

Men and women in their older ages suffer increased fragility, incapacity, chronic illness, and dependency. Several attempts of remote health monitoring can be found in the literature [5–7]. For example, Stikic et al. [8] present an effective and unobtrusive long term monitoring and recognition of activities of daily living based on the combination of the data from two different types of sensors: radio frequency identification (RFID) tag readers and accelerometers. A system based on wireless body sensors and smart phones was presented in [9] to offer remote monitoring and alert family and ambulance if detects an emergency. As was established by the authors, iCare is not only a real-time health monitoring system for the elderly, but also a living assistant.

Related to home automation and control, in the work of Ghazal and Al-Khatib [10], the authors propose the use of a single controller to command home appliances and sensors by using XBee transceivers. The remote controller has command buttons, alert LEDs and a LCD for showing messages. The unique master board toggles the ON/OFF switches of the appliances by means of relays.

Other works of Akanbi and Oladeji [11] use voice commands to control multiple home electrical or electronic appliances with maximum of 5 V using an Arduino Uno microcontroller. The design transmits voice command through a wireless microphone and a graphical interface. A systematic review of smart-home technologies to assist older adults can be found in [7], which concludes that smart-home technologies are readily accepted by older adults and their family members, and must be improved to enhancing safety and privacy. This work remarks the future challenge in aspects such as social and emotional well-being as well as outdoors interests and activities monitoring.

The system herein proposed has significant differences with these approaches, because of it was created especially for people with special needs and poor familiarity with technology. The system combines home monitoring of physiological and emotional states through a set of wearable's sensors, user-controlled (automated) home devices, and adapted human-computer interfaces (HCI) are used in order to provide a safe and friendly environment according to the limited capabilities of the users. The main objective is to create the easy, low-cost automation of a room or house to provide a friendly environment that enhances the psychological condition of immobilized or vulnerable users, improves their safety and allows living at home longer. Moreover, the complete interaction of the components provides an overview of the physical and emotional state of the user, building a behavior pattern that can be supervised by the caregiving staff.

The emotional content is included here, as one of the main concerns in elder and disabled people. We propose the use of emotion recognition from voiced speech algorithms in order to maintain the integrated emotional state of the patient and use the signals as indicator for certain behavior. It has been an author's effort through years to develop and offer the most possible accurate algorithms, and here we propose a data fusion of the best approaches. Moreover, from voice analysis can be possible to detect Parkinson's disease (PD) so our proposal allows for constant monitoring and early detection of this condition. In addition, there is an important feature added to our proposal such as a methodology for detecting movements of interest, i.e., fall detection. Consequently, we present a couple of methodologies that can be easily understood and implemented in an in-house application.

There is a wide variety of commercial domotic systems, almost focus in lights automation, blinds, air conditioning, and other predefined tasks, driven by ever-increasing needs for house comfort, user connection, energy saving, and security. Phone remote access or voice commands are the most common user interfaces, not always suitable for use by the elderly. House automation for elderly people has different needs and objectives, attempting to provide the minimal user intervention and maximizing the physical and emotional support.

With this aim, we present an integral assistive home care system (IAHCS), specially designed for elderly or chronically ill people, who present mobility difficulties and reduced decision-making capacity. The main objective is to provide a technological aid that balances promoting autonomy while protecting a vulnerable adult from harm. Along with this, the caring for the elderly and people with chronic diseases, have also improved emphasizing the need of preventive medicine and monitoring of these patients in their home.

The approach proposed in this chapter comprises a user wearable device, a domotic system's core installed in a personal computer (PC) and an ichnographic software (SICAA) that allows the interaction of the patient with the environment and peripheral devices. Besides, a microphone equipped with Wi-Fi connection record the user's voice and sends it to the processing unit, in order to recognize emotional states. This scheme is integrated in a control block, described in **Figure 1**.

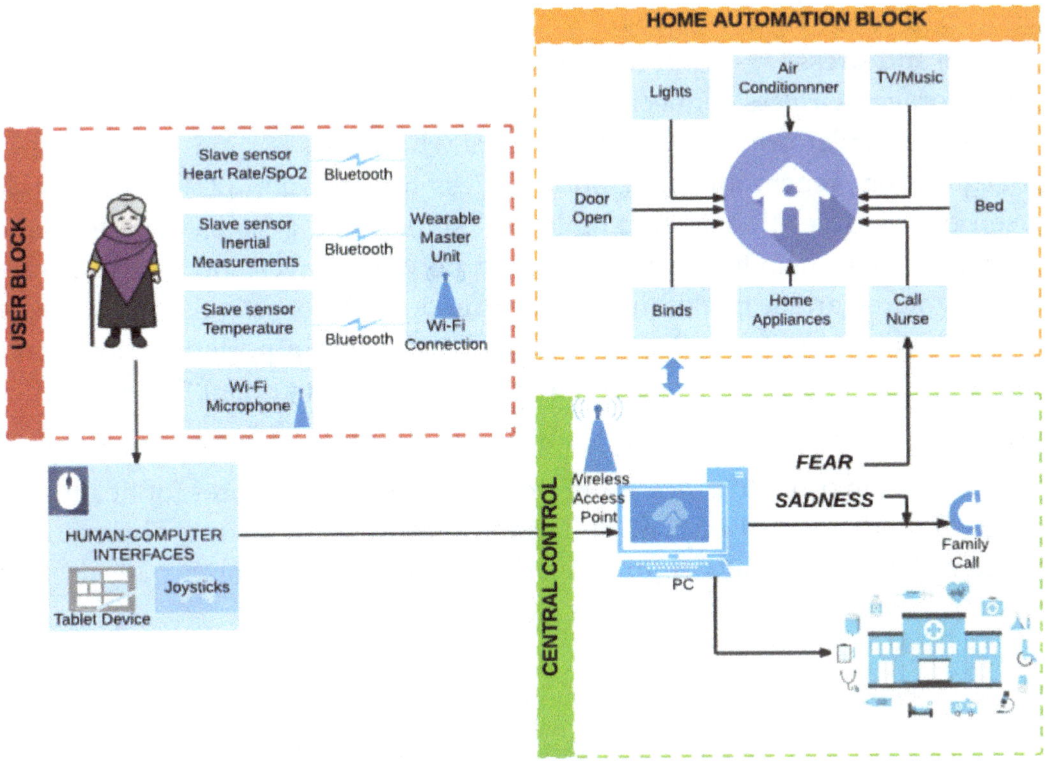


**Figure 1.** Overall scheme of the integral assistive home care system. The user block belongs to wearable sensors for health and voice acquisition. Home automation block includes the control board of relays and home appliances. Human-computer interfaces communicate the user with the central control. All communications are wireless.

## 2. Human-computer interface (HCI)

Regarding the HCI, the major requirements are noninvasiveness, low cost, robustness, and adaptability for a group of users with similar capacities. For many years, we have developed HCI that was essayed as control input with acceptable results, especially for disabled people needs, such as adapted keypads, head-mouse controllers, vision based Interfaces using hand or head position detection, electromyogram, and electrooculogram-based interfaces, among others [12–16].

For this system, a conventional mouse can be used, and also tablets, Wii commands or more sophisticated controls. Voice commands are eligible too, and preferred because they allow the emotion recognition processing as will be explained below.

In any case, the control input is configurable and versatile according with user's abilities, allowed by the modularity of the system.

## 3. Wearable monitoring

Wearable sensors are steadily becoming the most prevalent personal devices, playing a crucial role in the chronic patients monitoring [17, 18]. Biological variables such as heart rate and oxygen saturation are being used for self-monitoring and preventing health conditions such as hypertension and stress [19–21]. A wearable system should meet certain design conditions, such as data storage, wireless connection, power supply, portability and versatility, among others. We propose a platform of wearable sensors whose core is a master module that deals with data acquisition, synchronization, and wireless transmission [22]. This module is connected to sensors or slaves that acquire biological signals and process them to minimize the amount of data to be transmitted. The connection between slaves and master is intended to be in a properly wired article of clothing or via Bluetooth. Also, active sensors are selected to minimize battery consumption, and store data selectively. It is important to note that the communication protocol must be the same, independently of the nature of the acquired signal.

The data transmission from the master is carried out through Wi-Fi using TCP/IP protocol to a personal computer in order to process and extract descriptive features for health monitoring that will be used in the supervised control. The master board is shown in **Figure 2**, noting that the main core is the CC3200 microcontroller unit of Texas Instruments®

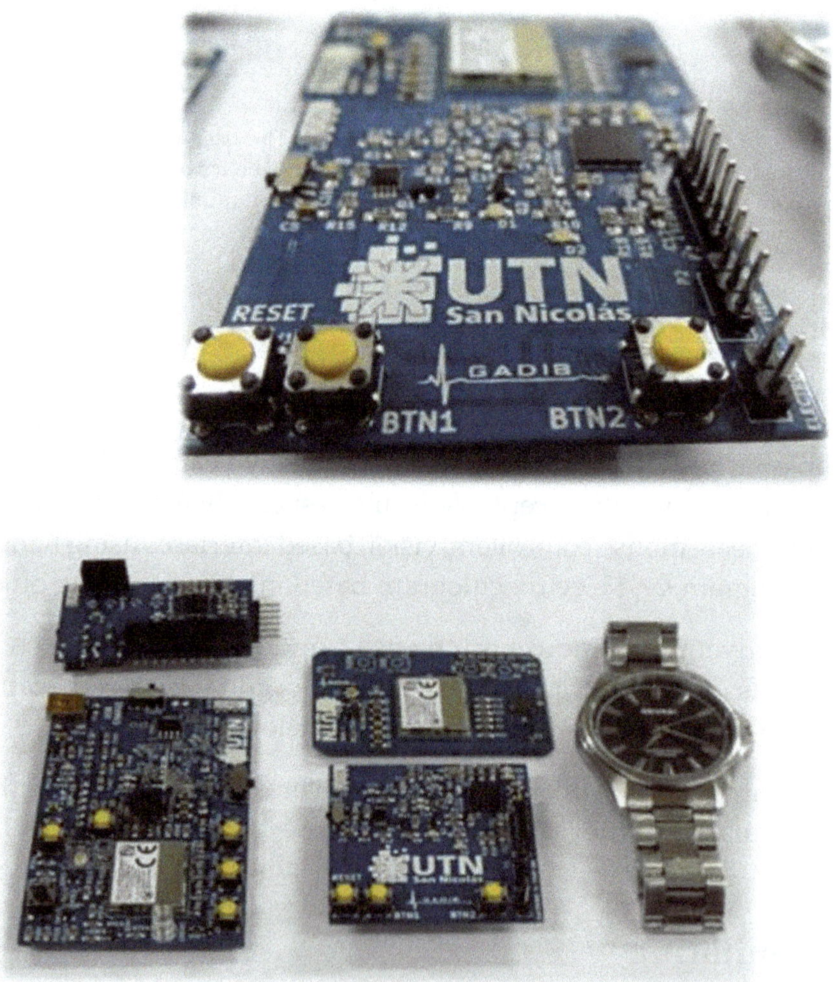


**Figure 2.** Wearable modules. Up: master module. Down: slaves modules for heart rate/SpO2, IMU, temperature, and microphone. It is important to note the size related with a wristwatch.

The sensors module or slave units consist of a base platform where the principal component is a microcontroller unit (MCU) with ARM architecture (Advanced Reduced instructions Machine) that allows the addition of different analog circuits according to the biologic variable that is intended to measure. This module meets specific requirements of consumption, inputs/outputs and radio-frequency transmission. Thanks to the ultra-low power consumption, it allows to operate for long periods of time, even with smaller batteries.

The biological variables (each with its own specific acquisition and preprocessing module) acquired are:

- Temperature module: It registers two temperature channels. Especially for chronic illness the body temperature is sensed and also the ambient temperature, to prevent hypothermia or excessive perspiration (this control is in a higher level that the domotic air conditioning, chosen by the user). This module is based on LMT70 sensor, ultra-small (0.88 by 0.88 mm) and with 0.1°C of accuracy, and the temperature was estimated with a first order approximation in the range of interest, from 30 to 45°C.
- Heart rate module and pulse oximetry: This module is of crucial importance in the monitoring of cardiac and respiratory patients. On the other hand, the module is useful to detect sedentarism in elderly and obese users. The module is based on the absortion of the red light (660 nm) for deoxygenated and infrared light (940 nm) for oxygenated hemoglobin. The sensors must be placed directly on the skin and a single circuit (AFE4403 based) detects the relation between absorbed light and the peaks related with cardiac pulse. The output is a signal for SpO2 and heart rate.
- Kinetics measurements module: This module has an inertial sensor inertial measurement unit (IMU), based on the MPU6050 that contains an accelerometer and a gyroscope. The information is processed to avoid singularities and both sources (an accelerometer and a gyroscope) are merged through a complementary filter reference. The output is processed to provide information related to the user's activity level and the algorithms explained in the next section are implemented for fall detection and alarm.
- Personal microphone module: To transmit human voice to the central PC, a commercial wireless Wi-Fi microphone is used and connected to the control unit. This module provides connection with the emotion processing unit.

The main software should be modular to suit the sensors chosen for each application, which give versatility to the system, functioning in an interchangeable way.

## 4. Fall detection algorithm

Using the data provided by the IMU sensor, we also analyze the problem of falls in independent elderly people. In Ref. [23], authors demonstrated that the consequences of a fall could be minimized by a portable automatic detection system, which sends an alarm right after an event. A dataset (SisFall) was created with 38 participants that conducted 19 activities of daily life and simulated 15 types of falls. This responded to the need of a fall detection dataset with a large number of activities determined after a literature review and our own survey; well documented acquisition conditions (authors recorded videos of each activity); and data from an embedded device fixed to the body (other datasets publicly available were recorded with smartphones). SisFall dataset consisted of 34 activities [falls and activities of daily living (ADL)] performed by 38 participants (15 of them had more than 60 years old). All files were made publicly available for the scientific community. The dataset was tested with the most widely used features to detect falls. With this work, it was demonstrated that a simple fourth order Butterworth filter with a cut frequency of 5 Hz is enough to detect falls without loss of information. Additionally, it was found that dynamic features based on statistical moments are the most accurate to classify among falls and ADL. However, it was also found that training algorithms with young people are insufficient to obtain acceptable accuracy with the objective population [24].

Preliminary tests with feature extraction algorithms commonly used in the literature to discriminate between falls and activities of daily living presented up to 96% of accuracy. They were implemented with a low computational cost threshold-based classifier, which can operate in real-time embedded systems. An individual activity analysis with each feature extraction algorithm demonstrated that some of them are complementary to each other. This analysis was used as a starting point to develop nonlinear discrimination metrics that improved the accuracy upto 99%. It is important to note that most false-positives are due to high acceleration periodic activities, and could be detected solely based on their period.

An energy-based fall detection algorithm was also implemented. The authors used a static feature extraction characteristic together with an energy-based feature. This algorithm was tested in data from a smartphone and the embedded device, with acceptable results [23].

Moreover, the most important finding was that the combination of different features provides higher discrimination capabilities than the individual ones. This result led to a second conclusion, a threshold-based classifier is enough to achieve accuracy levels of up to 99%. The importance of this final finding relays in the low complexity (and consequently energy consumption) that threshold-based classifiers require (**Figure 3**).

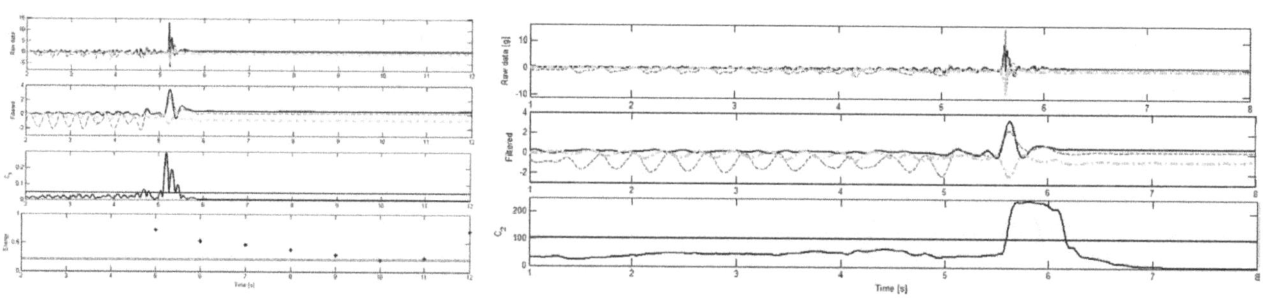

**Figure 3.** Example for acquisition and processing of IMU signals during jogging and fall detection. The raw data is initially filtered. Then, features are computed and if thresholds (horizontal lines) are crossed a fall is detected. Left: threshold algorithm, parameter C2 is the standard deviation magnitude. Right: Energy based detection (Figure from Ref. [23], with permission).

It was found that most of the errors in the threshold-based algorithms were focused in some individual activities, such as periodic ADL with high energy, namely walk, jog, or going up or down stairs. Consequently, was developed a novel methodology for detecting and characterizing walk and jog based on nonpeak-based acceleration features. It was demonstrated that with the Kurtosis of wavelet coefficients it was possible to obtain a measure to correctly identify these activities. However, the authors found that it was more stable to obtain the period of the acceleration signal using its autocorrelation. A posteriori statistical analysis demonstrated that the period provides statistical significant differences between walk and jog. This methodology proved to be sensitive enough to provide a "quality of the activity" measure. The authors were able to determine online the regularity of the activity when the subject walked or jogged. This result could be useful for sports, allowing the person to maintain a regular jog rhythm for long periods of time.

In order to guarantee that the developed methodology can be implemented on the IMU slave sensor without affecting their computational capability (and the consequent battery consumption), authors propose an algorithm based on a Kalman filter, with a preprocessing stage based on a fourth order Butterworth filter, a nonlinear feature based in two commonly used feature extraction characteristics, and a threshold-based classifier. This algorithm was implemented the module in the *in-situ* microcontroller and validated by simulating the same activities of the dataset acquired in this work, along with a pilot test in real conditions with elderly adults. Both tests presented an error rate below 1%.

The algorithm was tested with the wearable sensor in full-day tests with objective population (two females and one male, all over 60 years all). The volunteers were asked to do what they use to, including traveling in train and bus, making exercise and cooking or cleaning. With a sampling frequency of 25 Hz (lower than most works in the literature), It was obtained more than 17 continuous hours of acquisition (we recorded online, increasing the consumption) with encouraging results, just with a couple of false-positives due to hits of the device during cooking.

## 5. Home automation

The domotic SICAA software and control hardware were designed to achieve some automatic tasks, such as air conditioning, basic lights, environmental music, and alarms (related to the health and emotional monitoring). Through an ichnographic software (**Figure 4**) is possible to access to these and other functions: house control (that comprises blinds, lights, orthopedic bed, air conditioner, television, and intercom); medication alarm; carer communication (nurse call, voice synthesizer), and computer access (internet, chat, games, text processors). The software must accomplish several requirements, regarding the limited experience with technology or reduced capabilities of the users. An intuitive interface, big buttons and vibrant colors were chosen for the software. The software has a principal panel, (**Figure 3**) with date, hour, a control menu showing the outputs states, and icons representing the TV control, home control, internet access, voice synthesizer, nurse call, bed control, medication reminder, and diary. The icons of the menu are also easy to interpret and relative large in the screen, regarding the vision problems or essential tremor. Each main icon allows the access to another submenu or

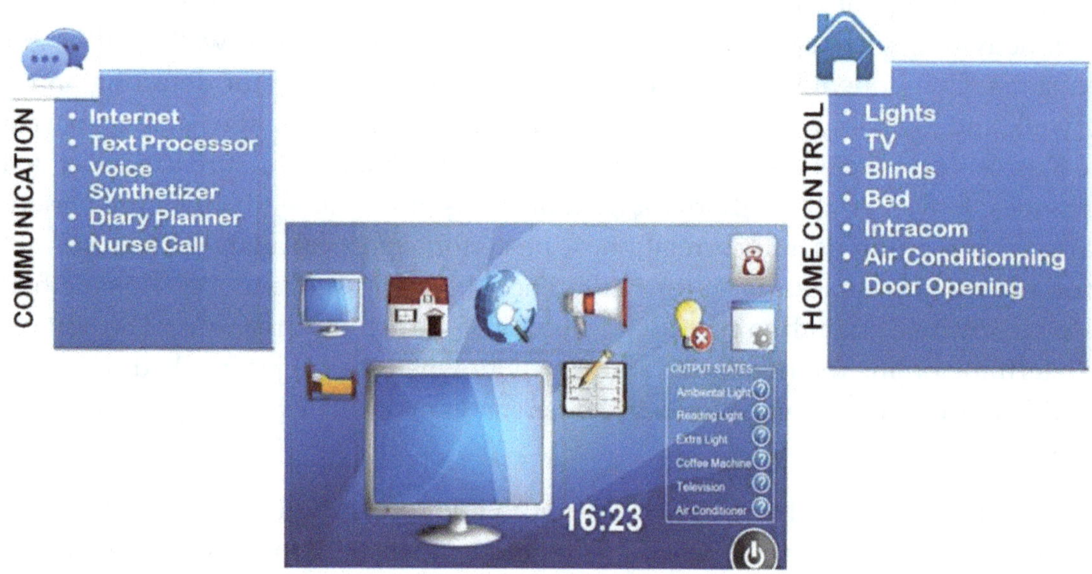
COMMUNICATION
• Internet
• Text Processor
• Voice Synthetizer
• Diary Planner
• Nurse Call
HOME CONTROL
• Lights
• TV
• Blinds
• Bed
• Intracom
• Air Conditionning
• Door Opening
OUTPUT STATES
Ambiental Light
Reading Light
Extra Light
Coffee Machine
Television
Air Conditioner
16:23

**Figure 4.** Principal panel of SICAA system and submenus with functions for communication and for home control. The icons, colors, and size were designed especially for people with poor contact with technology.

screen for specific tasks, such as ambient or home control, TV, and so on. All system configurations are accessible by the programmer or authorized personnel, in order to prevent system failures. The software is available in Spanish, English and Portuguese [25].

A custom-made electronic board was designed to control peripheral devices, including relays, analogical and digital inputs, isolation conditions, and an ATMega 8-16PU microcontroller of 1 MHz. A generic IR transducer was used for TV and air conditioning control, to prevent incompatibilities with previously installed devices, but door lock and intercom has to be adapted for electric opening.

The Aid Call is a luminous and sonorous alarm, interrupted only by hardware, assuring the presence of the caregiver. Other devices such as orthopedic bed and lights only need a minimum electrical connection to be controlled by the SICAA and other devices must be added without affecting the functioning. In the main menu a panel control shows the appliances activation state. As is possible to see, is a simple and low cost solution in order to enhance autonomy, improving the relationship of the elderly or ill users with family or caregivers. The home care system would provide elderly people more satisfied and autonomous behaviors and habits as well as more nominal care.

## 6. Voice speech emotion recognition

As we stated in introduction, the emotional status of the patient is one of the milestones of our work. Even if the physiological signals are constantly monitored in order to detect any physiological damage, we have demonstrated that emotion can be recognized from voice and developed specialized algorithms to be used in this kind of application.

Biomedical signal processing allows the identification of certain paralinguistic parameters in a speaker such as pathologies, nationality, gender, among others [26–28]. The interest in emotion recognition from speech has increased in the last decade because emotion recognition can improve the quality of services and the quality of life of people. It is possible to make predictions by using a supervised learning scheme, whose final scope is determining the health status of individuals [29]. Through a set of features, it is possible to identify and characterize states of people that can be as common as unpredictable such as emotional states.

Health status of a person has drawn the attention of researchers involved in several different branches of knowledge, such as psychology, cognitive sciences, economy, bioengineering, and medicine [31, 32]. In Ref. [33], we developed an algorithm to recognize certain regions on the emotional plane specialized on sadness and in Ref. [34], an algorithm for Parkinson's disease detection and monitoring was proposed. Another practical use is the monitoring of telephone interactions, i.e., call center, [35].

Here, we present a general framework methodology for the understanding of the reader, widely used in our developed algorithms. In particular, voiced-speech signals are initially processed using multiple techniques, e.g., filtering, Fourier transform, which allow revealing important information inside the signals [36–38]. Then, relevant features should be selected in order to find patterns that divide meaningfully the data in terms of the classes of interest, e.g., healthy person/sick person. Identified features are used to training machine learning algorithms that automatically perform the classification of new data, in this case voiced-speech signals, into the previously defined classes [39]. In traditional methodologies, spectrograms time-frequency representation have been used for identifying subtle cues related with utterance acoustics, providing the means to identify the speaker and his emotional [40, 48], or health status [41, 42].

Several works have used conventional features such as Mel Frequency Cepstral Coefficients, Renyi entropy, Fisher rate, Local Hu moments, and vocal source parameters, among others in order to find patterns inside audio-voice signals [30]. Additionally, these methods use classifiers with different schemes, some of them are K-nearest neighbor, Gaussian mixture models, hidden Markov models, multilayer-perceptron, and support vector machine [43–45]. One of the main problems in emotion recognition from speech is to find suitable features to represent the phenomenon. In Refs. [46, 47], new features based on the energy content of wavelet-based time-frequency (TF) representations to model emotional speech were proposed. Three TF representations were considered: (1) the continuous wavelet transform, (2) the bionic wavelet transform, and (3) the synchrosqueezed wavelet transform.

A simple methodology can be stated as signal acquisition, signal preprocessing, feature extraction, and classification. A summary can be found in the following steps:

(1) Windowing: Since the speech signal is quasi-stationary is necessary a windowing process. Blackman window is used, an overlap of 60% was done, and a window size of 16384 samples, near to 1 second.

(2) Wavelet decomposition: The wavelet decomposition was implemented using the stationary wavelet transform (SWT). The SWT can be considered as a filter bank, with low-pass and high-pass filter, that decomposed the input signal into two groups of subsignals,

which are approximation and detail signals [36]. Each filter bank is related to a mother wavelet, in this work Daubechies wavelet is used particularly the wavelet db1, db6, db8, and db10. Each segment taken from the signal on the windowing process is decomposed into five levels with each type of wavelet; for analyzing this signal a matrix was constructed for each type of wavelet and for each window size, with 5 coefficients of detail and the fifth coefficient approximation of the decomposed signal.

(3) Statistical features: Each subsignal obtained by the SWT was analyzed using the 12 features, some with a temporal approach: root mean square, absolute mean value, mean, variance, standard deviation, wavelength, standard wavelength, and kurtosis; and with a spectral approach, such as zero crossing, mean frequency, median frequency, and maximum power spectral value

(4) Features selection: In Ref. [49], a new set of features based on nonlinear dynamics measures obtained from the wavelet packet transform for the automatic recognition of "fear-type" emotions in speech was proposed. The experiments are carried out using three different databases with a Gaussian mixture model for classification. The results indicate that the proposed approach is promising for modeling "fear-type" emotions in speech. On the other hand, classification of sets with high dimensionality of descriptive characteristics is computationally demanding [50]. Subsets of features may be associated with elements of noise or information different from the state of health of the speaker. The feature selection was implemented, with a recursive elimination method that iteratively eliminates the feature that least contributes to the determination between the two states, using a classifier to assign weights. This process is carried out until obtaining the target number of features

(5) Classification: A simple Multilayer Perceptron (MLP) can be trained based on the new set of features obtain by the feature selection method. The final MLP structure called patternet must be configured as follows: the output layer has the number of neurons of the states to be determined, preferably only one hidden layer shall be considered to avoid problems of gradient backpropagation. The hidden layer must contain multiple numbers of neurons, i.e., 1, 2, 5, 10, 50, and 100 to find the best set to be used fulfilling the conditions of the problem. The suggested transfer function is the hyperbolic tangent sigmoid, and trained using a Bayesian regularization [9]. Also, other classifiers such as Gaussian mixture model (GMM) have been recently used [43]: the classification is performed using GMM supervectors. Different classification problems are addressed, including high vs. low arousal, positive vs. negative valence, and multiple emotions. The results indicate that the proposed features are useful to classify high vs. low arousal emotions, and that the features derived from the synchrosqueezed wavelet transform are more suitable than the other two approaches to model emotional speech.

In our approach, the emotion recognition is focused in sadness, joy, and fear detection, because they are the most critical emotional situations for the system's users. The election for the algorithm is based on the computational cost, since the data must to be classified and stored to construct an emotional pattern of behavior. Throughout the days, family or medical staff can study this pattern to rethink visits, or treatment support for the patient. Also, sadness and fear are connected to the SICAA block, activating nurse call for fear detection and selected music and family alarm for sadness. This simple connection elicits a safety sensation for patients and also for the family in the daily living.

On the other hand, the use of portable devices for the assessment of Parkinson's disease (PD) patients at home from voice analysis is feasible from the technical point of view; however, it could be relatively expensive either the patients or the health system. The information and communication technologies (ICT) allow thinking on doing telemonitoring of PD patients using different communication tools already existing in internet. There are several aspects in such new technologies and tools that have to be studied to analyze the feasibility of using them in real scenarios. For instance, there exist different communication systems that can be used for the remote evaluation of speech, e.g., the mobile communications network, the internet, and the landline, among others. All of these technologies compress the audio signals in order to transmit them through the communication channel. The compression rates depend on the technology and on the bandwidth available in the network.

In Ref. [34], a method was developed, addressing to discriminate between the speakers with Parkinson's disease (PD) and healthy controls (HC). It consists on the systematic segmentation of voiced and unvoiced speech frames. Each kind of frame is characterized independently. For voiced segments noise, perturbation, and cepstral features are considered. The unvoiced segments are characterized with Bark band energies and cepstral features. According to the results, the codecs evaluated do not affect significantly the accuracy of the system, indicating that the addressed methodology could be used for the telemonitoring of PD patients through internet or through the mobile communications network.

## 7. Conclusions

We have described the use of new technologies applied in the health monitoring and assistance for elderly and chronically ill people, focused in home care and independence for a better quality of life. Aging does not have to be a social limit, or a hospitalization cause. In the last years, technology has brought the major advances in elderly care, but the access is still limited. In the Latin America, most of the health systems financed the home hospitalization, but in specific cases and not for long time. Our proposal is exactly in the opposite paradigm, encouraging the use of technologies, in order to extend as much as possible the home care possibilities and family well-being. The main challenge in this area is the correct identification of user's needs, because the acceptation of the technology aid depends on this completely.

The system proposed has three main parts, the wearable block that accomplish with requirements of performance, autonomy, size, and low cost. The electronic parts are available in any country and in constant evolution.

Acquisition of real falls demonstrated that setting an algorithm with young adults does not perform well with falls of elderly people. So, even the methodology proposed seemed to solve this issue, it is necessary to increase the number of falls with elderly people to have a representative sample. However, with the impossibility of performing simulated falls with elderly people (the risk of accident is too high), with an average of one fall per year, it is unrealistic to expect acquiring confident data of real falls. Then, this remains as an open issue that must be solved in the near future.

Regarding emotion recognition, health status, and similar algorithms from voiced speech, we demonstrated that wavelet-based algorithms with the proper feature selection procedure could be easily trained and implemented to be merged with other devices within this integrated framework. We also can guarantee that algorithms performance can increase under data fusion schemes so far widely developed and implemented. Data fusion schemes will also include the physiological signals from the patient such as temperature, heart rate module, and pulse oximetry. Alerts are included for the transmission in order to ask for help in case of accidents or a "nonnormal state."

The second part, home automation, enables limited users to control their household appliances. This was achieved by using low-cost control interfaces and a customized board that interact with the central control block. For the target, user population of the system has shown great adaptability and the potentiality of increasing user independence.

The third block, central control, allows the integration of physiological and emotional measures, constructing a behavior pattern for the user and detecting risk or emergency situations. Alarms can be activated either by predefined levels of biological variables, by emotional risk detected by fear or sadness or by the user himself.

A further test with a control and an experimental group is needed in order to quantify the satisfaction and acceptation of this system by the users. Tests are needed in a controlled environment with emotions inducement or with physiologic and environment disturbances to valid the development and obtain data for a multimodal analyses of the signals. However, making a behavioral pattern must be customized. This requires a previous collection of data and a dynamic model of adjustment and learning for each patient.

As we have mentioned, it is a special group and several considerations are necessary to determine definitely the usability of our approach. Also, it is important to note that these technologies can help to improve communication, independence, and self-esteem, but it cannot replace the role of caregivers and medical staff.

## Acknowledgements

Authors acknowledge their colleagues and students for the collaboration and support during these years of work.

Natalia Lopez wants to thank Max Valentinuzzi, Paola Bustamante and Elisa Pérez.

Sergio Ponce wants to acknowledge David Piccinini, Nicolás Andino, Sofía Avetta, Alexis Sparapani, Martín Roberti, and Camilo García for the incomparable effort to deal with electronics.

Lucia Quintero deeply recognizes the contributions of Damian Campo, Manuela Bastidas, Alejandro Uribe and Alejandro Gómez for following carefully the insights for research.

Francisco Vargas wishes to thank his colleagues Rafael Orozco and José David López, and his students Angela Sucerquia, Nicanor García, and Juan Camilo Vásquez.

## Author details

Natalia López Celani[1,2]*, Sergio Ponce[1], Olga Lucía Quintero[3] and Francisco Vargas-Bonilla[4]

*Address all correspondence to: nlopez@gateme.unsj.edu.ar

1 Gabinete de Tecnología Médica, Universidad Nacional de San Juan – Consejo Nacional de Investigaciones Científicas y Técnicas, Argentina

2 GADIB, Facultad Regional San Nicolás, Universidad Tecnológica Nacional, Buenos Aires, Argentina

3 Mathematical Modeling Research Group, Universidad EAFIT, Medellín, Colombia

4 SISTEMIC Research Group, Universidad de Antioquia, Medellín, Colombia

## References

[1] World Health Organization. World Report on Ageing and Health. World Health Organization. Geneva, Switzerland; 2015. ISBN: 9789241565042

[2] Tang YP, Wang W, Fu YZ. Elder health status monitoring through analysis of activity. Chinese Journal of Computer Engineering and Applications. 2006;**43**(3):211-213

[3] He W, Goodkind D, Kowal P. U.S. Census Bureau, International Population Reports, P95/16-1, An Aging World: 2015. Washington, DC: U.S. Government Publishing Office; 2016

[4] Pan American Health Organization. Innovative Care for Chronic Conditions: Organizing and Delivering High Quality Care for Chronic Noncommunicable Diseases in the Americas. Washington, DC: PAHO, 2013

[5] Najafi B, Aminian K, Paraschiv-Ionescu A, Loew F, Bula CJ, Robert P. Ambulatory system for human motion analysis using a kinematic sensor: Monitoring of daily physical activity in the elderly. IEEE Transactions on Biomedical Engineering. 2003;**50**(6):711-723

[6] Xiang Y, Tang Y-P, Ma B-Q, Yan H-C, Jiang J, Tian X-Y. Remote safety monitoring for elderly persons based on Omni-Vision analysis. PLoS One. 2015;**10**(5):e0124068. DOI: 10.1371/journal. pone.0124068

[7] Morris ME, Adair B, Miller K, Ozanne E, Hansen R, et al. Smart-Home technologies to assist older people to live well at home. Aging Science. 2013;**1**:101. DOI: 10.4172/jasc.1000101

[8] Stikic M, Huynh T, Van Laerhoven K, Schiele B. ADL recognition based on the combination of RFID and accelerometer sensing. In: Pervasive Computing Technologies for Healthcare, 2008. Second International Conference on Pervasive Health 2008; 30 Jan–1 Feb 2008

[9] Lv Z, Xia F, Wu G, Yao L, Chen Z. iCare: A mobile health monitoring system for the elderly. In: IEEE Conferences: 2010 IEEE/ACM International Conference on Green Computing and Communications (GreenCom) & International Conference on Cyber, Physical and Social Computing (CPSCom). Hangzhou, China, October 30–November 1, 2010

[10] Ghazal B, Al-Khatib K. Smart home automation system for elderly, and handicapped oeople using XBee. International Journal of Smart Home. April 2015;**9**(4):203-210. DOI: 10.14257/ijsh.2015.9.4.21

[11] Akanbi CO, Oladeji DO. Design of a voice based intelligent prototype model for automatic control of multiple home appliances. Transactions on Machine Learning and Artificial Intelligence. 2016;**4**(2):23-30

[12] López NM, Orosco EC, Perez E, Bajinay S, Zanetti R, Valentinuzzi ME. Hybrid Human-Machine interface to mouse control for severely disabled people. International Journal of Engineering and Innovative Technology. 2015;**4**(11):164-171. ISSN 2277-3754

[13] Perez E, López N, Orosco E, Soria C, Mut V, Freire-Bastos T. Robust human machine interface based on head movements applied to assistive robotics. The Scientific World Journal. 2013;**2013**:11 pages. DOI: 10.1155/2013/589636. Article ID 589636

[14] Perez E, Soria C, López NM, Nasisi O, Mut V. Vision Based Interface applied to assistive robots. International Journal of Advanced Robotic Systems: Computer Vision and Ambient Intelligence. 2013;**10**(116):1-10. DOI: 10.5772/53996. Print ISSN 1729-8806; Online ISSN 1729-8814

[15] Orosco EC, López NM, di Sciascio F. Bispectrum-based features classification for myoelectric control. Biomedical Signal Processing and Control. 2013;**8**(2):153-168. ISSN: 1746-8094. Available from: http://dx.doi.org/10.1016/j.bspc.2012.08.008

[16] López NM, di Sciascio F, Soria CM, Valentinuzzi ME. Robust EMG sensing system based on data fusion for myoelectric control of a robotic arm. BioMedical Engineering OnLine. 2009;**8**(5). DOI: 10.1186/1475-925X-8-5, ISSN 1475-925X.

[17] Teng X-F, Zhang Y-T, Poon CCY, Bonato P. Wearable medical systems for p-Health. IEEE Reviews in Biomedical Engineering. 2008;**1**:62-74

[18] Bonato P. Wearable sensors and systems. From enabling technology to clinical applications. IEEE Engineering in Medicine and Biology Magazine. 2010;**29**:25-36

[19] Anzaldo D. Wearable sport technology – Market landscape and compute SoC trends. In: IEEE Conference Publications: International SoC Design Conference. 2-5 Nov. Gyungju, South Korea. 2015. pp. 217-218. DOI: 10.1109/ISOCC.2015.7401796

[20] Chen B, Patel S, Buckley T, Rednic R, McClure D, Shih L, Tarsy D, Welsh M, Bonato P. A web-based system for home monitoring of patients with Parkinson's disease using wearable sensors. IEEE Transactions on Biomedical Engineering. 2011;**58**(3):831-836

[21] Asada HH, Shaltis P, Reisner A, Rhee S, Hutchinson RC. Mobile monitoring with wearable photoplethysmographic biosensors. IEEE Engineering in Medicine and Biology Magazine. 2003;**22**:28-40

[22] Piccinini D, Andino N, Ponce S, Roberti M, López N. Wearable system for acquisition and monitoring of biological signals. Journal of Physics: Conference Series. 2016;**705**:012009. ISSN: 1742-6596. Available from: http://iopscience.iop.org/1742-6596/705/1/012009

[23] Vega LAS. Methodology for Detecting Movements of Interest in Elderly People. Colombia: Universidad de Antioquia UDEA Facultad de Ingeniería Medellín; 2016

[24] Sucerquia A, López JD, Vargas-Bonilla JF. SisFall: A fall and movement dataset. Sensors. 2017;**17**(1):198. DOI: 10.3390/s17010198

[25] López N, Piccinini D, Ponce S, Perez E, Roberti M. From hospital to home care. Creating a domotic environment for elderly and disabled people. IEEE Pulse, IEEE. 2016;**7**(3):38-41. DOI: 10.1109/MPUL.2016.2539105. ISSN 2154-2287

[26] Kumari M, Ali I. A new gender detection algorithm considering the Non-stationarity of speech signal. In: International Conference on Communication, Control and Intelligent Systems CCIS. IEEE Conferences: 18-20 Nov. 2016 Mathura, India Vol. 2. 2016.

[27] Martinez C, Rufiner H. Acoustic analysis of speech for de tection of laryngeal pathologies. In: Proceedings of the 22nd Annual International Conference of the IEEE Engineering in Medicine and Biology Society (Cat. No. 00CH37143). Vol. 3. 2000. pp. 2369-2372 Chicago, IL, USA.

[28] Bouselmi G, Fohr D, Illina I, Haton JP. Discriminative phoneme sequences extraction for non-native speaker's origin classification. International Symposium on Signal Processing and Its Applications, Vol. 9, 2007; 12-15 Feb 2007; Sharjah, United Arab Emirates: IEEE; 2007

[29] Orozco-Arroyave JR, Belalcazar-Bolaños EA, Arias-Londoño JD, Vargas-Bonilla JF, Skodda S, Rusz J, Daqrouq K, Honig F, Noth E. Characterization methods for the detection of multiple voice disorders: Neurological, functional, and laryngeal diseases. IEEE Journal of Biomedical and Health Informatics. 2015;**19**(6):1820-1828

[30] Sierra-Sosa D, Bastidas M, Ortiz PD, Quintero O. Double fourier analysis for emotion identification in voiced speech. Journal of Physics: Conference Series. Oct 2016;**705**:012035

[31] Cipriano PF, Bowles K, Dailey M, Dykes P, Lamb G, Naylor M. The importance of health information technology in care coordination and transitional care. Nursing Outlook. 2013;**61**(6):475-489. Available from: http://dx.doi.org/10.1016/j.outlook.2013.10.005

[32] Shin D-H, Biocca F. Health experience model of personal informatics: The case of a quantified self. Computers in Human Behavior. 2017;**69**:62-74. Available from: http://linkinghub.elsevier.com/retrieve/pii/S0747563216308391

[33] Bustamante PA, Lopez Celani NM, Perez ME, Montoya OLQ. Recognition and regionalization of emotions in the arousal-valence plane. In: Conference of the Proceeding IEEE Engineering in Medicine and Biology Society. 2015:6042-6045

[34] Orozco-Arroyave JR, García N, Vargas-Bonilla JF, Nöth E. Automatic detection of Parkinson's disease from compressed speech recordings. In: Král P, Matoušek V, editors. Text, Speech, and Dialogue. Vol. 9302. Lecture Notes in Computer Science. Cham: Springer. ISSN: 0302-9743 DOI: 10.1007/978-3-319-24033-6_10

[35] Vásquez-Correa JC, Orozco-Arroyave JR, Arias-Londoño JD, Vargas-Bonilla JF, Nöth E. Non-linear Dynamics Characterization from Wavelet Packet Transform for Automatic Recognition of Emotional Speech. Smart Innovation, Systems and Technologies. Springer Publishing Company, Inc.; 2016. Berlin, Germany pp. 199-207. ISBN: 2190-3018

[36] Campo D, Quintero OL, Bastidas M. Multiresolution analysis (discrete wavelet transform) through Daubechies family for emotion recognition in speech. Journal of Physics: Conference Series. 2016;**705**(1):12034. Available from: http://stacks.iop.org/1742-6596/705/i=1/a=012034

[37] Chen L, Mao X, Xue Y, Cheng LL. Speech emotion recognition: Features and classification models. Digital Signal Processing: A Review Journal. 2012;**22**(6):1154-1160. Available from: http://dx.doi.org/10.1016/j.dsp.2012.05.007

[38] Sun Y, Wen G, Wang J. Weighted spectral features based on local Hu moments for speech emotion recognition. Biomedical Signal Processing and Control. 2015;**18**:80-90. Available from: http://dx.doi.org/10.1016/j.bspc.2014.10.008

[39] He L, Lech M, Maddage NC, Allen NB. Study of empirical mode decomposition and spectral analysis for stress and emotion classification in natural speech. Biomedical Signal Processing and Control. 2011;**6**(2):139-146. Available from: http://dx.doi.org/10.1016/j.bspc.2010.11.001

[40] Vayrynen E, Toivanen J, Seppanen T. Classification of emotion in spoken Finnish using vowel-length segments: Increasing reliability with a fusion technique. Speech Communication. 2011;**53**(3):269-282

[41] Dang A, Likhar N, Alok U. Importance of economic evaluation in health care: An indian perspective. Value in Health Regional Issues. 2016;**9**(6):78-83. Available from: http://dx.doi.org/10.1016/j.vhri.2015.11.005

[42] Shepley MM, Watson A, Pitts F, Garrity A, Spelman E, Fronsman A, Kelkar J. Mental and behavioral health settings: Importance; effectiveness of environmental qualities; features as perceived by staff. Journal of Environmental Psychology. 2017;**50**:37-50. Available from: http://linkinghub.elsevier.com/retrieve/pii/S0272494417300051

[43] Lanjewar RB, Mathurkar S, Patel N. Implementation and comparison of speech emotion recognition system using gaussian mixture model (GMM) and K-Nearest neighbor (K-NN) techniques. Procedia Computer Science. 2015;**49**:50-57

[44] Albornoz EM, Milone DH, Rufiner HL. Spoken emotion recognition using hierarchical classifiers. Computer Speech & Language. 2011;**25**(3):556-570

[45] Truong KP, Van Leeuwen DA, De Jong FMG. Speech-based recognition of self-reported and observed emotion in a dimensional space. Speech Communication. 2012;**54**(9):1049-1063. Available from: http://dx.doi.org/10.1016/j.specom.2012.04.006

[46] Gomez A, Quintero L, Lopez M, Castro J, Villa L. Emotion recognition in single-channel EEG signals using Stationary Wavelet Transform. IFMBE Proceedings. 2016

[47] Gomez A, Quintero L, Lopez M, Castro J, Villa L. An approach to emotion recognition in single-channel EEG signals using Discrete Wavelet Transform. In: The 38th Annual International Conference of the IEEE Engineering in Medicine and Biology Society. Vol. 6. Florida, USA; August 17-20, 2016

[48] Gomez A, Quintero L, Lopez N, Castro J. An approach to emotion recognition in single-channel EEG signals: A mother child interaction. Journal of Physics: Conference Series. 2016;**705**(1):12051. Available from: http://stacks.iop.org/1742-6596/705/i=1/a=012051.

[49] Vasquez-Correa JC, Arias-Vergara T, Orozco-Arroyave JR, Vargas-Bonilla JF. Evaluation of wavelet measures on automatic detection of emotion in noisy and telephony speech signals. In: 48th IEEE International Carnahan Conference on Security Technology (ICCST)

[50] Vasquez-Correa JC, Arias-Vergara T, Orozco-Arroyave JR, Vargas-Bonilla JF, Noeth E. Wavelet-based time-frequency representations for automatic recognition of emotions from speech. Itg-Fachbericht. 2016;**267**:235-239. ISSN: 0932-6022 ed: fasc

4

# Effect of Phone Interviews and Anger Management Training Provided to Caregivers of the Patients with Breast Cancer in Turkey

Birgül Özkan, Selahattin Menteş and
Gökmen Zarasız

**Abstract**

**Background:** Psychosocial interventions involve anger management training and phone interviews to the family of the patients with breast cancer.

**Aims:** The present study aimed to measure the effect of phone interviews and anger management training provided to patients with breast cancer on the levels of emotional expression and caregiver burden.

**Study design:** The present study was conducted as a randomized-controlled experimental study (experiment-control groups with pretest and posttest design) between 2012 and 2013.

**Methods:** The study was conducted on caregivers of the patients with breast cancer who received radiotherapy in Radiation Oncology Center in Turkey. The experiment and control groups included 22 and 20 subjects, respectively. All subjects completed a survey about general features, Level of Expressed Emotion (LEE) Scale and Zarit Caregiver Burden Scale.

**Results:** A significant difference was found between study and control groups in terms of mean overall general expression emotion and Zarit Caregiver Burden scores ($P < 0.05$). A significant difference was found between measurements ($P < 0.05$).

**Conclusions:** It is recommended to provide home care (e.g. phone interviews, home visits) following anger management training in patients with breast cancer and to arrange education program for those who received radiotherapy.

**Keywords:** anger management, breast cancer, caregivers, support, telephone follow-up

## 1. Introduction

In recent years, shorter hospital stays, limited discharge planning, and expansion of home care technology have placed increased costs as well as increased care responsibilities on families [1–3]. As care has shifted from the hospital to the home, the role of the family caregiver has been transformed into a complex responsibility [2]. Unfortunately, involvement of family caregivers is essential for optimal treatment of cancer patients, especially in ensuring social support and patients in the home care [2, 4].

Caregivers function as home health aides and companions. They are expected to provide patients with emotional support, conversation, and other forms of distraction [5–7]. A major body of research indicates that household family who provide care to individuals with chronical situation are themselves at risk. Emotional, mental, and physical health problems result from complex caregiving situations and the strains of caring for weak or disabled relatives [5, 6]. The mental health of the family caregiver is negatively moved by providing care. Higher levels of stress, anxiety, depression and other mental health effects are common among family members who care for an older relative or friend [7, 8]. Several works have indicated that caregivers use recipe and psychotropic drugs more than noncaregivers [9–11]. Family caregivers are at greater risk for higher levels of hostility than noncaregivers [12]. Marriage caregivers who are at risk of clinical depression and are caring for a annulment with significant cognitive annulment and/or physical care needs are more likely to keep in detrimental behavior toward their beloved one [9–11].

In Turkey's health of oncology services, treatment and care of patients with breast cancer are provided only during hospitalization and home care cannot be provided after discharge. There are few work related to emotion expression and family burden in caregivers of patient with breast cancer in Turkey [13–15]. Therefore, these studies are needed.

Emotion expression is very important for the families of patients with cancer. Expressed emotion forward it to our needs and expectations of others is a way [16]. The concept of expressed emotion; be critical, hostile take extreme interest to hear, not intrusive, intimacy and includes positive comments. Expressed emotion includes some sub-terms. One of them is criticism; the nature of the other critics blame, resentment, contains statements such as dislike and disapproval hostile, often defined as a negative expressed emotion. Excessive not interested and not excessively intrusive protect and nurture, the restrictive, controlling and diver/refers to intrusive behavior [16, 17]. These studies show that there are a positive relationship between emotion, expression, and family burden.

Burden is the caregiver's response to the stressors engendered by caring for the patient with cancer that may result in negative role perception. Burden may be conceptualized as a multidimensional concept with objective and subjective components [18, 19]. Objective burden is defined as concrete cases, occurrences and activities related to caregiving, such as financial problems and personal activity limitations. Subjective burden is defined as sentimental answer to the caregiver experience, such as feelings and emotions related to fear, strain, or guilt [20–22]. It is important to reduce the burden and expression of emotions of caregivers with breast cancer. Apply to the study, interventions for families were restricted [18, 19].

Follow-up by phone is considered to be new and an innovative model that may facilitate home care for patients with cancers and caregivers, and difficulties in patient care may be reduced by this new paradigm model. There are studies which have indicated that phone based follow-up services can be used in clinical care, education and researches [20–22]. At the same time, follow-up services in home care for the patients with breast cancer may be provided through many ways; such as video conference, e-mail, website and phone. In this study, anger management, and telephone follow-up intervention effect for the caregivers of the patients were investigated.

This research was planned to determine the effect of anger management given to the caregivers of patients with breast cancer in the clinic and telephone follow-up provided by orderly phone, on their expression of emotions and family burden levels.

## 2. Material and methods

The present study was conducted as a randomized-controlled experimental study (including experimental and control groups with pretest and posttest design) in 2013. It was approved by Ethics Committee. The study conducted on patients with breast cancer who received radiotherapy in Radiation Oncology Center of a University, Oncology Hospital in ambulatory settings in Turkey. The experimental and control groups involved 22 and 20 subjects, in order of. After data collection, $\alpha$ value was found as 0.05 while power as 100% in the power analysis of all scales used in the research The research was carry out randomly with a sample set of criteria. After identifying the experimental and control group all the scales were applied to both groups.

In the present study, both experimental and control groups completed a survey about general characteristics, The Level of Expressed Emotion (LEE) Scale, The Zarit Family Burden Assessment Scale.

*Caregiver selection criteria for experimental and control groups:*

- Being aged between 18 and 65 years
- Having caregiver of patient with breast cancer
- Being graduated from primary school

*General survey sheet*

The survey sheet included 10 questions about demographic features of the subjects as well as another 10 questions about disease history

*The Level of Expressed Emotion (LEE) Scale,* developed by Cole and Kazarian and adapted to Turkish by Berksun [16] is applied to the caregivers. High scores indicate high level of negative expression of emotions. The Level of Expressed Emotion (LEE) Scale was developed to provide an index of the perceived emotional climate in a person's influential relationships. Unlike existing measures, the scale was constructed on the basis of a conceptual framework described by expressed emotion theorists. In addition to providing an overall score, the 60-item scale assesses the following four characteristic attitudes or response styles of significant others: Intrusiveness, emotional response, attitude toward illness, and tolerance/expectations.

*The Zarit Family Burden Assessment Scale* was developed by Martín et al. [17] and adapted to Turkish by Ozlu et al [18]. High scores indicate high family burden. The Zarit Family Burden Assessment Scale is 22-items instrument for measuring caregiver's perceived burden of providing family care. The 22 items are assessed on a 5-point likert scale ranging from 0 = "never" to 4 = "nearly always". Items score are added up to total score ranging from 0 to 88. High scores is indicated greated burden.

Phone-based follow-up of caregivers was carried out with the follow-up by phone form.

**Phases of investigation**

The patients in experimental group received anger management training during their radiotherapy period. Anger management trainings were given by two or three sessions. Each session was performed over 25–30 minutes. During this period, controls of caregivers underwent no intervention. After radiotherapy, follow-up by phone interview (weekly) were performed for 6 months in experimental group. Phone interviews included counseling. In the present study, supporting follow-up by phone was performed.

In all subjects, The Level of Expressed Emotion (LEE) Scale, The Zarit Family Burden Assessment Scale were completed by researchers via face-to-face interview during radiotherapy, one month after anger management training and 6-months follow-up period achieved by phone interviews.

The data acquire subjects in experimental and control groups were resolve by using chisquare significance test, t test and two-way analysis of variance for repeated measurements. Bonferroni and Least Significant Difference (LSD) tests were performed to identify the source of difference in the variables that are found to be significance in the analysis of variance. All statistical analyses were performed by using SPSS Statistics 20.0 (IBM SPSS Inc, Chicago, ILL, USA). $P < 0.05$ was well-considered as significant.

**The Content of Anger and Management Skills Training Anger;** the causes of anger in caregivers, effective and ineffective coping behavior with anger issues and the importance of emotional expression included.

## 3. Results

The experimental and control groups were composed of caregivers of patients' families. Randomization was performed according to certain characteristics of the caregivers. According to this; the age, educational status and pathological state of the patients were selected to be similar and no significant difference was found between experiment and control groups ($P > 0.05$).

**Table 1** submits mean scores in expressed emotion scales and subscales of the patients in experiment and control groups after anger management training and follow-up period. The group impact on mean overall expressed emotion score was found to be significant ($P < 0.05$). Measurement/time effect on mean expressed emotion score was also found to be significant ($P < 0.05$; **Table 1**). In the multiple comparisons performed to identify the source of difference in the experiment group, mean overconcern/over protectiveness score and criticim/hostility score after follow-up was establish to be lower compared to after training and before training ($P < 0.05$; **Table 1**).

In the multiple comparisons implement to identify the source of difference in the experiment group, mean overall expressed emotion score after follow-up was set up be lower compared to after training and increased before training. In the multiple comparisons performed to identify the source of difference in the control group, the difference was found to be significant in the comparison of mean expressed emotion score obtained after training to those obtained after follow-up, while no significant difference was found in other comparisons. In addition, significant difference was found between mean expressed emotion scores obtained before and after training in patients in the experiment group. Over again, significant difference was based on between experiment and control groups concerning mean overall expressed emotion score ($P < 0.05$). The group and time interactions of mean expressed emotion scores were found to be significant ($P < 0.05$; **Table 1**).

**Table 2** presents mean overall Zarit Family Burden scores of subjects in experiment and control groups found before and after training as well as those found after follow-up period. The group effect on mean overall Zarit Family Burden score was found to be significant ($P < 0.05$; **Table 1**). In the multiple comparisons performed to identify the source of difference in the experiment group, mean overall Zarit Family Burden score had after follow-up period was base upon be significantly lower crosscheck to those obtained both before and after training ($P < 0.05$). In the comparisons performed to identify the source of difference in the control group, no significant difference was found in mean overall Zarit Family Burden scores obtained after follow-up compared to those obtained both before and after training ($P > 0.05$; **Table 1**)

| **Groups** | **Time** | **Mean scores of overall Expressed Emotion Scale** | | |
|---|---|---|---|---|
| | | **Overconcern/over protectiveness** $\overline{x} \pm SS$ | **Criticim/hostility** $\overline{x} \pm SS$ | **General point** $\overline{x} \pm SS$ |
| Experimental | First hospitalized | $10.70 \pm 3.49^a$ | $7.65 \pm 3.01^a$ | $17.85 \pm 4.72^a$ |
| | After discharge | $11.50 \pm 3.45^b$ | $9.35 \pm 2.99^b$ | $20.35 \pm 5.61^b$ |
| | Sixth month follow-up | $10.35 \pm 3.74^a$ | $7.15 \pm 3.52^c$ | $18.00 \pm 4.67^b$ |
| Control | First hospitalized | $11.68 \pm 3.46^a$ | $10.31 \pm 2.96^a$ | $22.00 \pm 3.20^a$ |
| | After discharge | $15.45 \pm 4.17^a$ | $12.68 \pm 2.55^b$ | $28.40 \pm 5.28^b$ |
| | Sixth month follow-up | $15.00 \pm 2.29^a$ | $12.90 \pm 2.79^b$ | $25.90 \pm 2.92^c$ |
| Test | Time | | | |
| | Time + Group | | | |
| | Group | | | |
| | $P^*$ | <0.005 | <0.005 | <0.005 |
| | $P+$ | <0.005 | <0.005 | <0.005 |
| | $P\#$ | <0.005 | <0.005 | <0.005 |

$P^*$ = inter-group, $P+$ = between measurements/times, $P\#$ = group and time interaction.

The results of in-group multi-comparisons of the experimental and control groups were displayed with alphabethic superscripts; the same letters indicating an insignificant statistical difference between the measurement times and different letters indicating a statistically significant difference.

**Table 1.** The mean scores of Expressed Emotion Scale of the caregivers in the experimental and the control groups telephone follow-up.

| Groups | Time | Family burden general point $\bar{x} \pm SS$ |
|---|---|---|
| Experimental | First hospitalized | 73.31 ± 15.14[a] |
| | After discharge | 62.27 ± 8.25[b] |
| | Sixth month follow-up | 49.40 ± 6.74[c] |
| Control | First hospitalized | 57.65 ± 10.90[a] |
| | After discharge | 67.05 ± 9.19[a] |
| | Sixth month follow-up | 66.45 ± 8.20[a] |
| Test | | *F* |
| | Time | 0.56 |
| | Time + Group | 0.16 |
| | Group | 0.62 |
| | *P** | <0.001 |
| | *P+* | <0.005 |
| | *P#* | <0.001 |

*P** = inter-group, *P+* = between measurements/times, *P#* = group and time interaction.
The results of in-group multi-comparisons of the experimental and control groups were displayed with alphabethic superscripts; the same letters indicating an insignificant statistical difference between the measurement times and different letters indicating a statistically significant difference.

**Table 2.** The meanscores of Zarit Family Burden Scale of the caregivers in the experimental and control groups telephone follow-up.

## 4. Discussion

This study was designed to test the efficacy of a consultan intervention designed to improve caregivers with breast cancer patients. In addition to the issues that people with breast cancer face with; their relatives are experiencing some difficulties too. Related studies are expressing that the difficulties which patients and their relatives experience differ from each other [23]. The reason behind the problems of the patients is mostly their perception of disease and the disease itself whereas their relatives have problems related to the reactions that the patient gives. Even it is not adequate for the current health regulations on holistic treatments, it can be expressed that the patients are treated in a sufficient way whereas the treatments for their relatives are being limited with the researches. Therefore, the difficulties of the relatives of people with breast cancer must be determined and their abilities to overcome these difficulties must be improved. The primary problem of these relatives is the fact that they are constantly accompanying a patient and since they give care to this patient, there is a limitation of free time to spend for themselves or their family members [24]. Moreover, they are being forced to become caregiver. They often face with the difficulty of expression of feelings and suppression of anger, fury, etc. Design of this study is based on the reasons mentioned above.

This treatment is designed for the relatives of the patients in order to provide them an opportunity to express themselves and understand their patients more. The instruction that is given to the relatives of patients includes the ways of expressing fury and improvement of the methods of overcoming these feelings. With these instructions, relatives succeed in the expression of anger, fury and these kinds of feelings to the patient without feeling shame and guilt [25]. According to the results obtained from the study, it can be seen that total average of the expression of feeling values for the experimental group are significantly higher than the control group (**Table 1**) and it is determined that Zarit Caregiver Burden values are also decreased significantly (**Table 2**). When these results are considered together, it can be stated that with the increase of the ability to overcome expression emotion, relatives can express themselves easily and related to these, the burden they feel is being decreased. The current studies on this issue and our study have similar results [22, 26, 27]. For instance in a work admissibility and practicality of distant automated telephone follow-up annually, after breast cancer, as well as usual mammograms, the main objectives were to evolved the invention of psychosocial worry and of treatment-related lateral-effects among patients who had completed their adjuvant chemo-radiotherapy [20].

Conducting studies by telephone counseling to caregivers of cancer patients is very limited. The studies are related more patients with breast cancer. Therefore the results of similar studies in the discussion of our findings in the study were used coping with stress, to quality of life affecting comes among factors of the expression of mood and maintenance burden in caregivers. In studies conducted on this subject; the primary outcomes were psychological morbidity (state-trait anxiety inventory), general health questionnaire (GHQ-12), participants' needs for information, participants' satisfaction, clinical investigations ordered, and time to detection of recurrent disease. Caregivers in the intervention group decresed interest in over protectiveness compared to control caregivers. Our previous intervention research has shown decresed in ver protectiveness [28–30], even when delivered through a primary care setting (**Table 1**).

This result ensures support for forthcoming investigation that strictly evaluates these types of interventions. Not only is it possible to conduct efficacy studies in this setting, but also it is necessary to do so to enable later spreading of efficacious interventions to health and clinical settings [30]. We should use the same high standards of evaluation for electronic and interactive interventions that we use for print and other interventions. The positive effects of the intervention presented here pointed out that phone-based of follow-up interventions can change health attitude this lends support for design, development, and evaluation of future similar interventions in other applications and settings [28–30].

## 5. Limitation

There are many limitations to the present study that limit the generalization. Since our study is experimental and the sample group containing the relatives of patients is restricted with 20 people, number of sample group members is one of these limitations. This study is randomized controlled and it is suggested that the positive results of the sample group must be applied over a wider population. Second limitation of the study is the duration of monitoring and it is planned to have longer telephone based monitoring

## 6. Conclusion

If the results of the current studies on this issue and our findings are evaluated together, it can be stated that relatives of breast cancer patients must be approached similar to these patients and they should be taught about the skills of overcoming the difficulties related to their situation. In order to develop these skills, assistance groups must be developed for personal or collective improvement. If needed, these relatives must be supported to create their own groups. Sanitary crew must consider these patients and their relatives as a member of the crew and organize programs in order to prevent them from feeling alone and desperate at no step. Also, more planning should be done for the relatives of the patients in order to facilitate the expression of their feelings such as anger, fury and despair.

## Author details

Birgül Özkan[1*], Selahattin Menteş[2] and Gökmen Zarasız[3]

*Address all correspondence to: Ozkanbirgul7@gmail.com

1 Ankara Yildirim Beyazit University, Faculty of Health of Sciences, Turkey

2 Adana Numune Education and Research Hospital, Department of Radiation Oncology, Turkey

3 Department of Biostatistics, Faculty of Medicine, Erciyes University, Kayseri, Turkey

## References

[1] Rowland J, Holland J. Breast Cancer Handbook of Psycho-Oncology. London: Oxford University Press; 1989

[2] Miedema B, Tatemichi S, MacDonald I. Cancer follow-up care in new brunswick: Cancer surveillance, support issues and fear of recurrence. Canadian Journal of Rural Medicine. 2004;**9**(2):101-107

[3] Ferrario SR, Zotti AM, Massara G, Nuvolne G. A comparative assessment of psychological and psychosocial characteristics of cancer patients and their caregivers. Psycho-Oncology. 2003;**12**:1-7

[4] Grunfeld E, Coyle D, Whelan T, Clinch J, Reyno L, Earle CC, et al. Family caregiver burden: Results of a longitudinal study of breast cancer patients and their principal caregivers. Canadian Medical Association. 2004;**170**:1795-1801

[5] Macaraeg JC, Türk Smith S. Psychological distress and help-seeking attitudes of cancer caregivers on Guam. Pacific Asia Inquiry. 2013;**4**(1):121-135

[6] Northouse L, Williams AL, Given B, McCorkle R. Psychosocial care for family caregivers of patients with cancer. Journal of Clinical Oncology. 2012 Apr 10;**30**(11):1227-1234

[7] Kim Y, Wellisch DK, Spillers RL, Crammer C. Psychological distress of female cancer caregivers: Effects of type of cancer and caregivers spiritualty. Support Care Cancer. 2007;**15**:1367-1374

[8] Northouse LL, Katapodi M, Song L, Zhang L, Mood DW. Interventions with family caregivers of cancer patients: Meta-analysis of randomized trials. CA: A Cancer Journal of Clinicians. 2010;**60**(5):317-339

[9] Hewitt M, Bamundo A, Day R, Harvey C. Perspectives on post-treatment cancer care: Qualitative research with survivors, nurses, and physicians. Journal of Clinical Oncology. 2007;**25**(16):2270-2273

[10] Horning S. Follow-up of adult cancer survivors: New paradigms for survivorship care planning. Hematology/Oncology Clinics of North America. 2008;**22**:201-210

[11] Ganz PA, Casillas J, Hahn EE. Ensuring quality of care for cancer survivors: Implementing the survivorship care plan. Seminars in Oncology Nursing. 2008;**24**(3):208-217

[12] Montgomery DA, Krupa K, Cooke TG. Alternative methods of follow up in breast cancer: A systematic review of the literature. British Medical Journal. 2007;**96**:1625-1632

[13] Çayan S, Akbay E, Bozlu M. The prevalance of female sexual dysfunction and potential risk factors that may impair sexual function in Turkish women. Urologia Internationalis. 2004;**72**(1):52-57

[14] Kuscu MK, Dural U, Onen P, Yasa Y, Yayla M, Basaran G, et al. The association between individual attachment patterns, the perceived social support, and the psychological well-being of Turkish informal caregivers. Psycho-Oncology. 2009;**18**:927-935

[15] Babaoğlu E, Öz F. The relationship between psychological and social problems of the spouses who cared for the terminal cancer patients. Journal of Nursing Research Development. 2003;**2**:24-33

[16] Berksun OE. Family factors in schizophrenia: Expressed emotion (EE): Scale development and adaptation trial [thesis]. Ankara: Ankara University Institute of Health Sciences; 1992

[17] Martín M, Salvadó I, Nadal S, Miji LC, Rico JM, Lanz P, et al. Adaptación para nuestro medio de la Escala de Sobrecarga del Cuidador (Caregiver Burden Interview) de Zarit. Reviews in Gerontology. 1996;**6**:338-346

[18] Lewis R, Neal R, Hendry M, France B, Williams N, Russell D, et al. Patients' and healthcare professionals' views of cancer follow-up: Systematic review. The British Journal of General Practice. 2009;**59**(564):248-259

[19] Ganz P, Hahn E. Implementing a survivorship care plan for patients with breast cancer. Journal of Clinical Oncology. 2008;**26**(5):759-767

[20] Montgomery DA, Krupa K, Wilson C, Cooke TG. Automated telephone follow-up after breast cancer: An acceptability and feasibility pilot study. British Medical Journal. 2008. **99**(5):704-710

[21] Cox K, Wilson E. Follow-up for people with cancer: Nurse-led services and telephone. Journal of Advanced Nursing. 2003;**43**(1):51-61

[22] Montgomery DA. Follow-up by telephone after treatment for breast cancer. British Medical Journal. 2009;**337**:2753

[23] Stajduhar KI, Martin WL, Barwich D, Fyles G. Factors influencing family caregivers' abilty to cope with providing end-of-life cancer care at home. Cancer Nursing. 2008;**31**:77-85

[24] Duric V, Butow P, Sharpe L, Lobb E, Meiser B, Barratt A, et al. Reducing psychological distress in a genetic counseling consultation for breast cancer. Journal of Genetic Counseling. 2003;**12**:243-264

[25] Ryhanen AM, Siekkinen M, Rankinen S, Korvenranta H, Leino-Kilpi H. The effects of Internet or interactive computer-based patient education in the field of breast cancer: A systematic literature review. Patient Education and Counseling. 2010;**79**:5-13

[26] McMillan SC, Small BJ, Weitzner M, Schonwetter R, Tittle M, Moody L, et al. İmpact of coping skills intervention with family caregivers of hospice patients with cancer: A randomized clinical trial. Cancer. 2006;**106**:214-222

[27] Akpan-Idiok PA, Anarado AN. Perceptions of burden of caregiving by informal caregivers of cancer patients attending University of Calabar Teaching Hospital, Calabar, Nigeria. The Pan African Medical Journal. 2014;**18**:159

[28] Turkoglu N, Kılıc D. Effects of care burdens of caregivers of cancer patients on their quality of life. Asian Pacific Journal of Cancer Prevention. 2012;**13**(8):4141-4145

[29] Lewis R, Neal RD, Williams NH, France B, Wilkinson C, Hendry M, et al. Nurse led- vs conventional physician-led follow up for patients with cancer: Systematic review. Journal of Advanced Nurse. 2009;**65**(4):706-723

[30] Muttitt S, Vigneault R, Loewen L. Integrating telehealth into aboriginal healthcare: The Canadian experience. International Journal of Circumpolar Health. 2004;**63**(4):401-414

5

# Impact of a Parent's Neurodegenerative Disease and Care on the Daily Life of Children

Ulrika Ferm, Stefan Nilsson,
Margaretha Jenholt Nolbris, Petra Linnsand and
Annikki Jonsson

**Abstract**

The purpose of the study described in this chapter was to explore children's and parents' views of how a neurodegenerative disease in a parent influences the daily life of the child. Focus groups were carried out with nine families of children, adolescents and parents with and without Parkinson's disease, Multiple Sclerosis (MS) and Huntington's disease. Each group met twice over a period of 4 weeks. Data were transcribed and analysed using qualitative content analysis. The results explored the meaning of the two categories: consequences in daily life and influence of disease on children. These categories emerged out of the following subcategories: economy, responsibility, living with personal assistants, being and feeling, being different, activities and the symptoms of the disease. A parent's disease has an impact on the individual child who is affected emotionally and psychologically, and with regard to practical issues and basic needs. The parent's and the family's needs for support create a conflict between the child's rights for health, well-being and privacy and the needs and rights of the parent with the disease for high quality care. The negative impacts also relate to lack of information and knowledge about the disease and the family's need for economic support.

**Keywords:** neurodegenerative disease, child, parent, family, health, home environment, care, personal assistants

## 1. Introduction

According to the United Nation's Convention on the Rights of the Child (UNCRC) [1, 2], the child's best interests shall be of primary concern in all situations and actions relating to children. When a parent is affected by a neurodegenerative disease such as Parkinson's disease, Multiple Sclerosis (MS) and Huntington's disease, it may be particularly difficult to ensure the rights of the child. These diseases affect different body functions. As a result, the parent's ability to engage in daily activities and tasks may be limited. As the disease progress, the parent's personality may change and cognitive and communicative problems may further complicate everyday life and the parent's ability to maintain a healthy relationship with the child. Complex combinations of different symptoms, social factors and sometimes the long duration of the disease may be demanding for the child and the family. When a parent or other adults are affected by a disease or other serious difficulties such as drug abuse or violence, the whole family is influenced [3, 4]. Parental neurodegenerative illness may have a great impact on other family members' health and well-being. Approximately 17% of the children, aged 12–24, of parents with Parkinson's disease were classified as having a mild to moderate depression [5]. Having a parent with Parkinson's disease may have less negative impact than having a parent with MS [6]. The impact of parental MS on the child, in turn, depends on many factors including the family's social network [7]. The children of parents with MS were compared with their peers of similar age and gender whose parents had no physical illness, and the results showed that the children of parents with MS had greater emotional and behavioural problems [8]. Accordingly, children of parents with MS are at risk of developing mental health problems [9] and parental MS can have a negative impact on the child's social relationships as well as on his/her psychological well-being [10]. Similar results were found among children who grew up in a family where the parent was affected by Huntington's disease. These children could experience problems and were at risk of decreased psychological well-being [11].

Children of parents with a neurodegenerative disease may get extensively involved in domestic activities and may be expected to provide care for the parent who is ill. Children of parents with Huntington's disease have expressed changes in their family's everyday life. They sometimes have an adult role, could be expected to provide care for the parent [12] and could feel responsible for the family's functioning [13]. A recent survey showed that 7% of the 2424 responding adolescents in Sweden were involved in extensive care of a person close to them [14]. Health care professionals should acknowledge the impact of a neurodegenerative disease on families and support children and parents in finding strategies to cope with the situation [6]. Daily assistance for the affected parent is one kind of support that could be helpful for the entire family. In Sweden, where this study was conducted, the Act concerning Support and Service for Persons with Certain Functional Impairments [15] regulates the possibility for a person affected by a disease to get support in daily life. A person who has a neurodegenerative disease that affects his or her ability to manage activities related to basic daily needs has the right to be supported by personal assistants at home. The extent and type of support and care given is regulated by the law in relation to the person's needs and is assessed individually. When a family member receives assistance and care at home, the demands on the other family members may decrease. However, having other people than family members and friends at home may also intrude on the family's and the child's private life.

There is limited scientific documentation and a need for increased knowledge about the life situation of children in families affected by a neurodegenerative disease [16, 17]. Recognizing the situation of the people around the patient is relevant [18] and the children's views are important for the development of policy and intervention [19]. On behalf of the National Board of Health and Welfare and in collaboration with the Swedish Family Care Competence Centre, a project aimed at surveying the health and well-being of children and adolescents who have a parent with a neurodegenerative disease was carried out. The perceptions of younger children and adolescents as well as of parents with and without a neurodegenerative disease were examined and used to formulate a model of how public and private networks and non-profit organizations could support the individual child and family [20].

The present study had the above-mentioned project as its starting point but deepened the analysis and concentrated on the impact of the disease on the children's everyday life. A child centred perspective is held throughout and the purpose of the study is to explore the views of both the children and the parents, of how a neurodegenerative disease in a parent influences the daily life of the child. The perceptions of the children and the parents are discussed with regard to the children's rights and needs. Implications for rehabilitation, family support and care of a parent at home are also discussed.

## 2. Method

### 2.1. Participants

The families were recruited during the summer and autumn of 2013. The recruitment was conducted by doctors, counsellors and nurses at hospitals and centres for persons with neurodegenerative diseases. Patient organizations were also involved in the recruitment. A convenient sample of nine families affected by Parkinson's disease, MS and Huntington's disease participated in the project. In total, there were 23 participants; 10 children, 6 parents with a neurodegenerative disease and 7 parents without a neurodegenerative disease. Three of the families were represented with all family members. Three families were represented with all children and one parent. Two of the families were represented by one parent but no children. In one family, both parents and one of three children participated.

The participants' age and gender (**Table 1**) were: (a) four younger children, aged 8–11 years, two boys and two girls, (b) six adolescents, aged 13–16 years, four girls and two boys, (c) six parents with a neurodegenerative disease, four mothers (aged 42–51 years) and two fathers

| Participants | Boys Fathers | Girls Mothers |
|---|---|---|
| Children, aged 8–11 years | 2 | 2 |
| Children, aged 13–16 years | 2 | 4 |
| Parents with a neurodegenerative disease, aged 42–51 years | 2 | 4 |
| Parents without a neurodegenerative disease, aged 37–54 years | 4 | 3 |

**Table 1.** Description of the participants.

(aged 42 and 45 years) and (d) seven parents without a neurodegenerative disease, three mothers (aged 37–54 years) and four fathers (aged 41–49 years).

### 2.2. Data collection

Children and parents with and without a neurodegenerative disease were interviewed by two researchers (first and fourth authors). The interviews were based on an interview guide with predetermined themes, directly related to the purpose of the project. The themes concerned the children's everyday life situation. The interviews were conducted as five focus groups [21, 22], and the composition of the groups was based on the assumption that people with similar experiences inspire each other in a conversation. In this study, the similarities of experiences concerned experiences of being in a specific age as a child, to have a neurodegenerative disease and to be a partner to a person with a neurodegenerative disease. Accordingly, the groups were as follows: (a) younger children (8–11 years), (b) adolescents (13–16 years), (c) parents with a neurodegenerative disease to younger children and adolescents, (d) parents without a neurodegenerative disease to younger children and (e) parents without a neurodegenerative disease to adolescents.

No participant was excluded due to problems with communication, but one of the participants was interviewed individually using Talking Mats [23] due to communication difficulties. Talking Mats helps people with cognitive and communicative difficulties to express their opinions and has been used by people who have Parkinson's disease and Huntington's disease [24, 25]. The person who used Talking Mats also participated in the focus group. The interviews with Talking Mats were conducted towards the end of each focus group session by one of the interviewers who is certified in using Talking Mats with people with disability. The interviews took place in another room than the focus groups and the purpose was to give the participant an extra chance to tell his/her views. The subject areas in the Talking Mats interviews were the same as in the focus groups but simplified and presented with visual support.

Each focus group met twice over a period of 4 weeks. After each session, the researchers talked about their experiences and about issues to bring up during the second focus group session. Each session was allocated to 3 hours, starting with refreshments and socializing. The average time for each session was 1:23:18 (hours:minutes:seconds), ranging from 1:03:52 to 1:36:20. The duration of the interviews with Talking Mats was 21 min and 58 s and 18 min and 53 s, respectively.

An interview guide including the following nine subject areas was used to stimulate discussion in each focus group: (a) the disease, (b) mental and physical health, (c) home, (d) school, (e) leisure time, (f) social network, (g) peers, (h) communication and (i) support functions. The interviewers (researchers) took turns being the main and the more passive leader in the focus groups. Both interviewers made sure that all participants had a voice in the group. The more passive leader made sure issues were followed up. In the first session, a whiteboard was used to summarize factors identified by the participants as different when a parent has a neurodegenerative disease. The same interviewer, in collaboration with the participants, wrote on the whiteboard in all focus groups. The participants had the last say regarding the views and summary written on the board. All of the factors were reviewed and revised where necessary, i.e. a member check provided a possibility for the participants to correct data.

The participants were encouraged to discuss the subject areas in relation to the past, present and future time and it was the child that was of main concern. This meant that the younger children and adolescents talked about their own feelings and experiences and the parents talked about their views about the children's situation, i.e. the perspective was child centred [26, 27]. The children's feelings and dreams were discussed, as were theirs and the parents' thoughts about barriers and factors facilitating health, development and well-being. The younger children were asked to use crayons and paper to draw communication aids that they thought would make it easier for the parents with communication difficulties [28]. The drawings, and how the aids could support the communication, were discussed in the children's focus groups.

The focus group sessions were recorded with a digital voice recorder and a camera. The data on the whiteboard, and the children's drawings, were photographed. The Talking Mats interviews were recorded with a smartphone, and the mats were photographed. These photograph data were reviewed in the analysis.

One of the interviewers, a clinical psychologist, had follow-up telephone contact with all of the participants on two separate occasions. The purpose of the phone calls was to follow up the participants' emotional reactions to the focus groups. It was also an opportunity for the participants to ask questions. Data from the phone calls were not included in the analysis. The first call was made within 1 month after the focus groups and the second contact was taken after another 3–4 months. Ten months after the last focus group session was conducted the participants were invited to a meeting at which the study results were presented. The meeting was also an opportunity for the participants to express their views about the results.

### 2.3. Data analysis and presentation of findings

All recorded interview data were transcribed verbatim, and all drawings were saved as digital photos. The Talking Mats interviews were both audio recorded and saved as digital photos. All of the collected data became a unit of analysis according to the methodology of qualitative content analysis [29]. Each researcher individually chose meaning units from the unit of analysis, and coded and analysed these into subcategories. The subcategories were further analysed into categories. The researchers discussed their codes, subcategories and categories until consensus was reached in each step of the analysis. The analysis fulfilled the requirement of dependability and credibility because the researchers checked each other's analysis. The results were compared with the original data in each level of the abstraction to guarantee that trustworthiness was achieved [30]. In the results, categories related to the impact of the neurodegenerative disease on the children's daily life are treated. All main categories and subcategories are presented in Appendices 1 and 2.

### 2.4. Ethical considerations

The study was vetted and approved by the regional ethical review board. The voluntary nature of the study, as well as the right to withdraw from the study at any time without explanation and personal consequences, was highlighted. Written and oral information was provided to all of the participants. All participants gave their oral assent to participate. The adults gave their written consent. Written consent for the children's participation in the study was given by their parents.

## 3. Results

The children's and parents' perceptions of the children's health and well-being were condensed into nine categories of which two—*Consequences in daily life* and *Influence of disease on children*—concerned the direct effects of the parent's disease on the children's daily life (Appendices 1 and 2). These were further explored. Ten subcategories of which three were common between the children and the parents (*Economy, Responsibility* and *Living with personal assistants*), three were unique for the children (*Being and feeling, Being different* and *Activities*) and one was unique for the parents (*The symptoms of the disease*) emerged. The ideas shared in all focus groups concerned the children; the children's own experiences and views and the parents' thoughts about the children's experiences and views. We will refer to younger children and adolescents as well as parents with and without a disease. The word 'children' alone, from here onwards, refers to both younger children and adolescents.

### 3.1. Economy

Both the children and the parents talk about the family's economy as a problem.

> *and we cannot afford to buy because we are one that provides for the family* (parent without disease)

They cannot give the child the kind of things that other children get.

> *to feel that one may not have the same possibility to do these things that all the others can participate in and do* (parent with disease)

The adolescents think of their family's economy as worse than the economy of other families and have experienced difficult times with regard to money.

> *when dad became ill then there was like I hardly had any clothes I had to use the same pair of jeans for three years* (adolescent)

To lay aside money for travelling is difficult for the parent without disease. This means the children cannot see relatives and friends as often as they would like to and need. Economy is a sensitive issue and in order to avoid putting an extra burden on the parents the children work and earn their own money. One adolescent works for the parent who is ill.

> *one like feels a bit ashamed asking for money or anything* (adolescent)

### 3.2. Responsibility

The parents believe that their children have larger responsibilities than children in families that are not affected by a neurodegenerative disease. The responsibilities relate to practical duties but also imply that the children have to manage on their own in life situations where a parent, under other circumstances, would have been present. The children talk about having responsibilities for daily routines at home.

> *it meant I had to become more responsible at a young age* (adolescent)

> *I am like ready to become a dad at age sixteen* (adolescent)

Some have adult-like responsibilities for siblings without any real possibility to object.

> *not like that I could just ignore my little sister* (adolescent)

Responsibility with regard to siblings is also talked about as something positive, leading to closer relationships within the family. Having large responsibilities as a child may affect the possibility to do child things, like playing.

> *I wasn't the kind that played a lot* (adolescent)

Both the younger children and the adolescents talk about the burden of being responsible for telling others about the disease and give each other advice about how and whom to tell. One adolescent tried to get her parent to tell her friend about the disease. She arranged for this to happen naturally at a time when the parent usually took the medicine and was very disappointed when the parent hid the intake of the medicine by going in to the toilet.

> *so I tried to like get her to like tell but she like went to the toilet so that was also so oh no like why did you go to the toilet* (adolescent)

The children are well aware of the changed parental roles and the greater demands on the parent without the disease.

> *dad has done a lot of things too one could say that he also has had a bit of the role of a mother* (adolescent)

The children are concerned about easing the pressure on the parent who is not ill so that he or she remains healthy. Their concern is relevant.

> *because they know how mum is that she is ill and like that it is understandable that they nothing should happen to me* (parent without disease)

Some of the parents without the neurodegenerative disease have been affected by other diseases.

> *now my mother is also ill* (adolescent)

### 3.3. Living with personal assistants

Some parents have personal assistants by their side 7 days a week. This means that the child has to spend a considerable amount of time together with people that he or she has not chosen to be with. Having people at home almost all of the awake time is demanding and the issue was discussed in all focus groups.

> *since dad is sick we have assistants in our home who subs … who do everything that dad should have done sometimes I think this is quite demanding* (younger child)

The child needs to be aware, check where in the apartment or house the assistants are, and protect themselves by, for example, locking doors.

> *but really one is never alone* (adolescent)

> *it is like difficult if one wants to take a shower or something like that and walks into the bathroom one always has to lock or something like that because one doesn't want them to come rushing into the room and like do things* (younger child)

The children are also disturbed at night.

> *sort of very late at night when I am trying to fall asleep then the home care service comes and like wakes me up* (younger child)

> *I have to try to fall asleep again when one is like sleeping deeply* (younger child)

According to one of the parents, having personal assistants at home is the most difficult part of the disease.

> *but it (the presence of personal assistants) is actually the toughest of it all* (parent without disease)

Having personal assistants at home influences the child's sense of being able to be and act as 'oneself', as well as the possibility to be alone. The size of the apartment or house is important as well as guidelines regulating where in the home the assistants are allowed to be. A small home makes the situation even more difficult and having space and areas where only family members are allowed is perceived as valuable.

> *so one can never avoid them we have the kitchen together and we have some parts of the house together of course they think it (i.e., the personal assistants) is a lot sometimes* (parent without disease)

The fact that the family is involved in planning the assistance and the guidelines for its implementation, i.e. what the personal assistants should do and where they should be, is good but does not solve problems related to personal integrity. Having people at home, strangers from the beginning, who are paid to be there, triggers conventions about how to behave and makes the child feel uncomfortable.

> *to always be polite and not... like to never be able to just be in a bad mood and think that life is crappy but that you have to be polite to these people who are sitting in the kitchen smiling and being so nice* (adolescent)

The personality of the assistant is important.

> *they think a lot about which (assistant) is good or bad* (parent with disease)

The assistant should respect the family and know what to do and not to do with the child and the parent who is ill. The children use words such as compliance and natural when they describe the personality traits of a good assistant.

> *she knows when to leave she knows she is so nice and bloody good* (adolescent)

> *she is so natural with us it is not like if she is like not like if she is employed* (adolescent)

The way the assistants talk with the children about their presence in the children's home is also relevant and can make a big difference.

> *all the others talk about being staff and things like that but she (a "good" assistant) doesn't* (adolescent)

It is unnatural when an assistant takes the role of a parent but at the same time the assistant needs to be updated about the child's activities. The assistant needs to be able to talk with the parent about where the child is without having to call and ask the child. Frequent phone calls from the assistants can be annoying, especially if the child already has informed the parents and the assistant about his or her activities after school.

> *as soon as we are not at home they call* (adolescent)

> *also we have a calendar on which we write the whole week like that but they don't look there* (adolescent)

Both the children and the parents talk about how the assistants manage communication. The assistants could support the interaction between the child and the parent who is ill but often they do not. Rather, the children's stories indicate that some assistants have difficulties in understanding the speech of the person they work with, i.e. the parent with the disease, and lack knowledge about strategies that would support the communication. The child is sometimes more competent than the assistants in understanding the parent.

> *really I think that we perhaps are a bit better at understanding than them* (younger child)

The assistants' communicative style may also be burdensome for the child.

> *they start talking like this ... they sort of become a bit loud sometimes ... okay it is not like if they are screaming but they talk loud* (younger child)

The children understand the parent's need for assistance.

> *the assistants have to be there she cannot sit by herself* (adolescent)

Administrating assistance takes a lot of time and energy for the family and the children get tired by the fact that there is so much talk about care at home. This is particularly so when family members, for example grandparents, work as assistants as well.

> *I said that to dad at my birthday that today you are not allowed to talk about the assistants at all* (adolescent)

Spending time with family members only is appreciated.

> *those weekends you just long for* (adolescent)

### 3.4. Being and feeling

The adolescents have many thoughts and feelings about the disease and describe symptoms of psychological unhealthiness.

> *I was depressed from thirteen to fifteen* (adolescent)

> *so when I was twelve I thought about suicide* (adolescent)

The younger children are also affected psychologically.

> *one gets a bit worried about dad* (younger child)

### 3.5. Being different

A parent with a neurodegenerative disease is different. This makes the child different too. Not knowing anyone else who has a parent with a disease contributes to the feeling of being different.

> *I don't know anyone that lives that close like me who has a parent who is ill who has a disease* (younger child)

Aids are evident outward signs that make the parent and the family look different and strange.

> *in the beginning when mum started to use a walker we should walk in town with mum on our own then I was a child and I thought she was embarrassing* (adolescent)

Bringing friends home from school is difficult. The adapted home environment is a barrier.

> *in case I bring someone home... and our toilet is quite strange* (younger child)

The children do not like the way other people observe and speculate about the parent who is ill.

> *one of our friends Berra he like stands there and looks at him for a few seconds* (younger child)

A story about a parent leaving home in an ambulance is an example of how speculations can lead to rumours and affect the child negatively.

> *then some of our neighbours said the police got him and put him behind bars* (adolescents)

### 3.6. Activities

Physical, psychological and psychiatric symptoms hinder the parent with the disease from participating in activities in the way the children would like.

> *but like he can't swim with me and do things* (younger child)

> *she just sits there at home for the whole day* (adolescent)

Activities with friends at home are also affected.

> *then dad becomes a bit angry when one like plays in the living room* (younger child)

Family activities and holidays need to be planned in detail and yet everything could change in the last minute, like in this story about going to the swimming hall.

> *the MS was more difficult than usually the day we were going so we couldn't go* (younger child)

### 3.7. The symptoms of the disease

The parents without the disease talk about how different symptoms such as tiredness, anxiety, aggression and lack of empathy in the parent with the disease affect the children. Psychiatric problems are the most challenging to manage.

> *it is when she is not feeling well psychologically and anxiety and things like that when that comes it of course... now she has good medicines so things are working better ... I don't know if they think the physical really is hindering* (parent without disease)

Knowledge about the symptoms of the disease increases the children's understanding and gives them a possibility to gain control. The children get the knowledge from their parents. Yet, the parents are unsure about how much to tell.

> *my parents think it is awful they think we have been too open about it* (parent without disease)

> *why should I talk about it with her make her worried I could feel* (parent with disease)

## 4. Discussion and implications

The results are in line with existing research suggesting that a neurodegenerative disease in a parent affects the family and the children in particular [5, 10–13, 31, 32]. It is difficult to separate the needs of the children from the needs of other family members [33]. According to the parents and the children in this study, a parent's disease has a large impact on the everyday life of the child. Children are affected emotionally and psychologically with regard to practical issues and the fulfilment of basic needs.

One of the most obvious effects of a parent's disease on the child concerns the parent's need for support and care at home. The child is affected by the support their parent gets from people coming to their home. At the same time, as the present results also show, the families need this and other kinds of support. From a child perspective, paid external support such as personal assistance for a parent who is ill is both relieving and complicating. There is an evident conflict between the child's rights for well-being and privacy at home on the one hand and the needs and rights of the parent with the disease for high quality care on the other hand. The picture is that of a scalepan with external support in one of the bowls and the child's integrity in the other. Reaching a balance seems to be difficult. The aim of assistance is to support the person who is ill so that good health and living conditions are ensured [15]. This goal seems to be fulfilled, which could be relieving for the children who worry about both the parent who is ill and the parent without the disease. There is no evidence in the present data of children giving care by, for example, dressing or taking the parent who is ill to the toilet. Thus, it can be assumed that the support offered by the assistants is sufficient and prevents the children from becoming carers [14]. Well-functioning assistance for the parent who is ill also means reduced demands on the healthy parent and thus is positive for the child from this perspective as well. The responsibilities of the participating children, which are considerable according to the parents and the children, concern other issues such as having to do more practical work at home than is reasonable for a child, caring for siblings, worrying and being on their own in situations where a parent could have been involved.

Home is a central arena for the child's forming of identity and development, and therefore needs to be protected [1, 2]. A most noteworthy observation in this study concerns the lack of privacy for the children at home and the physical and mental space occupied by the disease. The children need free zones and the possibility to choose to be on their own and behave as they wish, without having to conform to social rules and etiquette. These children are under emotional pressure and show signs of unhealthiness. Having strangers around in the house and being woken up during the night, because of a parent's need for care, not only reflects lack of privacy but is a threat to the child's health. A calm and safe environment with well-known people, during the day and the night, is a right of the child. The institutionalization of the home, which becomes a combination of hospital and work place, also seems to be difficult to handle for the child but is good for the parent who does not have to move away to get care. It is not only the size of the house and the fact that there is little room to be on one's own or to play with friends that matter but also being surrounded with people who are at work, different instruments, aids and environmental adaptations. Some assistants, more than others, make the children understand that assistants are not a part of the family. This is redundant information for the child who may prefer when assistants behave as if they were members of the family, albeit with respect for the integrity of the child. Put differently, the child does not have to be reminded about the parent's disease but rather needs supportive adults. That home turns into a work place is evident also with regard to the administration and implementation of care on behalf of the parent without the disease and other relatives. Some parents and grandparents are part time employed for the parent who is ill. Thus, there may be a mess of roles and relations for the child at home.

Developing and maintaining a relationship with a parent who has a progressive neurological disease and deteriorating psychological and communicative functions is important but difficult for the child. Maintaining a relationship with the child is also a right of the parent, but difficult because of the disease. Other adults play a beneficial role in this regard. The parent and the child may need support to plan activities to do together. Economical support could also be valuable for a family where one parent has a neurodegenerative disease. To reduce stress on both the parent and the child, the parent with the disease needs to be updated about the child's activities. The parent will be content knowing where the child is and the child will not be disturbed by frequent phone calls from home, as was the case for one of the children in this study. Supporting communication is an issue along the same line. The children are negatively affected by the parents' deteriorating ability to communicate and by how communication is managed by others. The parents may have difficulties speaking as well as understanding when other people speak. The children often understand their parents better than other people and feel uncomfortable by the way others talk with their parents. They also may get the role of interpreter, at home and in society. This is a heavy duty and not in line with their rights [1, 2].

Working in the home and giving care to a parent with a neurodegenerative disease is difficult [34]. Specific education about the disease and different ways to support communication is important [35, 36]. Carers and health professionals also need to be aware of the fact that the person they work with is a parent with needs and obligations towards a child. Educated people in the child's network could support the child's health and well-being. For example, by informing people around the child about the disease, the kind of observations and rumours spread by other people, as reported of by the children in this study, could be avoided. It should not be the responsibility of the child to inform others about the disease and specific symptoms. There is also a need for the children to learn more about the disease, how it can fluctuate and how it will proceed. Increased knowledge about the disease and its sometimes unpredictable nature will increase the child's understanding of the parent's mood, activity level and behaviours and, as a result, his/her quality of life at home.

A child centred perspective will facilitate the child's well-being and development and implies listening to the wishes and needs of the child. These children are thoughtful and accommodative regarding their parents' needs. They understand and accept the situation, also because there is not much else for them to do. They carry out daily household tasks, care for siblings and work to earn their own money. Unnecessary burden on them should be avoided and they should not have to weigh their own needs against their parents'. Rather, adults in charge of the care need to consider how care can be given to the parent in a way that is minimally intrusive for the child. Taking the children's needs into account means asking them [27], given that their parent is ill, how would they like to organize their life at home? What is important for them in daily life? By asking the children about their situation and experiences, it will be possible to make life good for them at home and at the same time provide care for the parent.

Overall, the present findings point to the fact that children of families affected by a neurodegenerative disease need different kinds of support. Allowing the parent who is ill to attend a day care centre or a care home over the weekend, now and then, would give the child a temporary pause from the disease. Speech and language pathologists, social workers, psychologists and family nurses are other professionals, apart from personal assistants, who play important roles for the parent's rehabilitation as well as for the child and the family [37, 38].

## 5. Reflections about the study

Listening to the feelings and views of the children and the parents is important [19], and the present study is unique in involving children of different ages as well as parents with and without a disease. Children are not always willing to talk about their situation [19]. Both the children and the parents in this study expressed satisfaction about their participation in the larger project and 10 of the 23 participants came to the 10 months follow-up meeting. The meeting was an opportunity for the participants to get together with some of the other families and to reflect upon and give feedback on the findings and thus strengthened the credibility of the study. The participants attending the meeting agreed with and recognized the results as their own or the other focus group participants' views. The role of the health care system in supporting the children was discussed at the meeting, as was the important function of patient organizations.

Graneheim and Lundman [30] define transferability as the knowledge about whether the results can be transferred to other groups. This study describes the experiences of families living in Sweden and several of the participating families were recruited from patient-related non-profit organizations. Thus, there is a risk that the results not are transferable. However, the findings are in line with existing research [8–10] suggesting that the categories can be transferred to other families in western countries affected by a neurodegenerative disease. Furthermore, the findings should be treated in light of the fact that some of the families were known by the interviewers who also were experienced in talking with families living with progressive neurological conditions. Background knowledge may strengthen an interviewer's ability to ask relevant questions and to support the conversation in a group but may also make the interviewer to steer the conversation according to own interests and preferences.

## 6. Conclusions

A parent's disease has an impact on the individual child who is affected emotionally and psychologically, with regard to practical issues, and with regard to the fulfilment of basic needs. For example, the need for care of the parent at home creates a conflict between the child's rights for well-being and privacy and the needs and rights of the parent with the disease for good care. The presence of a personal assistant will influence the child's need for privacy, sometimes up to 24 hours a day. However, the assistant is also a valuable and necessary support for the family and the parent who is ill and prevents the child from becoming a young carer. The negative impacts also concern the child's lack of knowledge about the disease and economy. Professionals involved in the care and rehabilitation need thorough education and training in general care as well as in the symptoms, characteristics and consequences of specific diseases. In such training, the children's situation should be a focus area. Research involving more families as well as studies focusing the experiences of health care professionals and others in society supporting these families are needed in order to plan and carry out meaningful education and training programs.

## Appendices

| Main categories | Subcategories |
|---|---|
| The disease | How the disease is noticed |
| | Knowledge about the disease |
| | Heredity |
| | The progression of the disease |
| | Medicine |
| Consequences in daily life | Being and feeling |
| | Being different |
| | Economy |
| | Activities |
| | Responsibility |
| | Personal assistants |

| Main categories | Subcategories |
|---|---|
| Social relations | Close family |
| | Close family network |
| | Future relations |
| To cope with the situation | Accepting the situation |
| | Adjusting own behaviour |
| | Practical support |
| | To get knowledge about the disease |
| | Talking with someone |
| | Meeting people who are in a similar situation |
| | The role and function of school |
| | Communication aids and strategies |

**Appendix 1.** Younger children's and adolescents' perceptions of health and well-being.

| Main categories | Subcategories |
|---|---|
| Influence of disease on children in daily life | The symptoms of the disease |
| | The presence of the assistants |
| | Responsibility for domestic activities |
| | The family's economy |
| Interaction | Activities for the parent with the disease and the children |
| | The parent with the disease needs support to communicate |
| | Relations within the family |
| The role of the parents | The parents' roles change as a result of the disease |
| | Caring about the children's present and future life |
| Network | Friends |
| | Organizations |
| | School |
| | Health care and nursing |
| Being and feeling | Psychological and physical unhealthiness |
| | Thoughts about the disease |
| | Physical activity |

**Appendix 2.** Perceptions of the children's health and well-being by parents with and without a neurodegenerative disease.

## Author details

Ulrika Ferm[1]*, Stefan Nilsson[2], Margaretha Jenholt Nolbris[2], Petra Linnsand[3] and Annikki Jonsson[4]

*Address all correspondence to: ulrika.ferm@vgregion.se

1 DART Centre for Augmentative and Alternative Communication and Assistive Technology, Sahlgrenska University Hospital, Göteborg, Sweden

2 Institute of Health and Care Sciences, Sahlgrenska Academy, University of Gothenburg, Göteborg, Sweden

3 Dalheimers hus, Social Resursförvaltning, Göteborg, Sweden

4 Faculty of Caring Science, Work Life and Social Welfare, University of Borås, Borås, Sweden

## References

[1] Hall D. Children, rights, and responsibilities. Archives of Disease in Childhood. 2005;**90**:171-173. DOI: 10.1136/adc.2004.053017

[2] United Nations. Convention on the rights of the child document. 1989-1990. A/RES/44/25. Available from: www.ohchr.org/en/professionalinterest/pages/crc.aspx [Accessed: 27 January 2017]

[3] Socialstyrelsen [The National Board of Health and Welfare]. Barn som anhöriga. Konsekvenser och behov när föräldrar har allvarliga svårigheter eller avlider [Children as relatives. Consequences and needs when parents have serious difficulties or die]. 2013. Available from: www.socialstyrelsen.se/publikationer2013/2013-6-6 [Accessed: 27 January 2017]

[4] Storm Mowatt Haugland B, Ytterhus B, Dyregrov K. Barn som pårorende [Children as Relatives]. Oslo, Norway: Abstrakt förlag; 2012

[5] Schrag A, Morley D, Quinn N, Jahanshahi M. Impact of Parkinson's disease on patients' adolescent and adult children. Parkinsonism and Related Disorders. 2004;**10**:391-397. DOI: 10.1016/j.parkreldis.2004.03.011

[6] Jahanshahi M, Sheikh S. Long-term neurological illness in parents has a substantial impact on the lives of children. British Journal of Neuroscience Nursing. 2007;**3**:246-252. DOI: http://dx.doi.org/10.12968/bjnn.2007.3.6.23708

[7] Rintell D, Melito R. "Her illness is a project we can work on together": Developing a collaborative family-centered intervention model for newly diagnosed multiple sclerosis. International Journal of MS Care. 2013;**15**:130-136. DOI: 10.7224/1537-2073.2012-022

[8] Diareme S, Tsiantis J, Kolaitis G, Ferentinos S, Tsalamanios E, Paliokosta E, Romer G. Emotional and behavioural difficulties in children of parents with multiple sclerosis: A controlled study in Greece. European Child & Adolescent Psychiatry. 2006;**15**:309-318. DOI: 10.1007/s00787-006-0534-7

[9] Steck B, Amsler F, Grether A, Dillier AS, Baldus C, Haagen M, Romer G. Mental health problems in children of somatically ill parents, e.g. multiple sclerosis. European Child and Adolescent Psychiatry. 2007;**16**:199-207. DOI: 10.1007/s00787-006-0589-5

[10] Bogosian A, Moss-Morris R, Hadwin J. Psychosocial adjustment in children and adolescents with a parent with multiple sclerosis: A systematic review. Clinical Rehabilitation. 2010;**24**:789-801. DOI: 10.1177/0269215510367982

[11] Forrest Keenan K, Miedzybrodzka Z, van Teijlingen E, McKee L, Simpson SA. Young people's experiences of growing up in a family affected by Huntington's disease. Clinical Genetics. 2007;**71**:120-129. DOI: 10.1111/j.1399-0004.2006.00702.x

[12] Sparbel KJ, Driessnack M, Williams JK, Schutte DL, Tripp-Reimer T, McGonigal-Kenney M, Paulsen JS. Experiences of teens living in the shadow of Huntington Disease. Journal of Genetic Counseling. 2008;**17**:327-335. DOI: 10.1007/s10897-008-9151-6

[13] Williams JK, Ayres L, Specht J, Sparbel K, Klimek ML. Caregiving by teens for family members with Huntington disease. Journal of Family Nursing. 2009;**15**:273-294. DOI: 10.1177/1074840709337126

[14] Nordenfors M, Melander C, Daneback K. Unga omsorgsgivare - en kartläggning av ungdomar som ger stöd, vård och hjälp till en nära anhörig [Young carers—A survey of adolescents who support and give care to a close relative]. Nationellt kompetenscentrum anhöriga, Barn som anhöriga [The Family Care Competence Centre, Children as Relatives]. Kalmar, Sweden; 2014. Available from: http://www.anhoriga.se/Global/BSA/Dokument/Rapporter_kunskaps%c3%b6versikter/Nka_BSA_Rapport_2014-5_webb.pdf [Accessed: 28 January 2017]

[15] Swedish Code of Statutes. Act concerning support and service for persons with certain functional impairments. SFS 1993:387. S 1993. Available from: http://www.independentliving.org/docs3/englss.html [Accessed: 27 January 2017]

[16] Morley D, Selai C, Schrag A, Jahanshahi M, Thompson A. Adolescent and adult children of parents with Parkinson's disease: Incorporating their needs in clinical guidelines. Parkinson's Disease. 2011;**2011**:951874. DOI: 10.4061/2011/951874

[17] Morley D, Jenkinson C. Furthering our understanding of the needs of adolescent children of parents with Parkinson's disease. Adolescent Health, Medicine and Therapeutics. 2013;**29**:75-77. DOI: 10.2147/AHMT.S47878

[18] Bhimani R. Understanding the burden on caregivers of people with Parkinson's: A scoping review of the literature. Rehabilitation Research and Practice. 2014; Article ID 718527:1-8. DOI: 10.1155/2014/718527

[19] Aldridge J. All work and no play? Understanding the needs of children with caring responsibilities. Children and Society. 2008;**22**:253-264. DOI: 10.1111/j.1099-0860.2007.00094.x

[20] Ferm U, Jenholt Nolbris M, Jonsson A, Linnsand P, Nilsson S. Hälsa och välbefinnande hos barn och ungdomar som har en förälder med progredierande neurologisk sjukdom [Health and well-being in children and adolescents who have a parent with a progressive neurological disease]. Nationellt kompetenscentrum anhöriga, Barn som anhöriga [The Family Care Competence Centre, Children as Relatives]. Kalmar, Sweden; 2015. Available from: http://www.anhoriga.se/Global/BSA/Dokument/Rapporter_kunskaps%c3%b6versikter/BSA-rapport_2015-2.pdf [Accessed: 28 January 2017]

[21] Creswell J W. Qualitative Inquiry & Research Design. 3rd ed. Thousand Oaks, CA, USA: SAGE Publications; 2013. p. 472. ISBN: 9781412995306

[22] Wibeck V. Fokusgrupper: Om fokuserade gruppintervjuer som undersökningsmetod [Focus Groups: About Focused Group Interviews as a Method]. Lund, Sweden: Studentlitteratur; 2010. 178 p. ISBN 10: 914405856X

[23] Cameron L, Murphy J. Obtaining consent to participate in research: The issues involved in including people with a range of learning and communication disabilities. British Journal of Learning Disabilities. 2007;**36**:113-120. DOI: 10.1111/j.1468-3156.2006.00404

[24] Ferm U, Bloch S, Saldert S. Negotiating disagreement in picture symbol supported decision making. Journal of Interactional Research in Communication Disorders. 2015;**6**:131-156. DOI: 10.1558/jircd.v7i1.27534

[25] Ferm U, Sahlin A, Sundin L, Hartelius L. Using Talking Mats to support communication in persons with Huntington's disease. International Journal of Language and Communication Disorders. 2010;**45**:523-536. DOI: 10.3109/13682820903222809

[26] Coyne I, Hallström I, Söderbäck M. Reframing the focus from a family-centred to a child-centred care approach for children's healthcare. Journal of Child Health Care. 2016;**20**:494-502. DOI: 10.1177/1367493516642744

[27] Nilsson S, Bjorkman B, Almqvist A L, Almqvist L, Björk-Willén P, Donohue D, Hvit S. Children's voices—Differentiating a child perspective from a child's perspective. Developmental Neurorehabilitation. 2015;**18**:162-168. DOI: 10.3109/17518423.2013.801529

[28] Druin A. Children as codesigners of new technologies: Valuing the imagination to transform what is possible. New Directions for Youth Development. 2010;**2010**:35-43. DOI: 10.1002/yd.373

[29] Elo S, Kyngas H. The qualitative content analysis process. Journal of Advanced Nursing. 2008;**62**:107-115. DOI: 10.1111/j.1365-2648.2007.04569.x

[30] Graneheim UH, Lundman B. Qualitative content analysis in nursing research: Concepts, procedures and measures to achieve trustworthiness. Nurse Education Today. 2004;**24**: 105-112. DOI: 10.1016/j.nedt.2003.10.001

[31] Bogosian A, Moss-Morris R, Bishop F, Hadwin J. How do adolescents adjust to their parent's multiple sclerosis? An interview study. British Journal of Health Psychology. 2011;**16**:430-444. DOI: 10.1348/135910710X521492

[32] Williams JK, Driessnack M, Barnette JJ, Sparbel KJ, Leserman A, Thompson S, Paulsen JS. Strategies used by teens growing up in families with Huntington disease. Journal of Pediatric Nursing. 2013;**28**:464-469. DOI: 10.1016/j.pedn.2013.02.030

[33] Wihstutz A. Working vulnerability: Agency of caring children and children's rights. Childhood. 2011;**18**:447-459. DOI: 10.1177/0907568210394878

[34] Borreani C, Bianchi E, Pietrolongo E, Rossi I, Cilia S, Giuntoli M, Pe N. Unmet needs of people with severe multiple sclerosis and their carers: Qualitative findings for a home-based intervention. PLoS One. 2014;**9**:e109679. DOI: 10.1371/journal.pone.0109679

[35] Morris MA, Dudgeon BJ, Yorkston K. A qualitative study of adult AAC users' experiences communicating with medical providers. Disability and Rehabilitation: Assistive Technology. 2013;**8**:472-481. DOI: 10.3109/17483107.2012.746398

[36] Ghafari S, Khoshknab MF, Norouzi K, Mohamadi E. Spousal support as experienced by people with multiple sclerosis: A qualitative study. The Journal of Neuroscience Nursing. 2014;**46**:E15-24. DOI: 10.1097/JNN.0000000000000081

[37] Bell JM. Knowledge translation in family nursing: gazing into the promised land. Journal of Family Nursing. 2014;**20**:3-12. DOI: 10.1177/1074840714521731

[38] Benzein EG, Hagberg M, Saveman BI. 'Being appropriately unusual': A challenge for nurses in health-promoting conversations with families. Nursing Inquiry. 2008;**15**:106-115. DOI: 10.1111/j.1440-1800.2008.00401.x

# 6

# Using Information and Communication Technology in Home Care for the Elderly

Boštjan Kerbler

**Abstract**

Due to population aging, countries' financial capacities to maintain the current level and scope of services and institutional care for the elderly are decreasing, which is why there are increasing demands to rationalize services and residential care for the elderly as much as possible. The society has responded to such issues with the idea that the elderly should be able to remain in their home environment as long as possible, where they would be able to lead their lives with the best possible quality of life. People support the idea broadly because it meets the desires and needs of the elderly. Most want to stay at home, and in the same social environment, they want to maintain their autonomy as long as possible. To make to the elderly, the possibility to remain in their living environments and moving elder-care activities to their homes can be achieved with the help of information and communication technology (ICT) by which home care could be provided remotely.

**Keywords:** aging at home, the elderly, information and communication technology, smart homes, remote home care

## 1. Introduction

European countries as well as other western countries are dealing with an aging of population. The United Nations Department of Economic and Social Affairs [1] reports that in the 1960s (1950–2010), the population of the elderly almost doubled, and there was an increase from 8.2 to 16.2%. This rate of aging will also increase in the coming decades. According to Eurostat data [2], by 2060, the proportion of people over 65 years of age would constitute 29.3% of the total population in the Member States of EU, as well as Norway, Switzerland, Iceland, and Liechtenstein, if natural fertility continues to decline and will have no regular (or significant) entry of young immigrants. Because people will live longer, the demographic structure of seniors will also change: the number of seniors over 80 years will increase significantly; it should double by 2040, and by 2060, it will almost be three times more. As a result of the aging of the population, in particular, the rapid increase in the number of very elderly and sick people who generally need a lot of care and because families are finding it increasingly difficult to take care for older members due to a modern rhythm and lifestyle, there is increasing pressure to move them to social and medical institutions, where they receive appropriate services and care. This creates an increasing expenditure on health care and social protection systems. This is particularly problematic in countries that have by now developed only the institutional form of care for the elderly, which is the most expensive of all forms of housing care.

The financial security of services for the elderly is already a concern, and the European Commission [3] estimates that the future costs of pensions, health care, and long-term care will increase by 4–8% of gross domestic product (GDP), and total health expenditure and social services are expected to be doubled by 2050. By 2050, only social security costs in EU Member States are expected to account for around 35% of GDP [4] The effect of the generation of the baby boom generation should be revealed in the provision of care services to the elderly, as this generation will become a huge user of these services. Given the dynamics, in particular, the impact on social health expenditure or maintenance of use, the future fluctuation of the dependency ratio is very important. This ratio shows how many older people depend on the workforce. The forecasts suggest that in the future, there may not be enough workers to support the health and social care system. The relationship between age, which is the ratio between the number of workers (15 to 60 years old persons) and the number of retirees (over 65 years), rose from about 5:1 in 2000 to 1.9:1 in 2060 [2]. In the case of the unchanged growth rate of the elderly, the unchanged level of the right to productivity, and the unchanged employment rate, the increase in the share of GDP in aging-related public spending is the same as the dependence on the age [5].

Due to a decline in the financial capacity of countries to maintain the current level and scope of institutional services and care for the elderly, the need for rationalization of housing and services is rising. Since the home is of primary importance in later life [6], these requirements are possible, as the main idea is to stay older for the elderly and to move health and social care for the elderly. The idea includes the concept of "aging at home" or "aging in place". This concept has been the main topic of many research programs, strategic plans, and actions in some countries in recent years, for example, in the United States, the United Kingdom, Canada, Japan, etc. The aim is to reduce the rising costs of service delivery, thus reducing the pressure on public funds to meet the health and social needs of the aging population. The advocates of this idea derive from the preferences of the elderly. Studies show that elderly people stay as long as possible in their homes and in the same known environment and maintain their independence as long as possible [7–11]. Although the preferences of the elderly depend on cultural differences, in most regions, older people have a negative attitude toward institutionalization, and they feel that this is primarily a traumatic experience. Many times they find their last refuge, their last resort before their death. Such perception is deeply rooted in societies without diversification in institutions and in collective dwellings for the elderly. Extensive institutional care is as long as possible; therefore, it is in the interest of the elderly and is also in the public interest, it seeks to limit the demand for institutional care only for the elderly who really need this form of social assistance.

Moving elder-care activities to the homes of the elderly demands that effective service provision and service quality should be adapted to the living environment, as well as the implementation of new organizational procedures and technological solutions. With the development of the information society, the idea of moving elderly care activities to their living environment and implementing efficient and high-quality health care and social care services at home can be achieved with the use of information and communication technology (ICT), which can convert an elderly person's home into an innovative living environment and provide remote home care. This is a system that remotely connects the homes of the elderly with the control center and, via this center, with health care centers and other care facilities.

This chapter presents the role of ICT or their applications to the needs of offering remote home care support to the elderly. It discusses its importance and functioning, the efforts and achievements made to date in developing this innovation, and the premises for implementing it in practice based on opinions of the elderly about staying in these ICT environments. The chapter is an analysis form critical perspective of the relevant studies and scientific literature on the topic, as well as on our own research findings, and offers new knowledge, results, synthetic ideas, and critical perspectives. The chapter also sets questions for further consideration and scope for future research and applied work in this field.

## 2. Modern technologies used for providing an innovative living environment

Aging population and the development of modern technologies are parallel and interconnected processes in developed countries. A modern diagnosis of health and treatment methods is used to extend life, and modern technologies offer housing and life support to the elderly. This link has also been developed by new interdisciplinary areas, such as gerontechnology and domotics. Gerontechnology is a combination of the word "gerontology", the science of aging and age, and the word "technology". According to Ref. [12], the term was expressed by Graafmans and Brouwers in 1989. It explores and develops technologies based on researchers' findings on the aging process, with the aim of improving health and facilitating the daily lives of the elderly, enabling them being independent and participating in social activities [12–14]. Domotic derives from the Latin word domus "home" and the English word "informatics". It explores the use of information technologies that can be integrated into the living environment [15]. With regard to the development of technology for the elderly, it is possible to define two directions [16]: the improvement and development of assistive technologies that make everyday life easier for the elderly and develop and disseminate information technologies that exceed telecommunication beyond the limits of physical space.

"Assistive technology" means any device, equipment, product, or tool that maintains or improves the functional capabilities of persons with disabilities who may use them to facilitate and safely perform a particular task that they would otherwise be unable to perform or execute [17–19]. According to Ref. [20], assistive technologies allow the user to control the environment more efficiently with minimal physical effort. The environment in which support technologies are integrated should take into account not only the general standards but also the specific needs of individuals [21]. With the help of assistive technologies, differences are reduced between the individual's abilities and the environment, allowing an autonomous life [22]. We distinguish between low-, medium-, and high-tech technologies [23]. Low-level technologies include minor mechanical modifications or adjustments in a particular type of product (e.g., furniture); in contrast to the first, the second includes simple devices that require an energy for working (e.g., automatic alerts); and the third devices are programmed with integrated electronics [18].

The development of modern information and communications technology (ICT) opens new opportunities and solutions for assistive technologies. The term "information and communication technology" refers to the system of electronic integration of providers, hardware, software, and Internet users. It is used to obtain, save, manage, process, transmit, and disseminate data through the telecommunications system [24]. It reduces the physical distance and expands the social dimension of space. Together with computer hardware and software, ICT makes it possible to control and manage assistive technologies in the home. This reduces physical distance and expands the social dimension of space [25]. The concept is known as an ambient intelligence or a smart environment. According to Ref. [26], we use those terms for defining technologies and methods that are always prepared to perform for persons and their needs and wishes. Such environment is combining computing and advanced technologies (intelligent and innovative devices) and special interfaces (sensors) that detect and interact discreetly with users. The equipment must be environmentally nonintrusive and in the smallest measure, with the smallest possible use of space and energy, provided by intelligent materials, various nanotechnologies, etc. A complex and heterogeneous network (i.e., the telecommunication infrastructure) operates on the discrete manner in such environments. These environments recognize the presence of people in a room based on physiological characteristics (e.g., voices and gestures) and are always ready to respond to a request for environmental assistance. This enables the measurement of biological functions and safety of the user. Controlling the operation of environmental intelligence ensures security in terms of innovative technologies and ethics (e.g., the security of user personal data and other data) [27, 28]. A smart home is an application for the environment, which is an example of an innovative living environment.

It is a system that responds to desires, needs, and activities of people and is adapted to the abilities (cognitive and physical) of users. These homes are equipped with interconnected equipment, tools, and technologies. Electronic systems in smart homes monitor the living environment and can even perform certain tasks (shutters, opening and closing doors, and turning on and off heating) with minimal physical force using various methods (remote control, wheelchair, voice control, and even moving eyes). These homes have an integrated communication technology that allows electronic access and integration in different environments:

a living environment in the form of social buildings and infrastructure, a social environment (interaction with family, neighbors, and service providers), and a secondary environment (culture, politics, trade, ecology, etc.) [28]. Some authors [29] believe that these systems define the vision of the information society in the future—they will support a number of human activities transmitted electronically, will have access to many services and applications, and will make technologies less costly and the availability of different types of telecommunications. Therefore, smart home technology can support the health, safety, and independence of the elderly. While these technologies offer significant benefits to seniors and their families, seniors become the primary adoptive users of a new 24-hour lifestyle that monitors, manages, and maintains their health and well-being periodically [30]. However, smart homes cannot serve their purpose with the best technical and technological support if the living environment does not adapt physically from the start: without architectural barriers and adapted to the needs, capacities, and requirements of the elderly. When adapting the physical living space in an intelligent home, the principles of inclusive design [31] or design for all [32], also called universal forms [33–35], must be followed. The principles of such a concept are [33, 36] (1) equitable use for all users the same means must be provided, (2) flexibility of use—the design must correspond to many individual strengths and capacities, (3) simple and intuitive—the use must be easy to understand not looking for the knowledge, skills and experiences, (4) perceptible information: different forms (images, verbal, tactile) must be used for the redundant presentation of most important information for living, (5) tolerance for errors—the hazards and adverse consequences of random or unintentional acts must reduce, (6) low physical effort—effectively and comfortably with minimal fatigue must be provided, and (7) size and space for access and use—size and space must be provided for access, scope, handling, and use.

With these principles, the access of a living environment is emphasized. In such cases, layout must be functional and user-friendly as much as possible. Nothing should be complicated and difficult to use, and (at the same time) product should maintain their esthetic and practical value [37]. Some examples: the doors and halls must be wide, the passages between the rooms must be without thresholds, the furniture, electrical installations, and windows must be at an appropriate height, the floor must be level and not slippery, bathrooms must have handrails, seats, backrests, and appropriate furniture, rooms must be adequately lit, have adequate contrast between shades of bright and dark colors, and so on. Smart homes are therefore a combination of a living environment without architectural barriers and information and communication technologies that are integrated into such a living environment. The home environment in a smart home must always be accessible to everyone.

## 3. Four generations of ICT systems for enabling remote home care for the elderly

The ICT application for enabling remote home care is called telecare. The authors in Ref. [38] define this as the use of ICT to support health and social protection at a distance. Telecare is a mixture of telecommunications and computer technology and relevant information services to help individuals at home. All this have to be managed [39]. The most typical model is known as the business to customer (B-2-C) model. In this case, health and social services are provided directly to end-users (patients) at their homes [40]. According to Ref. [41], ICTs that are included in the remote home care system are divided into three generations.

The first generation of these systems is the most basic and simplest remote home care application. It was developed in some western European countries more than 25 years ago. The system was created in some countries of Western Europe more than 25 years ago. The system consists of a special telephone device. This is because users had a special phone for remote triggers that were wireless. The users worked with the trigger themselves and had them, for example, in the form of a pendant or bracelet. This enabled users to activate the wireless trigger anywhere in the apartment or house, as well as anytime (even if the phone could not be accessed). By pressing the trigger, the system automatically names the administrator (relative, neighbor, or friend) or calls the help center [42]. The system may also include a reminder. This is a feature that sends a reminder to the user at a certain time, in which the user has to perform a specific task. You can send reminders to one or more addresses at a time, including the user's caretaker. Users always had to confirm that they received a reminder. If this was not confirmed, the reminder was resubmitted, and the caretaker was informed that users did not confirm the reminder [43]. These simple versions of the safety alarm system are intended for elderly people with various health problems such as forgetfulness and various forms of disability [44]. The extent of usage differs and varies from one country to another. The ICT & Aging—European Study on Users, Markets and Technologies [45] showed that the share of users over 65 years was the highest in the United Kingdom and Ireland (around 15%), followed by Scandinavian countries—Denmark, Sweden, and Finland (up to 10%), and the United States, the Netherlands, Japan, Spain, Germany, Hungary, Italy, and France (up to 3%).

With the development of smart technologies, the system has evolved further. Today, there are already many providers of advanced information systems. These systems work by collecting information about the user's life functions by themselves. Systems send this information from users' homes to health and other help centers. This is facilitated by networks and broadband communication channels. The United Kingdom is at the forefront of the implementation of these advanced services for the elderly in the form of ambient intelligence. The British government has identified the implementation of these advanced systems as one of the most important national strategic priorities for sustainable development. According to Ref. [46], 175 million pounds was spent in England, Scotland, Wales, and Northern Ireland between 2006 and 2011 to carry out pilot projects aimed at obtaining as much practical experience and evidence as possible, on the basis of which smart homes can be implemented successfully and with greater certainty. The results were extremely good and encouraging. For example, in Scotland, for every pound that was invested in the establishment and implementation of this system, six pounds was saved (8 million pounds were invested and 48.4 million pounds saved) [47]. This included, inter alia, a reduction in the number of admissions of elderly people to elderly homes (47.5%), a reduction in the number of unnecessary hospitalizations for old people due to rapid hospital dismissal (42%), the reduction in unexpected hospitalization due to the rapid response of the system to injuries happened at the old man's home (9.1%), and reduction in the number of calls for quick home help and nightly shifts in hospitals. This is also the purpose of remote home care and advanced smart systems for the elderly.

These advanced systems of an innovative and smart living environment (second generation of remote care) operate in a way that different sensors are built into the user's home environment. The sensors are built into the user's home environment quite discreetly (e.g., on furniture handles, door handles, under carpets, in watches, etc.). The sensors measure and monitor the user's operation and its life cycle. They can measure the physiological functions of users (e.g., blood pressure, heart rate, and so on). They also monitor all activities of the user (e.g., when they go to the carpet next to the bed in the morning, how many times they go through the door, when they open the refrigerator, when they prepare meals, etc.). Sensors also warn those users who have different cognitive or sensory deficiencies (e.g., the system warns them to take medicines, also give users instructions on how to manage things and appliances in the dwelling). In addition to the devices that monitor and measure the health and psychic state of the users, they contain the smart domes of another device. These are the triggers/sensors that identify any unusual state or situation in a living environment that deviates from the normal. In this way, these devices provide security and control in the user's environment. These devices include detectors that detect motion (e.g., sensors for detecting falls of users, sensors that allow the lights to turn on and off automatically, sensors that allow the door to open automatically and close, etc.). In addition to sensors that detect movement, smoke detectors, fire sensors, gas sensors, water sensing sensors, and so on are also included among these devices. All the information recorded by the system in the user's smart home is transferred to the help and control centers via multipass telecommunication systems. If the system that is built into the home environment of users detects any changes that deviate from everyday or normal parameters, an automatic alarm is triggered. This alarm is transferred to a control center or help center (also to administrators). In the help centers, they immediately decide what to do. Some authors [24] therefore define such a system as a "response mode" or "r-mode". Within the descriptive supply system, control centers are a kind of intermediary between users and providers of services or services. They also provide information coordination between service providers and helpers (health and medical personnel, social workers, firefighters, relatives, neighbors, and so on). Depending on the problem and severity of the problem detected by the system at the user's home, the responsible person in the control center also provides the user with appropriate instructions (recommendations) or informs the service provider about the needs of users [48].

There is also the third generation of information and communication support systems for remote home care. This generation of systems includes the support of medical personnel. Doctors and other well-trained workers have occasional access to data recorded in users' homes and are transmitted and stored in the databases via broadband. Such access and monitoring of the health status of users enables the detection of different health patterns, which provides important information for the early detection of various diseases and deterioration of the state of health of an individual. This can help to adequately and effectively, and above all, adapt the treatment program and services to the user in due time. The data collected do not only allow monitoring the performance and health of the individual and improving the efficiency of the carrier but also provide better and more informed insight into the condition and understanding of the patients' needs or/and "intelligently" monitor the effectiveness of the care and the wellbeing of the elderly [49].

Users that wish to monitor the results of their health efforts can access their aggregated data outfitted with appropriate recommendations and advices any time through the ICT of the fourth generation of such systems. Audio-visual technology allows virtual or remote consultation between the user and doctors, nurses, or other health care personnel, thereby reducing the need for home visits, hospital appointments, emergency room visits, or hospital admissions [50]. In this way, the elderly could feel significantly empowered in day-to-day life [49] and they can actively and effectively participate in promoting health, care, and remote protection [51]. Authors in Ref. [24] define the third and fourth generation of remote home care system as a "preventive mode" or "p-mode," as it "emphasis on prediction, prevention, and early detection so as to prolong active and healthy independent living" [49].

The use of information and communication technologies offers an opportunity for older people. They allow them to live in their homes, in their familiar living and social environment for as long as possible, and to be able to live as independently as possible in such an environment. Such a life enables them to have a good quality of living; thus, institutionalization is not necessary or postponed for a later period. According to Ref. [38], the findings of the studies confirm that remote care at home reinforces the mental and physical condition of older people, and that it has been proven that there have been fewer hospitalizations. If hospitalization occurs, its duration is shorter than it would have been in cases for those people who were not involved in remote care. Remote care is better, more efficient, and cheaper. That is a fact. Therefore, telecare is one of the possibilities for a significant reduction in costs for health care and social services, especially in socially aging societies. However, the question arises as to how to include telecare in existing national health care and social care systems.

## 4. How to implement ICT systems for enabling remote home care for the elderly?

Despite successful pilot and test projects, advanced forms of an innovative living environment for the elderly are not yet widely implemented. It is very important that the technologies are reliable. It is also important that the living environment of the elderly person is appropriately included. Only in this way, it is possible to effectively implement remote home care as an application of information and communication technologies. However, one thing cannot be bypassed, namely that in order to facilitate the aging of the home, technologies cannot in themselves provide for the successful implementation of home care in a regular health care system and social care for the elderly. According to Ref. [24], implementation within the existing health and social systems is very complex. It is a combination of technological design on the one hand and organizational planning on the other. At the same time, this also includes a large number of groups of different people and individuals. Each of them has different ideas about what are the risks and the different systems of values that need to be met. The implementation of telecare also changes the existing relationships between the various stakeholders involved. Based on studies on integrating innovations into existing systems, some conditions or requirements for successfully implementing innovations can be defined, such as *ethical and legal acceptability, the suitability of the distribution of funds among the stakeholders, the technical reliability of an innovation*, and *the suitable arrangement of the living environment*. Beside these, some other conditions and requirements for successfully implementing innovations, such as implementing of remote home care into the regular health care and social care system, are important.

### 4.1. "Local" social surroundings and support of innovation in it

When introducing innovation into a "local" social environment (from a global social environment), the implementation of this innovation must be defined with the characteristics of the "local" environment. The acceptance of innovation in a local environment depends entirely on who is involved in introducing innovation, who is identified with innovation, and who takes the lead role as an initiator and mediator in the implementation process [39]. Implementation of innovation can be hampered by lack of support from the very beginning of the implementation process. This is mainly due to the lack of strategic support and decision-making by various (local) political and professional bodies. In those local environments where political will and decision-making are weak, information on innovation is insufficient. In such environments, the efforts to implement innovation must first focus on clearly determining the importance of introducing a specific innovation for the local environment. This includes the analysis of the existing state and the purpose, goals, and expected benefits of the new application. Efforts should be also focused on developing a collective "understanding of the innovation" through various forms of providing information and communicating [52]. The next step should focus on active involvement of politics. The author in Ref. [53] considers that this is the only true way and the only right way to determine the solid and clear legal frameworks that are indispensable to ensure that innovation is successfully implemented in a specific local environment. The political support needed to introduce a certain innovation into health and social systems is particularly important in the welfare countries. In such countries, systems are regulated in such a way that government policy regulates the social and health system on the basis of statutory acts. The governments of these countries also define policies and priorities, legal, and ethical rules of operation and are also the main provider of financial resources.

### 4.2. Mutual cooperation

As stated in Refs. [54, 55], successfully implementing more complex innovations requires coordinated, harmonized, and close cooperation between all groups of stakeholders; specifically, between and within individual groups (the vertical network of those involved) and with certain stakeholders also between the various levels of operation (the horizontal network of those involved). Mutual cooperation is essential for achieving high levels of awareness and recognizability, showing better cost effectiveness, increasing transparency while taking into account needs of a user, searching for solutions for adjusting legal frameworks, dividing risks in research and innovations, interoperability, and monitoring progress in general [3].

### 4.3. Readiness of organizations and the change of norms

When implementing innovations, the common obstacles are the compliance of the innovations and the resistance of organizations with values and "cultural" norms of an organization. Therefore, according to Ref. [56], it is important for the organization to create an innovation that abolishes and replaces some of the existing routines. In this, we have in mind various organizational routines, behavior patterns, and mental patterns. The organization should devote itself to the appropriate preparation that is related to the planning of the introduction of innovation. This is about developing different plans (strategic and business), developing different models, and evaluating and analyzing what the needs are. It should also be dedicated to determine who the providers of different services (e.g., health and social) and also to bark to those who are in high positions (in politics, businesses, etc.) to gain advocates. The organization should also be dedicated in preparing an appropriate working environment for the purposes of implementing the innovation, which involves training and education of personnel. As part of the preparation of the working environment, it must also carry out the reorganization of the working process of the process and often change the management of the business. Referring to Ref. [57], this activity of the organization represents creativity in action and thinking. The author of the same reference also warns that such reorganization of work, management, thinking, etc. need to be carefully planned. The author also points out that such reorganization procedures need to be prepared for the needs of each individual organization, and that the universal approach does not exist. As stated in Ref. [58], we must therefore act according to the principle "one approach for all," because this may lead to resistance, especially in organizations which are less flexible.

### 4.4. Evidence of the potential effectiveness of innovation

A certain environment will receive certain innovations only if the potential effects (and benefits) of implementing the innovation are proven, and if they are such that all the groups involved are satisfied with the effects and benefits. It is important that interested groups have measurable evidence of the effects and benefits. The groups affected by the implementation of innovation usually have the following questions: what will be the benefits of implementing a particular innovation and what costs will be related, how the costs will be distributed, how innovation can improve the effectiveness of existing systems (such as care systems for the elderly), and the investment in innovation will revert to how soon the new innovation-based system will become (financially) more effective than the existing one. Evidence of the effects of innovation must be gathered before the implementation of innovation. Evidence is obtained through testing and pilot studies. The effects collected in this way should also be critically analyzed and evaluated [59]. As the author says in the refinement [60], the exact scope of the test environment needs to be accurately determined. Only in this way, we can reduce the risk for potential users and help to make the probability of success in implementing the innovation more likely. However, it should be emphasized that in the control environment, it is very difficult to precisely define all the possible effects that the actual implementation will have. Pilot tests provide useful information about any problems that may arise during the implementation. If the pilot tests are well done and the results are properly evaluated, we can obtain fairly real evidence of the effectiveness of innovation. However, regardless of the credibility of the control tests, the obtained data must always be taken with reservations and critically. This is partly because it is difficult to implement large-scale projects that are truly representative and partly because we have many stakeholders in the actual implementation. These groups have different needs and different requirements, and these groups are those who ultimately make decisions about the usability and value of a particular innovation. It is also a fact that not all parameters of innovation can also be measured or displayed or converted into monetary values (e.g., better quality of life, people's well-being, less burden on informal caregivers, etc.). Many benefits and many effects are visible only over a long period of time [61]. Therefore, in Ref. [62], the authors emphasize that a more pragmatic approach is needed in demonstrating efficiency before the commercial product phase and innovation. In doing so, they have in mind, in particular, the implementation of innovations that are more complex (e.g., implementation in social care and health care systems, where high emphasis is placed on high standards). In this respect, pragmatism implies that the implementation of innovation must be carried out even if all evidence of the effectiveness of innovation is not yet available.

### 4.5. Needs and requirements of users

Technologies form the basis for the operation of smart-home systems, but any innovation can only be successfully implemented if the abilities offered by the new technology match users' needs and requirements. In order for an innovation to succeed, it is therefore necessary that the capacities offered by the new technology match the needs, requirements, and capacities of the users. Users are not interested in technological aspects of innovation. Users are only interested in their use. It is therefore very important how users take a particular innovation (e.g., how older people take a living environment in which information and communication technologies are implemented). From this, we can deduce the conclusion that the service and experience with the service (innovation) are those that are important to the user and which user is interested in, but not the devices and the system itself. The technical functioning is important, but it is not enough. The main question is thus what users like and what "works" for them [63]. As already mentioned by the author in Ref. [60], the lack of consideration for the needs of the users proved to be one of the major obstacles for implementing innovations in general as well as implementing medical technologies [64]. According to Ref. [20], we need to look for reasons for this in those who are suppliers and who carry out marketing according to the principle of "technological push strategy" rather than the "pull strategy" principle. In this way, they create a breakdown between users and their innovation requirements (e.g., requirements for innovative systems that help them carry out daily tasks) and products that are available for use. Author in Ref. [65] believes that ICT innovations in public services are also problematic because the suppliers are not always completely clear who the "leading users" are; specifically, the users, according to author in Ref. [66], have to find out what are the needs for new products and services ahead of others and in this way create demand for certain innovations. In order to ensure that innovation is successfully adopted, it is therefore most important that potential users are involved in the planning, development, and implementation process. This is especially true when it comes to innovations in the field of information-communication technologies. These must be designed for users and should be designed with users [67]. As stated by numerous researchers [68–71], the failure to consider the needs and requirements of the users is the reason why innovations are not accepted in society after implementation.

We assume that the process of developing and implementing innovative ICT systems for enabling remote home care for the elderly takes place more or less because of the need to rationalize health care and social-care services, but far too little attention is paid to users and their wishes and needs, which is also one of the conditions and requirements for successfully implementing innovations into existing systems. According to Ref. [72], a number of products were created to help the elderly, but the creators, in their design, took little account of the esthetic, social, and emotional relationships that older people would establish with the product. In any case, this is wrong. Today's rapid advances in technology provide sophisticated and smart solutions, but when designing and implementing ICT applications for older adults, we need to make sure that no technological advancement is what determines what should be created, but this determines the actual needs of users of these products [15]. Studies dealing with the creation of innovative living environments and their implementation in society should therefore focus more on people who use the products. Users are those who need to assess the properties and the effects of living in such an innovative environment. It must be evaluated on the basis of how they perceive, feel, and understand it, namely as a desired or unwanted form of living.

## 5. Attitudes of the elderly towards ICT systems for enabling remote home care

Technologists and developers of the smart environment would be very helpful if, on the basis of a sufficiently large number of pilot studies and on the basis of user experience, they could find out the user's attitude toward such environments and how they perceive them. This would probably increase the effectiveness of the implementation of such a living environment in practice. However, they should also enable users to be able to truly assess information and communication technologies and their use. We believe that, therefore, the main goal of the implementation process should be to provide users with meaning and increase understanding of the innovative living environment. User perceptions can be distorted for various reasons, which is especially relevant for innovations based on the most advanced forms of ICT and intended for the elderly. Studies [73–77] show that elderly people generally do not trust ICT. Authors in Ref. [78] report that among older people, one of the most common beliefs that discourages them is that life in a smart environment is too automated or that technology is perceived as a kind of substitute for personal contact with a person, who provides care and protection as well as communication, which could lead to a reduction of social contacts and loneliness or, as authors in Ref. [79] point out, a creation of a society of "high-tech hermits." According to Ref. [80], this means that the elderly suffer from "technophobia"; they are afraid of innovation and new technologies. Author in Ref. [81] believes this is because they do not know how to use these technologies, and authors in Ref. [82] believe this is because they do not have confidence in and doubt their own abilities due to sensory and cognitive deficiencies. The authors consider [83], and this also somehow justifies the opinion that older people are more conservative. This means that the elderly do not want their current lives and their life habits and patterns to change too much. In particular, they do not want to do this because of "external", less-known, or foreign factors that could affect their private life. In particular, as regards advanced technological systems of the living environment, older people, in the opinion of authors in Ref. [71, 84], fear to lose their privacy. In such smart environments, the elderly would appear to have an unpleasant sensation that they are constantly being watched and monitored (Big Brother syndrome). This is also proved by the studies carried out by the authors in Ref. [85–87].

In our own research, we proceeded from the assumption that elderly people have for the most negative attitude toward technologies, but also that (correctly) informing potential users, raising their awareness, and understanding of the usefulness and operation of remote home care are important for acceptance of this innovation among elderly and its implementation. We collected data for the analysis by directly interviewing people aged 50 years and more. We interviewed 114 of them in total. We divided the intrepid people into two groups. There were 57 people in each group. Prior to the interviews, both groups were informed about smart homes. However, the importance of information between groups was significant. In the first group, participants were generally informed about smart homes (what is their concept, how they operate, and what life is in them). In the second group of respondents, the concept of the living environment with information and communication technologies was explained in more detail and in a comprehensible and simple way. For this occasion, we prepared five short "scenarios" for the interviewees from everyday events from the lives of older people. On the basis of these scenarios, the interviewees wanted to make it as sensible as possible to present how the smart environment works, for what purposes it can be used, and what is the role of users. In this way, the interviewees could more easily and with more experience imagine how life in such a smart home is taking place. If they had any questions, interviewers could also ask the interviewer. The results of the survey revealed that there was a big difference between the groups in terms of what opinions and attitudes the interviewees had to smart homes. This reveals that it was very important how the interviewees were informed about smart homes. Interviewees in the first group had a very negative attitude toward innovative living environments and living in them. The other groups, on the contrary, had a very positive opinion about smart homes: nearly 80% of them responded that they would be willing to stay in an environment that is supported by information and communication technologies and which provides remote care. The reason that this group of elderly people has, in generally, expressed positive attitudes toward remote home care is the result of the fact that before the survey, the services were presented in detail in the most comprehensive manner to all respondents in this group. Most of those with very positive attitudes were "younger" elderly people (85.7%), aged 55–64 years. In the higher age groups, the share of the respondents with positive attitudes declined but was, nevertheless, still high (71.8%). We also made further analyzes. They have discovered that even those people who are properly and adequately informed about smart homes still have certain concerns about remote home care. The results show that half of the interviewees did not believe that the remote care system allows older people to stay in their homes for longer, and that institutionalization is postponed later. Furthermore, about one third of the respondents (34.5%) stated that they fear that they will lose their privacy. A little more than a fifth (22.4%) said they did not believe that remote care can provide security and an independent life. The least (11.7%) of them believed that such service could reduce visits of relatives, friends, and acquaintances in their homes. According to our opinion, therefore, unsuccessful implementation of ICT systems for enabling remote home care in the societies is not only because of technical inefficiency and price disadvantage but also because of the fact that public awareness of this service for older people was very low and information campaigns about this service were very ineffective. For this reason, we believe that better and more effective information could be provided in order for better and more effective information to help to better understand the operation of these services. Understanding would improve if potential users had the opportunity to learn about the opinions and positive feedback from those older people who already use the distance service. This would also reduce the negative opinion and attitude of older people to this service. We therefore consider that it is crucial to raise awareness among potential users of this service for the reception of a telecare in society.

The importance of assigning meaning to and understanding the concept of an innovative living environment for successful implementation was confirmed by the similar findings of the studies in which elderly people were asked about their views on remote home care. The analysis showed that studies like these do exist. Three of them are presented here in greater detail. In one of these, which is described in Ref. [88], the authors carried it out in the cities of Plymouth, Barnsley, and South Bucks in the UK. In this study, almost two-thirds (64%) of older people said they wanted to have a remote supply in their home environments. Most of the elders expressed this desire in Barnsley, with a share of as much as 81%. Almost all of the respondents (98%) thought that remote care would provide them with extended stay in their homes. This service would also make the respondents feel safer in their home environments, as all users in Barnley and almost all (96%) respondents in South Bucks were saying. There were a few more concerns about the surveillance, as only half (51%) answered that they would not interfere with their control in their homes. The control seems to be the biggest problem. In a survey conducted in the United States, older people had concerns about distance care [87]. What were the results? Almost two-thirds of respondents would not allow their homes to be watched by videos, but they strongly supported all other services provided by the remote control service. A large percentage of respondents (90%) supported the idea of transferring information to the control center about the health status of users. In this proportion, automatic alarms are also supported, which are disputed if necessary and offered by this service. It has also been suggested that users receive reminder for taking medicines through this service. More than 80% of respondents expressed support for monitoring unusual changes in older people's homes (e.g., fall detection). They also supported the possibility of monitoring the life cycle of users (e.g., measuring physiological functions) and recording daily patterns of behavior among older people and the possibility for users remotely to monitor collected information about their health and psychological status over the Internet, and that, according to the data collected, older people receive appropriate recommendations and advice. The authors in Ref. [89] also write about the very encouraging and positive views of the elderly about the Australian telecare system. Most of those elderly people who were included in the survey stated that they would be willing to accept this service. In their opinion, this would be very useful. They also emphasized that they could help such a service help users in an independent and quality life in their living environment. In their opinion, such a service would also enable them to participate in the management of their own health. It would also provide them with better access to health services and prolonging the stay of users in their homes. They also emphasized the relationship between users and administrators (doctors, medical staff, and others). According to Australian elderly people, this attitude should not be based solely on the exchange of information that would only be virtual but emphasized that these relationships should maintain personal contacts (at least occasionally and in more important matters). According to the respondents, this could have very positive psychological effects both on the health of the elderly and on their well-being.

As we can see, our research had the same results (the positive attitude of the elderly to the remote control system) as research in the United Kingdom, the United States, and Australia. What is the reason for this? The reason is attributed to the fact that this service was detailed and as comprehensive as possible and presented to respondents in an easy and picturesque way before the interviews. In all three of these studies, interviewees did not know the home care system or just heard it, but they did not know what it meant. For this reason, interviewers (just as in our survey), prior to the gathering of information, described this service accurately to older people (interviewees). For example, in Australia, video films were used. In the UK, scenarios were used, just as we did in our research. From this, we can therefore conclude that the proper information of future users is of key importance for the adoption of this innovation. Users need to understand how this service works, they need to get all the relevant information and answers to the questions, and they need to understand how the system works. All this can make an important contribution to the successful implementation of this service in society. All this has been confirmed by the results of the pilot exercise of the telecare service in Scotland. In this country, from 2007 to 2010, on the basis of effective information, 25% of new users decided to adopt ICT in their home environments and thus to integrate their homes into the remote control network. It should be stressed that the Scottish Government has invested a lot of resources into the information (both time and money). Potential users were thoroughly informed about the characteristics of remote care at home and why such a service is important [47]. In the case of Scotland, it also turned out that users' experience had an important role to play in understanding and raising awareness among older people and hence for later adoption of this innovation among users. As reported by the authors in Ref. [90], the information provided by informers to potential users was obviously sufficiently informative that they motivated a sufficiently wide circle of addressees, as well as that the information was realistic. Among the users who took over this service, 60.5% of new users felt that their quality of life had improved with the adoption of this innovation. As many as 93.3% of users felt that their stay in their home environments became safer. Almost 70% of them believed that they were more independent with this service. Nearly 90% of new Scottish users said that because of the new service, their other family members are less likely to work with them. The Scottish example also confirms the study described in the case of the United States, namely that the most positive views on the new service had been the older people who had already had some experience with the technologies.

It should be noted, however, that informing and raising awareness about the new service should not be limited to older people. It is true that these people are the main users, but others are involved in the use of these services, for example, carers, especially those informal carers. They also need to be informed, as they are also the target audience for living environments that include information and communication technologies. The term informal caretaker refers to an unpaid relative, friend, or neighbor "who provides care to an individual who has an acute or chronic condition and needs assistance to manage a variety of tasks" [91]. Due to a rapid population aging, the share of the elderly who rely only on family caretakers has increased dramatically in the last decades. According to the results of Seniorwatch [92], more than 80% of the elderly are assisted in their daily activities and tasks by one of their family members as informal caretakers and care providers. As the informal care can be very demanding in terms of volume, intensity and duration, the most commonly adverse fact to ensure the care of the elderly is a burden. The burden of the care provider is defined as its negative response, namely the influence that the provision of care on the social, professional and personal roles of the caregiver has to provide. This burden is also the predecessor or predictors of future depressive symptoms among caregivers [91]. From this point of view, new technologies can help not only older persons but also their caretakers; authors in Ref. [90] reported that 74.3% of relatives felt less burdened thanks to their use. But new technologies can also assist to formal caretakers (i.e., nurses, care assistants), who supports old peoples' independence through empowerment, developing flexible responses to their needs and supporting their formal carers [93]. The relationship between an older person and formal caretaker should base on trust, understanding, and compassion. However, as the number of elderly people increases, formal caregivers are also facing ever-increasing pressure. Authors in Ref. [94] report that health care workers are considered to be a particular risk of developing a negative age-related relationship because they are exposed to a disproportionate percentage of sick or dependent elderly people.

However, it is important to emphasize that for a realistic evaluation, the remote system at home should also be properly presented. They should be given the proper meaning of this system. The results of the studies show that the views of the caregivers can very often be misleading, due to various reasons. In the case of caregivers, fear and resistance to this service are often present in relation to distance provision. Sometimes, however, an exaggerated enthusiasm for such a service occurs among carers. Caregivers are against the service, because in their opinion, the care of the elderly by means of information-communication technologies is too impersonal. In Ref. [95], authors also state that caregivers fear that they will lose their role and mission (or partially or completely). So that technology will take over that role. Such an opinion should, in particular, be made by official carers, who feel that they are trained and qualified in the pursuit of this profession. Where does this fear of carers come from? According to scientists, fear was often caused by the fact that carers lack knowledge and understanding of the use of telecare-related technologies. Caregivers often treat training for new technologies as something that is an additional obligation that is unnecessary and perceived as very stressful. We can conclude that if the administrators knew and understood how information and communication technologies work and what they actually do, if they knew about the advantages and benefits of remote control services, and if they learned how to use these technologies, the fear would disappear and carers would be ICT service as part of their work. In addition to the fears and fear of new technology carers, there are also carers who are overly excited about such technological services. This, of course, leads to the fact that carers would objectively evaluate the concept of a smart home and successfully adopt and implement it. Authors in Ref. [95] write that the too enthusiastic perception of telecare is the most common feature of informal caregivers (i.e., family members). The modern rhythm of life and patterns of living are increasingly limited by family members to take care of their elderly family members. "In the European Union, in the last few years, the family, as the main provider of care for the elderly (family members), seems to be no longer carrying out its basic task" [96]. As family carers are overwhelmed, they often expect illusory expectations that new technologies will compensate for their lack of time for elderly members of the family or that they will completely relieve them of the care of older family members. This is, of course, completely impossible. It can also be dangerous. It is dangerous for older people who, with full exposure to technologies, can really become socially isolated. It is also dangerous to successfully implement the innovation of this technology service. Why? Informal carers would soon realize that new technology cannot completely replace them. There would be disappointment, which would lead to the spread of a negative opinion on the new service and the resistance to this innovation. This means that carers (especially informal) must always be thoroughly informed about what technologies really can do, what is the actual life in smart homes, and what the caregivers should actually expect about the remote care service.

## 6. Conclusion

We can conclude that the use of information and communication technologies truly represents the right direction to realize the idea that we will move health care and social services into the living environment of older people. This will increase the rationalization of public finances due to the aging process of the population. In the future, it is expected that such smart/intelligent home environments will become part of everyday reality. Modern society is becoming increasingly informative, the content of our life is determined by various supporting technologies and information, and communication technologies have become an irreplaceable part of our everyday life. But beware! We cannot and should not expect that the aging of the population and the increase in financial expenditures associated with this process will be simply resolved with new technologies. In particular, we should not allow, in view of the increasing financial pressures on the existing health care and social care system, that information and communication technology be put into the implantation and the living home environment of the elderly be included spontaneously, without planning. This would not be beneficial to our company and the premiere of users, but it would be in the first place harmful. Equally unacceptable and harmful would be the implementation of new technologies in the lives of older people and for the needs of their care due to rapid technological development. Implementation of information and communication technology supply services must, in the first place, be in line with the needs, habits, desires, and opinions of those who will use the new technologies and related services. Implementation of these innovations must therefore emerge from a model that actively involves users and identifies them as the main actors in this process. On the other hand, old people should come to the realization that innovative living environments can help old people to stay where their heart is long for. So that in their homes where their memories are, they can maintain their independence with the help of new technologies. Older carers also need to realize that new support technologies will never be replaced by their presence, that they will never be able to replace human contact and human proximity. They can, however, help them to relieve them from living with less burdens and more straightforward, as they know that those who nurture nothing are not missing and safe. This approach is called the participatory evaluation approach. Such an evaluation can actually lead to the realization of the set goals of all those who are directly or indirectly involved in the care of the elderly. Of course, the user aspect that we have presented (yet) cannot guarantee that the concept of using information and communication technologies to care for the elderly at home will automatically be accepted and become part of the system and society.

However, in promoting the idea of care with the help of information and communication technologies, it is necessary to know that the whole concept and process of implementation of this innovation is very demanding, that it should be carefully planned and that in addition to users, all other stakeholders should always be included in the implementation process (i.e., technologists, insurance companies, the state, municipalities, developers, broadband operators, etc.). Each of these stakeholders has its own function, its own way of thinking, and its perception of risks and a scale of values that need to be carefully studied and analyzed. All future research in this specific field must therefore take into account all these findings—that is, the different conditions and requirements of different stakeholders (not only the elderly)—and analyze and evaluate them. All this takes time. For this reason, we can conclude that rapid changes should not and cannot be expected in the implementation of care for the elderly through information and communication technologies. In order for the implementation to be as successful as possible and that an innovative service could indeed serve its purpose, it will be necessary to carefully examine everything that has gone wrong so far, that is all the shortcomings and mistakes, especially on the basis of case studies. We can expect, beforehand, that this innovative service for the elderly will become part of everyday life and part of our society, and we think that we could do something in that time without the need for such in-depth planning processes. It is about the fact that first, all spaces in which bivouac, in particular homes and homes in which elderly people reside, can be physically adapted according to the principles of design for all. This means that they would start to create a living space without obstacles. Therefore, where obstacles are (e.g., in the home environment of older people), these barriers would be removed and new buildings and spaces would be built without barriers. This would be a big step toward providing old people (and, last but not least, to us) to remain in their loving living environment for a long time. Such dormitories will be the basis for their further upgrading into smart homes, which provide care for elderly people remotely with the help of information and communication technologies.

## Acknowledgements

The study this chapter is based on was financed by the Slovenian Research Agency (Grant No. Z5-2062, title *A Telecare System for the Elderly*).

## Author details

Boštjan Kerbler

Address all correspondence to: bostjan.kerbler@uirs.si

Social Geography, Urban Planning Institute of the Republic of Slovenia Ljubljana, Slovenia

## References

[1] United Nations Department of Economic and Social Affairs. Population Divison, Population Estimates and Projections Section [Internet]. 2017. Available from: http://esa.un.org/unpd/wpp/unpp/panel_population.htm [Accessed: Aug 10, 2017]

[2] Eurostat. Europop2010: Population Projections. [Internet]. 2017. Available from: http://epp.eurostat.ec.europa.eu/statistics_explained/index.php/Population_projections [Accessed: Aug 10, 2017]

[3] European Commission. Ageing Well in the Information Society. An i2010 Initiative Action Plan on Information and Communication Technologies and Ageing [Internet]. 2007. Available from: http://eur-lex.europa.eu/legal-content/EN/TXT/HTML/?uri=LEGISSUM:l24292&from=EN [Accessed: Aug 10, 2017]

[4] Jespen M, Leschke K. Social protection and the social reality of Europe. In: Jesepen M, editor. Benchmarking Working Europe 2008. 1st ed. Brussels: ETUI-REHS Documentation Centre; 2008. p. 58-66

[5] Dimovski V, Žnidaršič J. Economic aspects of population ageing in Slovenia: How to mitigate the consequences with the approach of active ageing. Kakovostna starost. 2007;**10**: 2-15

[6] Heywood F, Oldman C, Means R. Housing and Home in Later Life. 1st ed. Buckingham Open University Press; 2002. 185 p

[7] Callahan J. Aging in place. Generations. 1992;**16**:5-6

[8] Rojo Perez F, Fernandez-Mayoralas Fernandez G, Pozo Rivera E, Manuel Rojo Abuin J. Ageing in place: Predictors of the residential satisfaction of elderly. Social Indicators Research 2001;**54**:173-208. DOI: 10.1023/A:1010852607362

[9] Sabia JJ. There's no place like home: A hazard model analysis of aging in place among older homeowners in the PSID. Research on Aging. 2008;**30**:3-35. DOI: 10.1177/0164027507307919

[10] Costa-Font J, Mascarilla-Miró O, Elvira D. Ageing in place? An examination of elderly people housing preferences in Spain. Urban Studies. 2009;**46**:295-316. DOI: 10.1177/0042098008099356

[11] Wilesa JL, Allena RES, Palmera AJ, Haymana KJ, Keelingb S, Kersea N. Older people and their social spaces: A study of well-being and attachment to place in Aotearoa New Zealand. Social Science & Medicine. 2009;**68**:664-671. DOI: 10.1016/j.socscimed.2008.11.030

[12] Fozard JL, Rietsema J, Bouma H, Graafmans JAM. Gerontechnology: Creating enabling environments for the challenges and opportunities of aging. Educational Gerontology. 2000;**26**:331-344

[13] Harrington T L, Harrington M K. Gerontechnology: Why and How. 1st ed. Maastricht: Shaker Publishing; 2000. 225 p

[14] Bouma H, Fozard JL, Bouwhuis DG, Taipale VT. Gerontechnology in perspective. Geron. 2007;**6**:190-216. DOI: 10.4017/gt.2007.06.04.003.00

[15] Demiris G, Hensel BK. Technologies for an aging society: A systematic review of "smart home" applications. IMIA Yearbook of Medical Informatics. 2008:33-40

[16] Rudel D, Premik M, Hojnik-Zupanc I, Kogovšek M, Ličer N. Caring network based on community social alarm centres in Slovenia. Informatica Medica Slovenica. 1993;(Suppl. 1): 227-234

[17] Cowan D, Turner-Smith A. The role of assistive technology in alternative models of care for older people. In: Tinker A, editor. Royal Commission on Long Term Care. 1st ed. London: King's College London; 1999. pp. 325-346

[18] Cavanaugh T. The need for assistive technology in educational technology. AACE Journal. 2002;**10**:27-31

[19] Edyburn DL. Rethinking assistive technology. Special Education Technology Practice. 2004;**5**:16-23

[20] Barlow J, Venables T. Will technological innovation create the true lifetime home? Housing Studies. 2004;**19**:795-810. DOI: 10.1080/0267303042000249215

[21] Heywood F. The health outcomes of housing adaptations. Disability & Society. 2004;**19**:129-143. DOI: 10.1080/0968759042000181767

[22] McCreadie C, Tinker A. The acceptability of assistive technology to older people. Ageing & Society. 2005;**25**:91-110. DOI: 10.1017/S0144686X0400248X

[23] Kaye HS, Yeager P, Reed M. Disparities in usage of assistive technology among people with disabilities. Assistive Technology. 2008;**20**:194-203. DOI: 10.1080/10400435.2008.10131946

[24] Barlow J, Bayer S, Curry R. Implementing complex innovations in fluid multi-stakeholder environments: Experiences of telecare. Technovation. 2006;**26**:396-406. DOI: 10.1016/j.technovation.2005.06.010

[25] Hojnik-Zupanc, I. Independence of the Elderly in the Social and Spatial Contexts. Ljubljana: Faculty of Social Sciences; 1999. 224 p

[26] Remagnino P, Shapio D. Artificial intelligence methods for ambient intelligence. Computational Intelligence. 2007;**23**:393-394. DOI: 10.1111/j.1467-8640.2007.00312.x

[27] Rodriguez MD, Favela J, Preciado A, Vizcaíno A. Agent-based ambient intelligence for healthcareAI Communications–Agents Applied in Health Care 2005;**18**:201-216

[28] Zupan A, Cugelj R, Hočevar F. IRIS home (Independent residing enabled by intelligent solutions). Rehabilitacija. 2007;**6**:101-104

[29] Emiliani P L, Stephanidis C. Universal access to ambient intelligence environments: Opportunities and challenges for people with disabilities, IBM System JournalSpecial issue on Accessibility. 2005;**44**:605-619

[30] Coughlin JF, D'Ambrosio LA, Reimer B. Older adult perceptions of smart home technologies: Implications for research, policy & market innovations in healthcare. In: Proceedings of the Annual International Conference of the IEEE Engineering in Medicine and Biology Society; Aug 23-26, 2007. Lyon. Lyon: IEEE; 2007. pp. 1810-1815. DOI: 10.1109/IEMBS.2007.4352665

[31] Imrie R, Hall P. Inclusive Design: Designing and Developing Accessible Environment. 1st ed. New York: Spon Press; 2001. 187 p. DOI: 10.4324/9780203362501

[32] European Institute for Design and Disability. The EIDD Stockholm Declaration 2004 [Internet]. 2004. Available from: http://dfaeurope.eu [Accessed: Aug 10, 2017]

[33] Mace R, Hardie G, Place J. Toward universal design. In: Preiser W, Vischer J, White E, Van Nostrand R, editors. Design Intervention. Toward a More Humane Architecture, 1st ed. New York: Routledge; 1991. p. 155-175

[34] Danford GS, Tauke B, editors. Universal Design New York. New York: Vanguard Direct; 2001. 145 p

[35] Erkiliç M. Conceptual challenges between universal design and disability in relation to the body, impairment, and the environment where does the issue of disability stand in the philosophy of UD? 2011;**28**:181-203. DOI: 10.4305/METU.JFA.2011.2.9

[36] Warsson S, Stahl A. Accessibility, usability and universal design positioning and definition of concepts describing person-environment relationships. Disability and Rehabilitation. 2003;**25**:57-66. DOI: 10.1080/dre.25.2.57.66

[37] Kervina D, Pustinšek M, Bešter J. Informacijske in komunikacijske tehnologije za e-vključenost. In: Hočevar F. editor. Praktični vidiki in možnosti e-vključenosti in

dostopnosti za invalide, starejše in za osebe z manjšimi možnostmi. Ljubljana: Slovenian Institute for Rehabilitaion; 2007. pp. 13-21

[38] Barlow J, Bayer S, Curry R. Flexible homes, flexible care, inflexible organisations? The role of telecare in supporting independence. Housing Studies. 2005;**20**:441-456. DOI: 10.1080/02673030500062467

[39] Rudel D. Je telecare tehnologija za pomoč na daljavo rešitev za krč države pri reševanju problema socialno zdravstvene pomoči starejšim v Sloveniji? In: Vaupotič M, editor. Evropska unija – priložnost tudi za starejše 1st ed. Ljubljana: Zveza za tehnično kulturo Slovenije. 2004. p. 23-24

[40] European Telecommunications Standards Institute. Human Factors (HF); Telecare Services; Issues and Reconmiendations for User Aspects. 1st ed. Cedex: European Telecommunications Standards Institute; 2005. 68 p

[41] Porteus J, Brownsell S. Using Telecare: Exploring Technologies for Independent Living for Older People. 1st ed. Kindlington: Anchor Trust; 2000. 67 p

[42] Miskelly FG. Assistive technology in elderly care. Age and Ageing. 2001;**30**:455-458. DOI: 10.1093/ageing/30.6.455

[43] Cimerman P, Borštnar T, Rudel D, Obrežan D. E-reminder for selfhealth care – Presentation of a solution. Informática Medica Slovenica. 2010;**15**:51-52

[44] Ocepek J, Zupan A. Dom IRIS – An innovation in rehabilitation medicine. Journal of the Metrology Institute of the Republic of Slovenia. 2008;**18**:12-17

[45] Kubitschke L, Cullen K. ICT & Ageing – European Study on Users, Markets and Technologies. 1st ed. Brussels: Directorate General for Information Society and Media; 2010. 223 p

[46] Barlow J, Hendy J. The challenges of adopting integrated mainstream telecare services: Lessons from the UK. Eurohealth. 2009;**15**:8-10

[47] Joint Improvement Team. An Assessment of the Development of Telecare in Scotland: 2006-2010. 1st ed. Edinburgh: Scottish Government; 2010. 38 p

[48] Rudel D. Information and communication technologies for telecare of a patient at home. Rehabilitacija. 2007;**6**:94-100

[49] Authority of the House of Lords. Ageing: Scientific Aspects. Vol. II. Evidence. London: The Stationery Office Limited; 2005. 133 p

[50] Young & Elderly Secure Group. Telecare Information [Internet]. 2017. Available at: http://yesgroup.eu/telecare-information-2 [Accessed: Aug 10, 2017]

[51] Jelenc J, editor. Strategic Development Plan of Technological Platform I-TECHMED: Innovative and Assistive Technology in Medicine 2007-2013. 1st ed. Podnart: Iskra Techno; 2007

[52] Edmondson A. Framing for learning: Lessons in successful technology implementation. California Management Review. 2003;**45**:34-54. DOI: 10.2307/41166164

[53] Goodwin N. The state of telehealth and telecare in the UK: Prospects for integrated care. Journal of Integrated Care. 2010;**18**:3-10. DOI: 10.5042/jic.2010.0646

[54] Norris A. Essentials of Telemedicine and Telecare. 1st ed. London: John Wiley & Sons; 2002. 188 p

[55] Hailey D, Crowe BA. rofile of success and failure in telehealth-evidence and opinion from the Success and Failures in Telehealth conferences. Journal of Telemedicine and Telecare. 2003;**9**:22-24. DOI: 10.1258/135763303322596165

[56] Weick K, Sutcliffe K. Hospitals as cultures of entrapment: A reanalysis of the Bristol Royal Infirmary. California Management Review. 2003;**45**:73-84. DOI: 10.2307/41166166

[57] Faife D. Reflections on developing an assistive technology/telecare service as a model for change management, creative thinking and workforce development. Housing, Care and Support. 2008;**11**:34-42. DOI: 10.1108/14608790200800033

[58] Barlow J, Bayer S, Curry R, Hendy J, McMahon L. From care closer to home to care in the home: The potential impact of telecare on the built environment. In: Kagioglou T, editor. Improving Healthcare Through the Built Environment. 1st ed. London: Wiley-Blackwell; 2010. pp. 131-138. DOI: 10.1002/9781444319675.ch9

[59] Brownsell S, Blackburn S, Aldred H, Porteus J. Implementing telecare: Practical experiences. Housing, Care and Support. 2006;**9**:6-12. DOI: 10.1108/14608790200600010

[60] Rogers E. Diffusion of Innovations. 5th ed. London: Free Press; 1962. 576 p

[61] Bayer S, Barlow J, Curry R. Assessing the impact of a care innovation: Telecare. System Dynamics Review. 2007;**23**:61-80. DOI: 10.1002/sdr.361

[62] Finch T, May C, Mair F, Mort M, Gask L. Integrating service development with evaluation in telehealthcare: An ethnographic study. British Medical Journal. 2003;**327**:1205-1209. DOI: 10.1136/bmj.327.7425.1205

[63] Saranummi N, Korhonen I, Kivisaari S, Ahjopal H ramework for developing distributed ICT applications for health, distributed diagnosis and home healthcare. In: Conference Proceedings – 1st Transdisciplinary Conference on Distributed Diagnosis and Home Healthcare 2006 – D2H2; Apr 2-4, 2006; Arlington. New York: IEEE; 2006. pp. 137143

[64] Shaw B. The role of the interaction between the user and the manufacturer in medical equipment innovation. R&D Management. 1985;**15**:283-292. DOI: 10.1111/j.1467-9310.1985.tb00039.x

[65] Wyatt S. ICT innovation in central government: Learning from the past. International Journal of Innovation Management. 2000;**4**:39-416. DOI: 10.1016/S1363-9196(00)00021-4

[66] von Hippel E. The Sources of Innovation. 1st ed. Oxford: Oxford University Press; 1988. 218 p

[67] Milligan C, Roberts C, Mort M. Telecare and older people: Who cares where? Social Science & Medicine. 2011;**72**:347-354. DOI: 10.1016/j.socscimed.2010.08.014

[68] Sixsmith A, Sixsmith J. Smart care technologies: Meeting whose needs? Journal of Telemedicine and Telecare. 2000;**6**:190-192. DOI: 10.1258/1357633001934636

[69] Levy S, Jack N, Bradley D, Morison M, Swanston M. Perspectives on telecare: The client view. Journal of Telemedicine and Telecare. 2003;**9**:156-160. DOI: 10.1258/135763303767149960

[70] Demiris G, Rantz M, Aud M, Marek K, Tyrer H. Older adults' attitudes towards and perceptions of 'smart home' technologies: A pilot study. Medical Informatics and the Internet in Medicine. 2004;**29**:87-94. DOI: 10.1080/14639230410001684387

[71] Percival J, Hanson J. Big brother or brave new world? Telecare and its implications for older people's independence and social inclusion. Critical Social Policy. 2006;**26**:888-909. DOI: 10.1177/0261018306068480

[72] Forlizzi J, Disalvo C, Gemperle F. Assistive robotics and ecology of elders living independently in their homes. Human-Computer Interaction. 2004;**19**:25-59. DOI: 10.1207/s15327051hci1901&2_3

[73] Hanson VL. Web access for elderly citizens. In: Proceedings of the 2001 EC/NSF Workshop on Universal Accessibility of Ubiquitous Computing: Providing for the Elderly, May 22-25, 2001; Alcácer do Sal. New York: ACM; 2001. pp. 1418. DOI: 10.1145/564526.564531

[74] Marquié JC, Jourdan-Boddaert L, Huet N. Do older adults underestimate their actual computer knowledge? Behaviour & Information Technology. 2002;**21**:273-280. DOI: 10.1080/01449290210000020998

[75] Richardson M, Weaver CK, Zorn TE. 'Getting on': Older New Zealanders' perceptions of computing. New Media & Society. 2005;**7**:219-245. DOI: 10.1177/1461444805050763

[76] Lee SY, Phippen A. The state of elderly in ICT adoption at rural areas. Advances in Network & Communication Engineering. 2006;**3**:241-249

[77] Richardson MA. Interruption events and sensemaking processes: A narrative analysis of older people's relationships with computers [thesis]. Waikato: University of Waikato; 2006

[78] Tetley J, Hanson E, Clarke A. Older people, telematics and care. In: Warren T, Warren L, Nolan M, editors. Care Services for Later Life: Transformations and Critiques. 1st ed. London: Jessica Kinglsey Publishers; 2001. pp. 243-258

[79] Wylde M, Valins MS. The impact of technology. In: Valins MS, Salter D, editors. Futurecare: New Directions in Planning Health and Care Environments. 1st ed. Oxford: John Wiley and Sons; 1996. pp. 5-24

[80] Sponselee A, Schouten B, Bouwhuis D, Willems C. Smart home technology for the elderly: Perceptions of multidisciplinary stakeholders. Communications in Computer and Information Science. 2008;**11**:314-326. DOI: 10.1007/978-3-540-85379-4_37

[81] Pečjak V. The Third Age Psychology. 1st ed. Ljubljana: Free Press; 1998. 201 p

[82] Czaja S, Charness N, Fisk A, Hertzog C, Nair S, Rogers W, Sharit J. Factors predicting the use of technology: Finding from the Center for research and education on aging and technology enhancement (CREATE). Psychology and Aging. 2006;**21**:333-352. DOI: 10.1037/0882-7974.21.2.333

[83] Cheverst K, Clarke K, Dewsbury G, Hemmings T, Hughes J, Rouncefield M. Design with care: Technology, disability and the home. In: Harper R, editor. Inside the Smart Home. 1st ed. London: Springer; 2003. pp. 163-179. DOI: 10.1007/1-85233-854-7_9

[84] Fisk M. Social Alarms to Telecare: Older people's Services in Transition. 1st ed. Bristol: Policy Press at the University of Bristol; 2003. 304 p. DOI: 10.2307/j.ctt1t8951n

[85] Kaplan D. Access to technology: Unique challenges for people with disabilities. American Society. 1997;**21**:24-27

[86] Glueckauf RL, Ketterson TU. Telehealth interventions for individuals with chronic illness: Research review and implications for practice. Professional Psychology: Research and Practice. 2004;**35**:615-627. DOI: 10.1037/0735-7028.35.6.615

[87] Bertera EM, Tran BQ, Wuertz EW, Bonner AA. Attitudes towards health technologies for telecare and their relationship to successful aging in a community-based older minority population. Forum on Public Policy: A Journal of the Oxford Round Table. 2007:1-22

[88] Hanson J, Percival J, Aldred H, Brownsell S, Hawley M. Attitudes to telecare among older people, professional care workers and informal carers: A preventative strategy or crisis management? Universal Access in the Information Society. 2007;**6**:193-205. DOI: 10.1007/s10209-007-0075-y

[89] Rahimpour M, Lovell NH, Celler BG, McCormick J. Patients' perceptions of a home telecare system. International Journal of Medical Informatics. 2008;**77**:486-497. DOI: 10.1089/15305620050503889

[90] Beale S, Truman P, Sanderson D, Kruger J. The initial evaluation of the Scottish telecare development program. Journal of Technology in Human Services. 2010;**28**:60-73. DOI: 10.1080/15228831003770767

[91] Reinhard CS, Given B, Petlick N H, Bemis A. Supporting family caregivers in providing care. In: Hughes RG, editor. Patient Safety and Quality. An Evidence-Based Handbook for Nurses. 1st ed. Rockville: Agency for Healthcare Research and Quality; 2008. pp. 341404

[92] European Commission. Seniorwatch 2: Assessment of the Senior Market for ICT Progress and Developments. 1st ed. Brussels: Information Society and Media Directorate General; 2008. 185 p

[93] Mandy D, Mitchell A E, O'Neill S. Attitudes of healthcare workers towards older people in a rural population: A survey using the Kogan Scale. Nursing Research and Practice. 2011;1-7. Article ID 352627. DOI: 10.1155/2011/352627

[94] The Nursing and Midwifery Board of Ireland. Working with Older People: Professional Guidance. 1st ed. Dublin: The Nursing and Midwifery Board of Ireland; 2009. 31 p

[95] Raappana A, Rauma M, Melkas H. Impact of safety alarm systems on care personnel. Gerontechnology. 2007;**6**:112-117. DOI: 10.4017/gt.2007.06.02.006.00

[96] Ministry of Labour, Family and Social Affairs. Strategy of Care for the Elderly Till 2010 – Solidarity, Living Together and Quality Ageing of the Population. 1st ed. Ljubljana: Government of the Republic of Slovenia; 2007. 50 p

# 7

# Caregiver Burden and Responsibilities for Nurses to Reduce Burnout

Birsel Canan Demirbağ, Çiğdem Gamze Özkan,
Betül Bayrak and Yeter Kurt

**Abstract**

The world has been aging, and technology has been advancing. Increasing population and chronic diseases indicate that importance of home care will continue. Many important chronic diseases in the world-such as chronic obstructive pulmonary disease (COPD), hemodialysis and heart failure-affect the daily life and quality of life of the individual negatively. The patient needs help and support from the caregiver in many ways, such as using medicines, maintaining health checks, and maintaining daily living activities. In particular, in the home care process of the disease, there are difficulties in the physical, social, emotional and economical areas for both individuals and caregivers. Through the role of educator, the nurse can help to share the burden of care with family members, to give equal responsibility for each individual in the family and to plan the care period.

**Keywords:** burnout, caregiver, common diseases, home care, nurse

## 1. Introduction

Home care services are included in general health and social services in many countries as well as in developed countries. These services refer to care activities that are provided to those in need by conventional caregivers such as family, friend or neighbors, by formal home caregivers and by volunteers. Depending on the structure of general health and social service systems of countries, these services may be given by governmental, private or voluntary institutions, and primary, secondary and tertiary health institutions can design organizations in order to provide home care services [1]. Home care services are more economic than institutional health care in the short term or are more acceptable care model on behalf of those in need of care and their significant others. However, in the case of prolonged care, home care may not produce the same benefits due to different difficulties on behalf of those who provide these services at home. It is necessary to construct legal and financial background to provide home care services as well as education programs to be given by health professionals to those who will receive the care and will give the care and material background so that home care services can be offered.

### 1.1. Some definitions for home care

**Scope of home care system:** Similar to general health system, home care system also targets home preventive care, home diagnostic care, home therapeutic care, home rehabilitative care, long-term home care and home hospice care.

**Home health care (HHC):** HHC, broadly defined, refers to all the services and products provided to clients in their homes to maintain, restore, or promote their physical, mental and emotional health.

**Purpose of home health care:** The aim is to maximize clients' level of independence and minimize the outcomes of existing disabilities via non-institutionalization services. Its primary objective is to use these supportive services to reduce hospitalization and prevent or delay institutionalization.

**Home health nursing (HHN):** HHN is an expert area of nursing practice roots of which have firmly been placed in community health nursing [2].

**Types of home care personnel:** Home care providers are generally characterized as either informal or formal caregiver. Informal caregivers are family members and friends who give care in the home and are unpaid. Formal caregivers are professionals and para-professionals who are compensated for the homecare they provide.

**Caregiver burden:** Caregiver burden has been explained as a multidimensional response to the negative appraisal and perceived stress resulting from caring sick individuals. Caregiver burden threatens the physical, psychological, emotional and functional health of caregivers [3–6].

**Difficulties about heath care for family caregivers:** Family caregivers encounter numerous problems and at present families are mostly alone with their own coping strategies. Psychosocial problems are widespread among the caregivers. Knowledge deficits are observed correlated with physical care, diet, medications, the disease, exercise, function of the system. Additionally, caregivers suffer from fatigue and sleep disorders. They experience problems in affording medications and in taking the patients to check up. Some caregivers have financial problems so they prefer to hospitalize their patients in a government facility.

**Perceived social support in caregivers:** All interpersonal relations—which influence individuals' lives and provide emotional, physical and cognitive assistance to them whenever needed—are defined as "Social Support Systems" that support the state of health [7]. It has been stated that social support, which is conceptualized as the support given to any person in a troublesome or burdensome situation by family members, relatives as well as resources exerted by social connections, helps promote physical health and feeling oneself good [8].

There are some studies reporting that caregivers who get social support feel less care burden and that there exists a negative relation between the increase in social support and intensity of care burden [9, 10]. It has also been reported that social support level perceived by caregivers is among the primary factors affecting the health state of caregivers. For health professionals, it is highly important to protect the health state of caregivers providing service to long-term patients in particular and to save them from the negative effects of the treatment process.

### 1.2. Positive and negative aspects of home care

Home care has spread widely in the world, but it is known that there are negative and positive aspects of this care.

#### *1.2.1. Positive aspects of home care*

- The patient still continues to be a part of family life, and thus, family integrity is maintained.
- The patient keeps his/her comfort in a place to which he/she is accustomed.
- The patient can maintain previous activities and relations.
- Social isolation is prevented.
- Disease control can be enhanced because the patient feels independent.
- Quality of life of patients increases; recovery accelerates.
- The patient is protected against hospital infections.
- Cost of home care is relatively lower than the cost of hospital care and other institutions.
- Stress experienced by caregivers is reduced and their satisfaction increases because they are able to arrange and to plan health services.

#### *1.2.2. Negative aspects of home care*

- The patient may feel that his/her private life is intervened.
- The patient may be disturbed by too many family members, visiting relatives at home and interventions of medical devices depending on his/her condition.
- The patient in need of care may feel that his/her condition is more serious than he/she thought.
- Increasing economic, emotional and physical pressure may be exerted on family during caregiving procedure.
- Knowledge and skill deficit of home care providers in terms of medical tools and devices may lead to problems.
- Lack of professionals who can instantly intervene in an emergent case may be considered as a disadvantage of home care [11–13].

### 1.3. Home care team

Because home care is a team work, it necessitates interdisciplinary collaboration. This collaboration starts when the patient is at the hospital. Patient who is considered to need home care, physician who plans hospital discharge, physician who carries out observation of home care and caregiver who carries out home care should act together. The patient is discharged from home care in line with instructions (i.e. home care settings may be institutions or patients' own houses in some countries.). The physician in charge of home care team takes all responsibilities legally. Responsible caregiver must always be in contact with home care physician even if the patient receives these services through family members. Realization of home care depends on the willingness of the patient to receive these services and consent of his/her significant others to answer patient's needs. Basically, tasks expected to be realized by care providers are as follows:

1. To provide emotional support to patient
2. Make observation of patient
3. To provide physical support to patient
4. To help patient maintain housework
5. To participate in treatment plan
6. To seek assistance

To realize these functions, it is necessary for caregivers to receive education and training about these issues, which will enhance patient satisfaction and reduces care burden of caregivers.

***Importance of home care givers***: A basic component of home care is caregivers. In cases where care is necessary and if there are not any caregivers at home, it is impossible to continue home care. In economically underdeveloped or backward countries, the only care source for those who are functionally dependent on others is composed of care providers arranged with patients' significant others (husbands, wives, children, relatives or friends). Additionally, it is known that those who undertake caregiving responsibilities do not have enough education and training. These people receive education and training from the doctors or nurses about what to do at home for patient and emergency aid institutions in case of emergent situations. Besides, caregivers undergo personal, economic and social problems due to deficiency of healthcare system. The studies done identified that most of the care providers are female in the developed countries such as the USA, the UK, Canada and other countries [14].

The world has been aging, and technology has been advancing. Increasing population and chronic diseases indicate that importance of home care will continue. It should be considered as a necessity that from each family, those who are voluntary, are trained and are able to improve skills should be trained about caregiving. From each family, those who are voluntary and can improve knowledge and skills should be selected for caregiving. It should be considered as a necessity to provide these caregivers with education and training about caregiving. Besides, through programs designed for caregivers, care burden of those who want the responsibility of care will be lightened. When these interventions are developed with social actions and government supports, economic burden will go down and satisfaction of care providers will go up.

## 2. Home care of patients with COPD and caregivers

### 2.1. Introduction

Chronic obstructive pulmonary disease (COPD), a widespread preventable and treatable disease, is characterized by persistent airflow limitation that is usually progressive and associated with an enhanced chronic inflammatory answer in the airways and the lung to noxious particles or gases. Exacerbations and comorbidities contribute to the overall severity in individual patients [15].

According to World Health Organization (WHO) estimations, COPD, ranking fifth among the most common death causes today, will be in the third place in 2030, whereas according to DALY (Disability Adjusted Life Year) incidence/prevalence, it is estimated that COPD will rank seventh in 2030 [16, 17].

The characteristic symptoms of COPD are chronic and progressive dyspnea, cough, and sputum production that can be variable from day to day.

*Dyspnea*: Progressive, persistent and characteristically worse with exercise.

*Chronic cough:* May be intermittent and may be unproductive.

*Chronic sputum production*: COPD patients commonly cough up sputum [15].

Patients suffer from a cough, sputum/mucus, dyspnea as well as hemoptysis, chest pain, anorexia, lack of appetite and weight loss [18–20].

COPD patients undergo serious limitation/incompetence in physical and social functions, dependence, loss of productivity, social isolation and—therefore—need assistance and support of caregivers in many areas such as leading daily life, using medications, and attending medical checks. The disease socially isolates families from the society and deteriorates friendships and neighborhood relations. Those who provide care in the post-disease period experience physical, emotional, economic and professional difficulties. These difficulties turn the social life of families/care provider's upside-down. It is highly critical to give professional support by identifying these difficulties so that anxiety of caregivers can be decreased.

### 2.2. The importance of caregivers in COPD patients

Patients with COPD undergo limitedness/incompetencies, dependency, loss of productivity and social isolation and therefore are in need of help and support from a caregiver in many aspects such as continuing daily life, using medications, and maintaining health checks [21, 22]. Caregivers involved in answering these requirements are responsible for many aspects such as determining the needs of the patient, monitoring disease symptoms and maintaining treatment, preventing unexpected medical problems, repetitive hospital admissions and maintaining contact with healthcare providers [23–25].

### 2.2.1. *Difficulties of home care providers in COPD patients*

Since ambulatory treatment and home care have been accepted for today's health system, care burden of primary care providers who give care to patients with chronic diseases has been intensified. Family-based long-term care is an expensive process for caregivers, changing responsibilities and roles [26, 27]. Since many of the caregivers have to maintain their professional and social roles, the responsibilities of the patient along with care are expanding [28, 29]. Changes occur in intrafamilial roles and lifestyles and quality of life of caregivers worsens due to fear to lose patient, economical difficulties, poor sources and inadequate services, inability to answer basic needs satisfactorily and modified recreational and professional activities, all of which leads to burnout [23, 25, 29–31].

Quality of life of caregivers is physically, psychologically, socially and economically affected negatively and caregivers have difficulties in these areas. *Physical difficulties* may produce such negative outcomes as nutrition and digestion disorders, headache, muscle pain, increase or decrease in body weight, sleep disorders, concentration difficulty, wearing careless clothes and caregivers start to spare less time for self-care [32–34]. *Emotional difficulties* are uneasiness, sleeplessness, a decrease in self-esteem, social isolation, depression, sarcastic behaviors, increase in alcohol consumption and medication use and difficulty with problem-solving [35]. Time for ease and relaxation, leisure and free time activities of primary caregivers are restricted due to social difficulties, and they sacrifice from friendships or social activities, which—in turn—reduces social support, causes loneliness feeling in caregiving role and increases the risk for social isolation [33]. *Economic and profession-related difficulties* cause individuals to arrange their jobs in line with caregiving roles, and therefore, they generally have more difficulties and may give up advantages and benefits of work life and retirement, personal satisfaction and financial profits [33, 34].

In literature; it was identified that care providers of COPD patients begin caregiving without preparing for caregiving role, and—as a result—taking care responsibility affects the life of half of the caregivers negatively. Besides, observing new symptoms or taking new responsibilities and patients' loss of ability to care himself/herself create the biggest stress for caregivers [24, 36, 37].

It is very important to detect difficulties of caregivers in reducing pressure and anxiety related to their caregiving role [33, 38, 39]. In order to reduce difficulties of care providers of COPD patients, giving the necessary professional support, sharing caregiving burden with family members, assigning equal responsibility to each family member and detecting social support mechanisms will help them realize caregiving roles and enhance their quality of life [40–42].

## 2.3. Nursing care in COPD patients and training of caregiver

Disease course limits patient's activities and leads to incapacity. It is necessary to meet physiological needs of individuals so that they can continue their lives. As long as these needs are not met, it is difficult for them to live in a healthy way. The basic objective of home care is to help a patient maximize independent functions and to increase his/her quality of life.

Nurses play a critical role in controlling symptoms—dyspnea in the first place—and in implementing both pharmacological and non-pharmacological treatment modalities during treatment process [43]. As a part of the nursing care at hospital and home of COPD patients, such general and patient-specific nursing interventions as—quitting smoking, disease course, nutritional habits, maintaining activities, infection signs and symptoms, preventing environmental and professional problems, teaching medication principals and effective inhalation methods, preventing and detecting exacerbations early, oxygen treatment, strategies to decrease dyspnea feeling, opening respiratory way and increasing gas change, learning daily respiratory exercises and bronchial hygiene techniques, reducing activity intolerance and anxiety, preventing feeding which is less than the amount body needs, providing sleep routine, realizing routine medical checks, realizing hygienic home environment and clear air circulation, keeping body weight at a proper level, assessing free time and travel-related, psychological, social and behavioral interventions and causes of attending health institutions—are planned and implemented [44–48].

COPD affects not only patient but also his/her family and friends, too. Therefore, that patient can take responsibility in his/her life, his/her personal care ability can be increased and they can possess a more productive, satisfactory, happier and more quality life is possible only with an effective home care program that will provide patient and his/her care provider with specific knowledge and skills. Caregiving is a multi-dimensionally perceived experience on behalf of caregiving individuals. As a part of the trainer role, the nurse can increase the success of treatment by determining learning potential of care provider and improving the quality of care of patient through the training and education she will give. During the education and training planned for caregiver—particularly when disease and symptom management begins—such topics as quitting smoking, oxygen use, treatment, energy preventive techniques, sexuality, sleep, feeding, respiration exercises, coping with anxiety/depression and end-of-life care should be emphasized [15, 48, 49].

*Respiration exercises:* Care provider should encourage patient to cough through pursed-lip and diaphragmatic respiration exercises. Thus, secretion clearance becomes easy, and respiration difficulty of the patient may be lessened.

*Exercises*: Aerobic and strength exercise done by COPD patient reduce the energy needed for many activities by elevating exercise tolerance. Caregiver and the patient should determine duration, frequency, mode and intense of exercises considering data of the initial tests and severity of the disease.

*Feeding:* Headache manifested in the mornings and abnormally elevated carbon dioxide in the blood (hypercapnia) may affect COPD patients negatively in terms of preparing foods and feeding (malnutrition). However, such conditions as increased energy need for respiration, $CO_2$ retention and respiration inflammation augment energy need of patient [50]. Therefore, it is necessary to raise awareness of caregiver about preparing a proper diet for COPD patient and to maintain the diet. A dietary program designed with the help of a dietician and by taking patient expectations into consideration should be employed and feeding support should be provided.

*Sleep:* COPD patients are more hypoxemic than daytime relaxation and under risk for sleep apnea-hypoapnea syndrome. Therefore, patients should be watched by caregivers during sleep periods, and caregivers should be trained about ventilator devices.

*Psychological, social and behavioral interventions:* Anxiety and depression often accompany with COPD. Caregivers should motivate patients about psycho-social and behavioral therapies, training and stress management, progressive muscle relaxation techniques and panic control [51].

*Sexuality*: Sexuality is an issue that should be discussed because it leads to anxiety, embarrassment and fear feelings. Since caregivers are generally spouses, this issue should be discussed with spouses. Those special topics such as taking bronchodilators before sexual activity and using energy saving positions should be explained to individuals [49].

*End-of-life care:* Family and patients should receive support so that they can cope with this process positively. In decision-making process of end-of-life period, everything should clearly and explicitly be determined by paying the due respect to decisions of patients and family [49]. Caregivers should be informed of end-of-life care of the patient. Resources of palliative and hospice care centers should be explained and individuals should be directed taking decisions of family into consideration.

## 3. Home care of hemodialysis patients and caregivers

### 3.1. Introduction

With the technological advancements today, lifespan has increased, which results in an increase in the incidence of chronic diseases [52, 53]. Chronic diseases require long-term treatment and care, cause permanent changes that limit activities of daily life, and produce socio-economic problems for patients, families, and economy of the countries [54, 55]. Chronic renal failure (CRF), one of the significant chronic diseases in the world, may create deficits in the daily life of individuals and affect the quality of life of individuals negatively, aggravate impairment in renal functions and progress into end-stage renal disease [55, 56]. According to the statistics of 2004, it was reported that there were 1,783,000 CRF patients over the world, and CRF and end-stage renal failure (ESRF) prevalence were 1505 per 1,000,000 in North America, 2045 in Japan, 585 in Europa, 70 in Asia (Japan not included), 70 in Africa, 380 in Latin America and 180 in the Middle East [57]. According to findings of Turkish Society of Nephrology (TND) 2011, it is reported that end-stage renal failure (ESRF) prevalence is 809 per 1,000,000 and 60,443 patients that receive renal replacement therapy are ESRF patients [58]. In chronic renal failure, patients are treated with peritoneum dialysis or hemodialysis methods until they receive renal transplantation [59]. Both in Turkiye and Europe, hemodialysis is known to be the widest renal replacement therapy [60]. Besides, according to 2011 data, 49,404 patients received hemodialysis treatment in Turkiye, and the number of these patients was higher as compared to those receiving peritoneum dialysis [58].

### 3.2. What is hemodialysis?

Hemodialysis—one of the life-saving treatment methods in renal failure—is defined as the process in which a suitable vascular route of entry named fistula, graft or catheter is used, patient's blood is cleared from waste products through a semi-permeable membrane that is called dialyzer that functions like an artificial kidney and returns blood again to patient by providing suitable fluid-electrolyte replacement [59, 61, 62].

According to Turkish Language Association (TLA), hemodialysis refers to "clearance of circulating blood from waste agents through pumping it into a machine named dialyzer when kidneys do not function" and "a treatment method used to clear blood and to remove toxic agents by filtrating them in a permeable membrane" [63]. Hemodialysis treatment is the process in which metabolic waste products are removed from the body with the help of dialyzer by using diffusion, osmosis and ultrafiltration methods of dialysis solution and regulating fluid-electrolyte balance [60, 64]. Hemodialysis patients are taken to dialysis therapy given at hemodialysis unit by healthcare team on certain days, at certain hours of the week organized by doctors in a certain manner depending on their general conditions [65, 66]. Hemodialysis therapy—determined according to patients' existing renal function and protein amount in their diets—is generally given 2–3 times a week in 4–6 h [55, 67]. The basic objective of hemodialysis therapy is to relieve patients' uremic symptoms, to establish body homeostasis and therefore to protect their quality of life and to decrease mortality and morbidity [53, 67].

### 3.3. The importance of caregivers in hemodialysis patients

Chronic renal failure patients come to a turning point in their lives with hemodialysis therapy. In the beginning, patients and their families have difficulty accepting and thus adapting into the disease and this treatment modality, and therefore, they react [68]. Reactions demonstrated by patients against the disease, and hemodialysis therapy and their adaptation process vary depending on so many factors such as age, sex, educational level, residential place, religious life, family structure [69]. Patients in adolescence period resist against dialysis and dietary dependence more, while adult patients do not experience so many difficulties in terms of adaptation thanks to family support [70]. Patients, who are challenged by the inability to do activities of daily living, become more dependent on others and have more difficulties [71]. Toward last phases of adaptation into the disease and treatment process, patients perceive that they are saved from death by hemodialysis, and hemodialysis has changed their lifestyles and are now in need of various alternatives that will enhance their quality of life [64]. Besides, since they alleviate disease symptoms, add meaning and energy into life, doctors, nurses and other healthcare personnel and significant others of patients should show an optimistic attitude toward patients and give hope them [72]. Not only healthcare professionals but also care providers should demonstrate a sincere, reliable, supportive attitude toward patients in the struggle against the disease and adaptation into new lifestyles created by hemodialysis therapy.

Home care providers are defined as formal caregivers (professionals who are compensated for the homecare they provide) or informal caregivers in charge of supporting patients physically, socially, economically, emotionally by functioning as a bridge between medical treatment and psycho-social curing process [66, 73, 74]. People who provide assistance to the unable individuals who cannot self-care due to a disease, disability or elderliness or who regulate this assistance are called care-providers [75]. Those who stay with patients during all processes—from diagnosis process, treatment process to home care process—owing to limitedness caused by CRF therapy, support and help them and are mainly composed of family members are called "Primary caregivers" [53].

During hemodialysis therapy, one family member who acts like patient's dialysis partner is accepted as a primary caregiver [76]. When a family member suffers from a serious disease such as renal failure and dialysis therapy, the homeostatic balance of the family is broken, emotional energy reduces, and changes in intrafamilial roles and tasks occur [77]. Therefore, the disease may seriously impair quality of life of both sick individuals and their caregivers [78, 79].

Due to numerous physical and psycho-social problems caused by hemodialysis therapy among patients such as fluid-dietary restriction, medication intake, loss of work, functional disorders, change in body image, their healthy life cycle is broken [66, 80]. Individuals whose normal life cycle is broken owing to hemodialysis therapy, renal failure disease and the other factors affecting the disease (other chronic diseases) undergo various physical, psychological and social problems and become partially or fully dependent [81]. To these people, who become dependent, care services are provided by professional nurses at hemodialysis unit, while care responsibility out of dialysis units is taken by those being in the social environment and domestic places of the patients [55]. Caregivers who are in charge of the primary care of hemodialysis patients should mutually be in contact with healthcare team when they provide these services.

### 3.3.1. *Difficulties of home care residents in hemodialysis patients*

Caregiving, caregiving difficulty and care burden are significant problems for the families with chronic and progressive patients. Care burden is considered as emotional and financial difficulties encountered during care process [9, 33, 82]. While giving care to those with a chronic disease or disability, a family member or a significant other may experience difficulties, get nervous and undertake too heavy care burden to tolerate; which creates care burden and difficulties [83, 84].

On the one hand, the transition to hemodialysis during a chronic disease affects patients' quality of life and depression level negatively, and on the other hand, primary caregivers that take home care burden are negatively affected and undergo some problems [80, 85]. Primary caregivers may face various problems and experience difficulties at a different level [86, 87]. According to the studies in literature, it is identified that care providers who care patients during treatment process undergo such problems as anxiety, depression, fatigue, social isolation, deteriorated family relations and financial problems [86, 88, 89]. Caregivers have difficulty coping with helping patients do activities of daily living depending on patients' dependency level, routine transfer of patients to the dialysis unit, symptoms, medications, diet, body image changes, depression, social and economical problems [80, 90]. It is emphasized that in addition to these difficulties, caregivers undergo troubles in fulfilling their tasks and responsibilities owing to excessive medication use caused by depression, fatigue and other health problems, negative perception of physical health, gradual deterioration in their health status and quality of life [91]. Continually being engaged with their patient's care, changed life routines, fatigue, weariness, burnout, unhappiness, development of their own health problems, negligence of their own care and social relations contribute to impairment of their quality of life [55, 92].

Health professionals who are aware of these difficulties patients and their care providers may have help caregivers to adapt into changed domestic, family and social roles and lifestyles, to improve coping skills and thus contribute to quality of care given by those in charge of home care, which will result in a holistic care [74, 93].

### 3.4. Nursing care in hemodialysis patients and training of caregiver

Individuals can cope with diseases and changes in their life, keep up with changes caused by the diseases and live happily with hemodialysis as long as they are able to adapt themselves into these outcomes. It is healthcare professionals that will first help individuals who receive hemodialysis therapy as a result of chronic renal failure to adapt into modified lifestyles caused by the disease, to cope with existing or possible problems. Since it is nurses that spend the most time and interact with hemodialysis patients in the healthcare team, with the training and education, they support patients so that they can adapt into their new life [62]. During this process, patient and his/her family undergo, nursing care to be provided as training, implementation and research in relation to nursing model and theories are very important [94]. Nurses—developing a close communication with patients, answering their needs instantly and intervening them—take significant tasks and responsibilities [95, 96].

The objective of the nurses, who provide treatment and care services to hemodialysis patients in an interpersonal manner, is to provide individual, family, and society with health promoting, disease preventing experiences and help sick people and their caregivers to increase their own potentials [97]. To this end, nurses are supposed to provide patients' significant others who are together with the patient during hemodialysis process with training programs about hemodialysis and troubles created by it. Through patient-family group meetings, self-support groups and training programs, details about the disease should be explained to patients and their caregivers and considering life conditions in which patients and their caregivers are, a positive rehabilitation program should be initiated; thus, patients and their caregivers are prevented from having depression, their quality of life can be enhanced, and they can see future more positively and hopefully [53, 92]. Rehabilitation plays a crucial role in enabling hemodialysis patients and their families to overcome concurrent problems and other problems. This rehabilitation should include such issues as protection and promotion of general health, self-care education, physical therapy, feeding education, medication training, transport, domestic arrangements, job rehabilitation, sexual rehabilitation, talk-rehabilitation [98].

That hemodialysis patients and their caregivers are able to manage home treatment and care activities during their education and training is an important component in terms of continuity of care. If medications are delivered to patients' home or are given to patients by hand, it should be assured that caregivers in charge of home care should keep these medications properly and administer the correct medications to patients at the correct time and doses. In the training of patients and their caregivers, implementation phases of such care practices as feeding, excretion, hygiene, fistula or catheter care should be explained with visual materials and they should practice under the supervision of a health professional [99].

## 4. Home care of patients with heart failure and caregivers

### 4.1. Introduction

Heart failure is a clinical and life-threatening syndrome in which sufficient amount of blood that meets metabolic needs of the body is not pumped due to a structural or functional disorder of the heart and basic complaints of which are shortness of breath and fatigue [100, 101]. Because heart failure requires a long care process and treatment since its diagnosis phase, it affects patients as well as their families physically, psychologically, socially, economically and morally [102]. Public care is substituted with home care in developed countries. In home care; all aspects such as physical, emotional, social, economic and environmental factors are discussed. Home care burden is taken on by those who provide patients with care and answer their needs; therefore, they are named as a caregiver/care provider. The role of caregiver is to meet patients' physical, emotional, cultural and social needs and to maintain the health service relation with healthcare organization and healthcare professionals [103–105].

### 4.2. What is heart failure (HF)?

#### *4.2.1. Definition of heart failure*

HY is a clinical syndrome characterized by typical symptoms (shortness of breath, ankle swelling, and fatigue) accompanied by such signs as elevated jugular venous pressure, pulmonary and peripheric edema by causing structural and/or functional cardiac anomaly [101].

#### *4.2.2. Prevalence of heart failure*

Heart failure is a major public health problem that has now reached epidemic proportions in the United States and many other countries [106]. Recent estimates indicate that heart failure affects nearly 5 million Americans or approximately 1.9% of the general population and that more than 400,000 new cases are diagnosed each year [107, 108]. Heart failure (HF) afflicts nearly 6 million Americans and more than 1 million annual hospital discharges [109]. By 2030, an estimated 25% increase in HF prevalence will result in an additional 3 million affected individuals [109, 110]. Heart failure accounts for nearly 1 million hospitalizations annually, and it is the leading cause of hospital admission in individuals older than 65 years of age [107, 111]. Heart failure is also a leading cause of death in the United States, listed as the primary cause in 43,000 deaths each year and as a contributory cause in another 220,000 cases [107, 108].

#### *4.2.3. Symptoms of heart failure*

Clinically, HF results from structural or functional disorders in heart and patients typically experience such physical and emotional disturbances as dyspnea (shortness of breath–air hunger), fatigue, edema, sleep disorders, depression and chest pain. Among other physical symptoms, night coughing, wheezing, feeling of swelling, loss of appetite, confusion (particularly among elders), tachycardia, dizziness, and syncope are important [101].

#### *4.2.4. Symptoms that patients manifest because of heart failure and descriptive characteristics of these symptoms*

*Dyspnea:* Dyspnea is a syndrome with choking sensation leading to fear of death among patients. The presences of such accompanying diseases as edema in lungs, lung infections, pleural effusion, pulmonary embolism, neoplasm and chronic obstructive pulmonary disease may lead to dyspnea [112].

*Fatigue:* Failure and low exercise tolerance in heart failure are generally caused by reduced cardiac output. Anemia, use of diuretics and depression, may also lead to or elevate fatigue [113].

*Edema:* Accumulation of fluid spreads in HF and periphericedema is evident in feet, legs, and abdomen (hepatomegalia, pulmonary crepitation, pleural effusion, and acid). In particular, in patients who sit for a long time, bilateral edema develops in feet [101].

*Sleep disorders:* Patients with symptomatic HF may largely suffer from sleep-related respiratory disorders (central or obstructive sleep apnea) [101].

*Depression:* Patients with heart failure often suffer from depression and depression influences heart failure morbidity and mortality seriously [112]. Depression reduces patients' adaptation and may lead to social loneliness, and therefore, it should be included in HF management as a part of self-care and of care provided by family/caregivers [101].

*Pain:* Pain affects 80% of end-stage heart failure patients. In last days, patients complain about as much pain as cancer patients. Pain in heart failure may be associated with ischemia, diabetic neuropathy or osteoarthritis [114].

#### *4.2.5. Treatment process of heart failure*

Heart failure requires life-long treatment, leads to frequent hospitalization by causing high cost in economies of countries due to complicated and expensive treatments with technologically advanced medical devices. In chronic heart failure, the basic objective of the treatment includes interventions that decrease mortality and re-hospitalization, correct symptoms and signs, increase functional capacity and improve the quality of life [111, 115]. For most of the patients—especially for the elders— leading an independent life, not experiencing disturbing symptoms and not having hospitalization may mean the wish to maximize lifespan. Preventing heart failure and repressing its progress constitute the main two objectives [116]. In the ESC guidelines of heart failure diagnosis and treatment, three concepts are discussed in classifying heart failure: these are new onset heart failure (heart failure developing for the first time, acute or slow onset), transitory heart failure (heart failure with recurrent course or course with attacks), chronic heart failure (heart failure persistent, stabile, severe or decompensed heart failure) [116]. In acute periods, patients' clinical status and symptoms are assessed and hemodynamic status is balanced. In subacute period; cardiac function is evaluated, a suitable chronic pharmacologic treatment is commenced, and patients' treatment strategy is optimized. In the chronic period, patients' symptoms, their adaptation into treatment and prognosis are evaluated, and pharmacological treatment and use of medical devices are optimized. In the end-stage period, patients' worries and symptoms are found. It is recommended that patients' symptomatic treatment and long-term care should be planned, and their families should be supported [116].

### 4.3. Lifestyle changes recommended for home care given to those with heart failure

A successful management of HF often necessitates adaptation into lifestyle changes on behalf of both patients and their families. Main lifestyle changes projected for home care of those with heart failure are symptom control, daily weight monitoring, activity program, quitting smoking and alcohol, low salt diet and adaptation into treatment [117].

*Symptom control*: It is highly critical that the most commonly seen symptoms of heart failure patients should be controlled, patients and their care providers should recognize the symptoms of which they should see physicians and should know what to do for the symptoms. For pain, dyspnea, and fatigue, recommendations to be considered in symptom control are as follows [101].

*Pain:* In heart failure, pain may be associated with ischemia, diabetic neuropathy or osteoarthritis. In pain management, methods used in other chronic pains are used. Analgesics, sedatives, nitrates and opioids are some of the drugs used [114].

*Dyspnea*: In the respiratory management of the patients, the objective is to reduce dyspnea through oxygen treatments, pharmacological treatments, and non-pharmacological interventions. The position in which the patients feel comfortable for respiration is taken. Controlled respiration and relaxation techniques are among the helpful techniques to decrease dyspnea [113, 114].

*Fatigue*: Planning diuretics hours and sleep history are important factors in fatigue management. For example, making patients sleep by lifting their feet slightly so that they can sleep better, giving oxygen treatment as a support to periodic respiration, administering opiates of small doses before bedtime, nocturnal non-invasive ventilation if there is sleep apnea are among useful techniques [112].

*Daily weight monitoring*: Since sudden weight gain may be correlated with edema, it is crucial to watch patients' weight at home. Daily fluid intake restriction of 1.5–2 lt. may be considered in HF patients in order to reduce excessive fluid intake, signs and congestion. The hypotonic fluid restriction may correct hyponatremia. Fluid restriction proportional to weight (30 ml/kg; if > 85 kg 35 ml/kg) may produce less thirst [101].

*Activity program*: It is necessary to get rid of worries about physical activity, to relax and to understand benefits of exercises [101]. Regular exercise that consists of a 30-minute exercise program 5 days a week by increasing duration gradually is recommended. Patients with heart failure can be advised moderate continuous aerobic exercises (brisk walking, cycling slight running). Exercises that are adjusted to 3–5 grades of Borg scale, raise heart rate by 65–85% and produce an oxygen consumption of 50–75% can be considered [118].

*Smoking and drugs*: An expert opinion should be asked for to quit smoking and illegal drugs. For those patients who are unable to stop these dangerous habits, a coordination with relevant healthcare disciplines (seeking for mental, behavioral, psychological assistance and supports) should be sought for [101].

*Use of low-salt diets*: If recommended by a physician, sodium restriction includes a daily salt consumption of 5–6 g (a teaspoon of 2300 mg sodium). For those with severe HF symptoms, the salt restriction should be lower than 2 g sodium [118]. To the patients and caregivers, it is explained that salt causes accumulation of fluid in the body and if saltless foods are consumed edema in lungs and body will decrease and extra salt should not be added to food while cooking or eating. Also, it may be recommended to take salt away from dining tables and to use spices to flavor foods. Fresh fish, chicken, fatless beef, legumes should be consumed. Instead of canned and take-home foods, home-made foods should be preferred and directions on take-home foods should always be observed [117].

*Adaptation into treatment*: It should be clarified how to take medicines, what side effects medicines produce and which signs require medical help [101]. In particular, it is highly important to understand indications, doses and prescriptions of medicines, to notice common side effects of each prescribed medicine, to watch blood pressure in hypertension, to follow a strict glucose control in diabetes, to learn treatment options if suitable, to understand importance to observe treatment recommendations and to continue determination to implement treatment plan [118].

*Sexuality:* It is explained that a normal sexual life can be continued with a proposed diet, medicine treatment, and regular check-ups. After consuming heavy meals, when patients suffer from any bodily fatigue, are nervous, stay in extreme hot or cold weather conditions, and are drunk, it is advisable not to have a sexual relation. During sexual intercourse, if patients feel pain in the chest, back, arm, feel bad, shortness of breath, dizziness, excessive tachycardia, the sexual relation should be stopped and patients should rest. If these complaints go on, seek medical assistance [119].

*Conditions for which patients/care providers should consult the doctor are:*

- Sudden weight gain (2 kga day or 5 kg a week)
- Increasing dyspnea
- Elevated swelling in foot, legs and abdomen
- Need for more pillows while sleeping
- Waking up due to difficulty breathing
- Newly occurring or worsening dizziness
- Increasing heart beat or irregular heart beat
- Any problem with heart failure medicines (Interview)

*Conditions for which patients/care providers should call Emergency Aid Center and seek help are:*

- Increase in the severity of difficulty breathing
- Pink foamy mucus/sputum when coughing
- The pressure in the chest and/or feeling of pressure, pain not relieved by sublingual pills [119]

### 4.4. Nursing care in heart failure and role of home caregivers

Nursing care to be used in heart failure should be planned in a way to cover the patients and their families and is realized through patients' direct participation in their care. In order to enhance the quality of life of the patients, education and training programs including patients and their families should be designed, and they should regularly be watched. Nurses in charge of heart failure care management should improve and assess self-care skills by providing a detailed and comprehensive patient and family education in order to maintain physical stability, to avoid of acts that will aggravate the condition and to detect symptoms that indicate aggravation of the condition at an early period [118]. In particular, the target should be to correct lifestyles of HF patients and their families, diet and activity-related changes, to achieve regular drug intake and to realize symptom control, to quit smoking and alcohol consumption and to monitor weight on daily basis [116].

Self-care contribution of patients and contribution of caregivers are really of high importance. As a health care and disease management process, basic components of self-care—defined as the ability to promote health—are care, monitoring, and management. Care includes those behaviors demonstrated to improve health through reducing risk factors and adapting into advice (e.g., follow dietary restrictions, take medicines prescribed, and do exercises regularly). Monitoring refers to the observance of heart failure symptoms routinely/being careful (e.g., daily pains, edema control) and recognition of changes when they occur. Management includes assessment of changes in symptoms and determining necessary interventions (e.g., call a healthcare personnel) and assessment of the efficacy of actions [120].

Self-care in heart failure generally refers to necessary behaviors that will protect health, maintain or improve lifestyle changes and manage symptoms and outcomes created by living with heart failure. Care providers mostly make significant contributions to activities of self-care of patients and generally are in the same position in all care processes as are patients.

### 4.5. Difficulties experienced by home care providers to patients with heart failure

Symptoms of heart failure are generally insidious and worsen in time. The course of the disease is generally unpredictable, and signs may change from day to day. Therefore, patients with HF should change lifestyle habits by adapting themselves to life, prioritizing and re-directing life. In this case, these may lead to negative changes in physical and emotional roles of patients [111].

Because heart failure requires a long care process since its diagnosis, caregivers are affected physically, psychologically, socially, economically and spiritually as much as patients themselves and undergo a heavy economic burden in addition to intense stress [111]. It is stated that those who provide home care suffer from higher mental burden than other members of the family and therefore are more inclined to depression [121]. Care providers experience stress, helplessness, worry, loneliness, inability to spare time for themselves and disappointment with life. It is reported that female caregivers are under bigger risk than male caregivers [122]. Besides, it is emphasized that caregivers who are not experienced with HF acute affective disorders are considered as psycho-social care burden [123].

HF causes evident changes and difficulties in the daily life of patients' care providers. To increase knowledge level of health experts about risk factors of caregivers and to know factors that facilitate care will reduce risks in patients' and caregivers' health [124].

## Author details

Birsel Canan Demirbağ[1]*, Çiğdem Gamze Özkan[2], Betül Bayrak[2] and Yeter Kurt[2]

*Address all correspondence to: cdemirbag@gmail.com

1 Public Health Department, Faculty of Health Sciences, School of Nursing, Karadeniz Technical University, Trabzon, Turkey

2 Fundamentals of Nursing Departmant, Faculty of Health Sciences, School of Nursing, Karadeniz Technical University, Trabzon, Turkey

## References

[1] Yurtsever S, Özge A, Kara A, et al. The relationship between care burde and social support in Turkish Alzheimer patients family caregivers. Journal of Nursing Education and Practice. 2017;**3**(9):1-6. DOI: http//dx.doi.org/10.5430/jnep

[2] ANA. American Nursing Assaociation (internet) (avaible access: 01.11.2016), 1998

[3] Zarit SH, Reever KE, Bach-Peterson J. Relatives of the impaired elderly: Correlates of feelings of burden. The Gerontologist. 1980;**20**(6):649-655. DOI: https://doi.org/10.1093/geront/20.6.649

[4] Parks SM, Novielli KD. A practical guide to caring for caregivers. American Family Physician. 2000;**62**(12):2613-2622. PMID: 11142468

[5] Etters L, Goodall D, Harrison BE. Caregiver burden among dementia patient caregivers: A review of the literature. Journal of the American Academy of Nurse Practitioners. 2008;**20**(8):423-428

[6] Carretero S, Garces J, Rodenas F, Sanjose V. The informal caregiver's burden of dependent people: theory and empirical review. Archives of Gerontology and Geriatrics. 2009;**49**(1):74-79

[7] Kahriman F, andZaybak A. Caregiver burden and perceived social support among caregivers of patients with cancer. Asian Pacific journal of cancer prevention. 2015;**16**(8):3313-3317. PMID:25921137

[8] Ardahan M. Social support and the nursing. J Ataturk University School of Nursing. 2006;**9**:68-75 (in Turkish)

[9] Edwards NE, Scheetz PS. Predictors of burden for caregivers of patients with parkinson's disease. The Journal of Neuroscience Nursing. 2002;**34**:184-190

[10] Chiou CJ, Chang HY, Chen P, Wanga HH. Social support and caregiving circumstances as predictors of caregiver burden in Taiwan. Archives of Gerontology and Geriatrics. 2009;**48**:419-424. ISSN: 0167-4943. DOI: http://dx.doi.org/10.1016/j.archger.2008.04.001

[11] Gamez B, Calanzani N, Higginson IJ. Benefits and costs of home pallative care compaired with usual car efor patients with advanced illness and their family caregivers. JAMA. 2014;**311**(10):1060-1061. DOI: 10.10001/jama.2014.553

[12] Sayan A. Home care in today. Journal of Anatolia Nursing, 2004;**7**(3):91-96

[13] Drummond MF, Sculpher MJ, Claxton K, et al. Methods for the economic evaluation of home health care programss. 4th Ed, United Kingdom: Oxford Press; 2015. ISBN:978-0-19-966587

[14] Keefe J, GubermaN N, Fancey P, et al. (2014) "Policy Brief No. 19–Caregiver assessment: An Essential Component of Continuing Care Policy," Population Change and Lifecourse Strategic Knowledge Cluster Research/Policy Brief: 2014;**1**(5):7. DOI: http://ir.lib.uwo.ca/pclc_rpb/vol1/iss5/7

[15] GOLD. Global Strategy for the Diagnosis, Management and Prevention of COPD 2017 [updated 11.02.; cited 2017 11.01]. DOI: http://goldcopd.org/gold-2017-global-strategy-diagnosis-management-prevention-copd/

[16] Association TT. Agreement report of COPD diagnosis and treatment. Turkish Thoracic Association. 2010;**11**

[17] WHO. Chronic respiratory diseases Burden of COPD 2017 [updated 11.02.2017; cited 2017 11.02.207]. DOI: http://www.who.int/respiratory/copd/burden/en/

[18] ME COPD: Clinical and Diagnostic Approaches. In: Özlü T MM, Karadağ M, Kaya A (editors), editor. Respiratory System and Diseases. İstanbul: Medical Bookstore; 2010. pp. 693-700

[19] M. T. Frequency of Anemia and the correlated factors in COPD. İstanbul: Ministry of Health, Dr.LütfiKırdarKartal Education and Research Hospital; 2009

[20] Pauwels RA, Rabe KF. Burden and clinical features of chronic obstructive pulmonary disease (COPD). The Lancet. **364**(9434):613-620. PMID: 15313363

[21] Currow DC, Ward A, Clark K, Burns CM, Abernethy AP. Caregivers for people with end-stage lung disease: characteristics and unmet needs in the whole population.

International Journal of Chronic Obstructive Pulmonary Disease. 2008;**3**(4):753-62. PMID: 19281090. PMCID: PMC26505958

[22] Van Manen JG, Bindels PJE, Dekker FW, IJzermans CJ, van der Zee JS, Schadé E. Risk of depression in patients with chronic obstructive pulmonary disease and its determinants. Thorax. 2002;**57**(5). PMID: 11978917

[23] Bergs D. 'The Hidden Client'–women caring for husbands with COPD: their experience of quality of life. Journal of Clinical Nursing. 2002;**11**(5):613-621. PMID: 12201888. DOI: 10.1046/j.1365-2702.2002.00651.x

[24] Leff B, Burton L, Mader S, Naughton B, Burl J, Clark R, et al. Satisfaction with hospital at home care. Journal of the American Geriatrics Society. 2006;**54**(9). PMID: 16970642 DOI: 10.1111/j.1532-5415.2006.00855.x

[25] Pinto RA, Holanda MA, Medeiros MM, Mota RM, Pereira ED. Assessment of the burden of caregiving for patients with chronic obstructive pulmonary disease. Respiratory Medicine. 2007;**101**(11):2402-2408. DOI: 2402-2408.10.1016/j.rmed.2007.06.001

[26] Blumenthal JA, Keefe FJ, Babyak MA, Fenwick CV, Johnson JM, Stott K, et al. Caregiver-assisted coping skills training for patients with COPD: Background, design, and methodological issues for the INSPIRE-II study. Clinical Trials. 2009;**6**(2):172-184. PMID: 19342470. DOI: 10.1177/1740774509102565

[27] Kim JH, Kim EK, Park SH, Lee KA, Hwang YI, Kim EJ, et al. Burden of COPD among Family Caregivers. Tuberc Respir Dis. 2010;**69**(6):434-441. DOI: https://doi.org/10.4046/trd.2010.69.6.434

[28] Langa KM, Fendrick AM, Flaherty KR, Martinez FJ, Kabeto MU, Saint S. Informal caregiving for chronic lung disease among older americans. Chest. 2002;**122**(6):2197-2203. PMID: 12475863. DOI: 10.1378/chest.122.6.2197

[29] Cain CJ, Wicks MN. Caregiver attributes as correlates of burden in family caregivers coping with chronic obstructive pulmonary disease. Journal of Family Nursing. 2000;**6**(1):46-68. DOI: 10.1177/107484070000600104

[30] Hasson F, Spence A, Waldron M, Kernohan G, McLaughlin D, Watson B, et al. Experiences and needs of bereaved carers during palliative and end-of-life care for people with chronic obstructive pulmonary disease. Indian Journal of Palliative Care. 2009;**25**(3):157-163. PMID: 19824276

[31] Montgomery R, Kwak J. TCARE: Tailored caregiver assessment and referral. Journal of Social Work Education. 2008;**44**(sup3):59-64. PMID: 18797229

[32] Beaudreau SA, Spira AP, Gray HL, Depp CA, Long J, Rothkopf M, et al. The relationship between objectively measured sleep disturbance and dementia family caregiver distress and burden. Journal of Geriatric Psychiatry and Neurology. 2008;**21**(3):159-165. PMID: 18503035

[33] İnci FH, Erdem M. Validity and reliability of the burden interview and its adaptation to Turkish. Journal of Anatolia Nursing and Health Sciences. 2008;**11**(4):85-95. ISSN: 1309-5471

[34] Saunders MM. Factors associated with caregiver burden in heart failure family caregivers. Western Journal of Nursing Research. 2008;**30**(8):943-959. PMID: 18612092. DOI: 10.1177/0193945908319990

[35] Kasuya RT, Polgar-Bailey MP, MPH Robbyn, Takeuchi M. Caregiver burden and burnout a guide for primary care physicians. Postgraduate Medicine. 2000;**108**(7):119. PMID: 11126138. DOI: 10.3810/pgm.2000.12.1324

[36] Kanervisto M, Paavilainen E, Heikkilä J. Family dynamics in families of severe COPD patients. Journal of Clinical Nursing. 2007;**16**(8):1498-1505. PMID: 17655538. DOI: 10.1111/j.1365-2702.2006.01804.x

[37] Spence A, Hasson F, Waldron M, Kernohan G, McLaughlin D, Cochrane B, et al. Active carers: Living with chronic obstructive pulmonary disease. International Journal of Palliative Nursing. 2008;**14**(8):368-372. PMID: 19023952. DOI: 10.12968/ijpn.2008.14.8.30771

[38] Schulz R, Sherwood PR. Physical and Mental Health Effects of Family Caregiving. Journal of Social Work Education. 2008;**44**(sup3):105-113. DOI:10.5175/JSWE.2008.773247702

[39] Sherwood PR, Given CW, Given BA, Eye Av. Caregiver burden and depressive symptoms: analysis of common outcomes in caregivers of elderly patients. Journal of Aging and Health. 2005;**17**(2):125-147. PMID: 15750048. DOI: 10.1177/0898264304274179

[40] AkgünŞahin Z. Determine burden care and depression for caregivers of chronic obstructive pulmonary patients. Medicine Reserches Journal. 2014;**12**(3):113-119

[41] Selçuk KT, Avcı D. The care burden of caregivers caring for elderly with chronic diseases and affecting factors. Süleyman Demirel University Health Sciences Journal. 2016;**7**(1): 1-9

[42] Tel H, Demirkol D, Kara S, Aydın D. Care burden and quality of life Among the caregivers of patients with COPD. Turkish Thoracic Journal. 2012;**13**(3):87-92. DOI: 10.5152/ttd.2012.21

[43] Upton J, Madoc-Sutton H, Sheikh A, Frank TL, Walker S, Fletcher M. National survey on the roles and training of primary care respiratory nurses in the UK in 2006: Are we making progress? Primary Care Respiratory Journal. 2007;**16**:284. PMID: 17906825. DOI: 10.3132/pcrj.2007.00068

[44] Coultas D, Frederick J, Barnett B, Singh G, and Wludyka P. A randomized trial of two types of nurse-assisted home care for patients with copd. Chest. 2005;**128**(4):2017-2024. PMID: 16236850. DOI: 10.1378/chest.128.4.2017

[45] Kara M, Aşti T. A home care of the chronic obstructive pulmonary disease. Eurasian Journal of Medicine. 2002;**34**:75-81

[46] Karadakovan A. Chronic obstructive pulmonary disease. In: Akbayrak NSEİ, Ançel G, Albayrak A, editors. Nursing Care Plans. Ankara: Alter; 2007; pp. 201-205

[47] Ovayolu N, Ovayolu Ö, Ateş Ç. COPD and nursing care. Fırat Health Services Journal. 2008;**3**(9):3-16

[48] Özkaptan BB, Kapucu S. The importance of home care to improve self-efficacy of people with chronic obstructive pulmonary disease. Cumhuriyet Nursing Journal. 2015;**4**(2): 74-80

[49] Fadıloğlu Ç. Home care in respiratory system diseases. In: ÇiçekFadıloğlu FD, GülErtem, editor. Home care. İzmir: Meta Basım; 2006

[50] Çiftçi H, Akbulut G, Mercanlıgil SM. Respiratory system diseases and nutrition treatment. Ankara: Ministry of Health Publications. 2008. Available from: http://beslenme.gov.tr/content/files/yeterlibeslenme/hastaliklarda_beslenme/c9.pdf

[51] Paz-Díaz H, Montes de Oca M, López JM, Celli BR. Pulmonary rehabilitation improves depression, anxiety, dyspnea and health status in patients with COPD. American Journal of Physical Medicine & Rehabilitation. 2007;**86**(1):30. PMID: 17304686. DOI: 6.10.1097/PHM.0b013e31802b8eca

[52] Aydemir Ç, Kasım İ, Cebeci S, Göka E, Tüzer V. Ouality of life and psychiatric symptoms in the caregivers of chronic renal insufficiency patients. Journal of Crisis. 2002;**10**(2):29-39

[53] Kaya Akı M, Demir Y. A review on caregiver burden and quality of life of primary family caregivers for hemodalysis patients. Journal of Duzce University Institute of Health Sciences; 2012;**2**(3):24-28. ISSN: 2146-443X

[54] Deeken JF, Taylor KV, Mangan P, Yabroff KR, Ingham JM. Care for the Caregivers: A review of self-report instruments developed to measure the burden, needs, and quality of life of informal caregivers. Journal of Pain and Symptom Management. 2003;**26**(4): 922-953

[55] Hacımusalar DG. The identification of the problems of caregivers responsible for the nursing of hemodialysis patients. 2005; Master Thesis, Kayseri: Erciyes University Institute of Health Sciences

[56] KaradakovanA, Aslan FE. Care in the medical and surgical diseases. 2nd Ed. Adana: Nobel Medical Bookstore. 2011; ISBN:978-605-397-055-2

[57] Grassmann A, Gioberge S, Moeller S, Brown G. ESRD Patients in 2004: Global overview of patient numbers, treatment modalities and associated trends. Nephrology Dialysis Transplantation. 2005;**20**(12):2587-2593

[58] Süleymanlar G, Altıparmak MR, Seyahi N, Trabulus S. Türkiye'de Nefroloji-DiyalizveTransplantasyon Registry Raporu 2011. İstanbul: Türk Nefroloji DerneğiYayınları; 2012

[59] SezenA, Arslan H. Renal Failure. In A. Sezen (Ed.) Dialysis Nursing. Istanbul: Nobel Medical Bookstore. 2014; pp. 113-142

[60] Ören B. Investigation of factors affecting the quality of life and self care agency of patients receiving hemodialysis and peritoneal dialysis. (PhD Thesis), 2010; Istanbul: Istanbul University Institute of Health Sciences

[61] Daugirdas JT, Blake PG, Ing TS. Handbook of Dialysis. (Vol. Fourth Edition). Philadelphia: Lippincott Williams & Wilkins. 2010

[62] VicdanAK, Karabacak BG. The use of patient education Roy adaptation model hemodialysis. Journal of Human Sciences, 2014;**11**(2):209-220. ISSN:1303-5134. DOI: http://dx.doi.org/10.14687/ijhs.v11i2.2729

[63] TDK (Turkish Language Association), Great Turkish Dictionary. Access Date: 06.02.2017 http://tdk.gov.tr/index.php?option=com_bts&arama=kelime&guid=TDK.GTS.589860a3652b79.04938173

[64] Asan, T. The evaluation of people whose family members have chronic kidney diease. 2007; Master Thesis, Istanbul: Haliç University Institute of Health Sciences

[65] Demirbilek H, Ciğerli Ö, Yakupoğlu Ü, Turhan F, Erman AM, Köse A, et al. Sign of burnout and depression in relatives or caregivers of dialysis patient. Göztepe Medical Journal. 2011;**26**(3):103-107. ISSN 1300-526X. DOI: 10.5222/J.GOZTEPETRH.2011.103

[66] Kekeç, M. Determination of burden of caregivers to patients under hemodialysis therapy and affecting factors. (Master Thesis), Kayseri: 2011;Erciyes University Institute of Health Sciences

[67] AkpolatT, Utaş C. Common Problems in Hemodialysis Patients. Hemodialysis Nurse Handbook. 2000; Istanbul: GüzelSanatlar Printing House

[68] Güler Ö, Yüksel Ş, Acartürk G, Emül HM, Özbulut Ö, Çölbay M, et al. Psychosocial assessment in patients with end-stage renal disease treated with hemodialysis. Anatolian Journal of Psychiatry. 2007;**8**(3):173-178

[69] Günler OE. Social role change, expectations and challanges in hemodialysis patients due to the disease: A study of health sociology. 2011; Master Thesis, Konya: Selçuk University Institute of Social Sciences

[70] YeğenağaBakioğlu I. Fundamentals of hemodialysis. 1995;Istanbul: Nobel Medical Bookstore

[71] Levendoğlu F, Altıntepe L, Uğurlu H. Disability, depression and quality of life among older hemodialysis patients. Turkish Journal of Geriatrics; 2004;**7**(4):195-198. ISSN: 1307-9948

[72] Gordon T, Edwars WS. Doctor-Patient Cooperation. Aksay, E. (translator) Istanbul: Sistem Publishing. 1997

[73] Karahan A, Güven S. Homecare for elderly. Turkish Journal of Geriatric; 2002;**5**(4):155-159. ISSN: 1307-9948

[74] Suri RS, Larive B, Garg AX, Hall YN, Pierratos A, Chertow GM, et al. and FHN Study Group. Burden on caregivers as perceived by hemodialysis patients in the Frequent Hemodialysis Network (FHN) trials. Nephrology Dialysis Transplantation, 2011;**26**(7):2316-2322. PMID: 21421590. DOI: https://doi.org/10.1093/ndt/gfr007

[75] Küçükgüçlü Ö. The reliability and validity of the caregiver burden inventory in Turkey. (PhD Thesis), 2004; İzmir: Ege University Institute of Health Sciences

[76] Ferrario SR, Zotti AM, Baroni A, Cavagnino A, Fornara R. Emotional reactions and practical problems of the caregivers of hemodialysed patients. Journal of Nephrology. 2002;**15**(1):54-60. PMID: 11936427

[77] Könezoğlu B. The family and family protection. (Master Thesis), 2006; Ankara: Ankara University Institute of Social Sciences

[78] Tüzer V. Systemic family approach to chronic illness and disability. Turkish Journal of Clinical Psychiatry; 2001;**4**:193-201. ISSN 1302-0099 https://www.journalagent.com/kpd/pdfs/KPD_4_3_193_201.pdf

[79] İlaslanArıkan E. The problems and burn out level experienced by caregivers responsible for the care of hemodialysis patients. 2009; Master Thesis, Istanbul: Istanbul University Institute of Health Sciences

[80] Aydemir Ç, Kasım İ, Cebeci S, Göka E, Tüzer, V. Ouality of life and psychiatric symptoms in the caregivers of chronic renal insufficiency patients. Crisis Journal. 2002;**10**(2):29-39

[81] Ünsar S, Dindar İ, Zafer R, Kumasoglu Ç. The self-care agency and affecting factors in hemodialysis patients. Journal of the Fırat Health Services; 2006;**1**(3):70-80

[82] Lee JE, Shin DW, Cho J, Yong HK, Kim SY, Yoo SH. Caregiver burden, patients' self-perceived burden, and preference for palliative care among cancer patients and caregivers. Psycho-Oncology; 2015;**24**(11), pp. 1545-1551. Published online in Wiley Online Library. PMID: 25920720. DOI: 10.1002/pon.3827 http://onlinelibrary.wiley.com/doi/10.1002/pon.3827/full

[83] Ilse IB, Feys H, De Wıt L, Putman K, Weerdt WD. Stroke caregivers' strain: prevalence and determinants in the first six months after stroke. Disability and Rehabilitation. 2008;**30**(7):523-530. PMID: 18365864

[84] Urizar AC, Maldonado JG, Garcia MF, Molina PD. Burden of care in Aymara caregivers of patients with schizophrenia. Revista de Psiquiatría y Salud Mental; 2012;**5**(3):191-196. ISSN: 2173-5050. DOI: 10.1016/j.rpsmen.2011.07.004

[85] Shanks-McElroy HA, and Strobino J. Male caregivers of spouses with Alzheimer's disease: Risk factors and health status. American Journal of Alzheimer's Disease and Other Dementias. 2001;**16**(3):167-175. PMID: 11398566

[86] Gülpak M, Kocaöz S. The care burden and the affecting factors of individuals receiving hemodialysis treatment. TAF Preventive Medicine Bulletin. 2014;**13**(2):99-108. ISSN:1303-734X. DOI: 10.5455/pmb 1-1359391140

[87] Atagün Mİ, Balaban ÖD, Atagün Z, Elagöz M, Özpolat AY. Caregiver burden in chronic diseases. Current Approaches in Psychiatry. 2011;**3**(3):513-552. DOI: http://dx.doi.org/10.5455/cap.20110323

[88] Schneider RA. Fatigue among caregivers of chronic renal failure in patients: a principal components analysis. Nephrology Nursing Journal. 2003;**30**(6):629-633. PMID: 14730783

[89] Cukor D, Cohen SD, Peterson RA, Kimmel PL. Psychosocial aspects of chronic disease: ESRD as a paradigmatic illness. Journal of the American Society of Nephrology. 2007;**18**(2):3042-3055. DOI: 10.1681/ASN.2007030345

[90] Bülbül E. Quality of life of hemodialysis patients according to patients, family members and healthcare personnel. 2010; Master Thesis, Istanbul: Haliç University Institute of Health Sciences

[91] Belasco A, Barbosa D, Bettencourt AR, Diccini S, Sesso R. Quality of life family caregivers of elderly patients on hemodialysis and peritoneal dialysis. American Journal of Kidney Diseases. 2006;**48**(6):955-963. ISSN: 0272-6386. DOI: http://dx.doi.org/10.1053/j.ajkd.2006.08.017

[92] Gayomali C, Sutherland S, Finkelstein FO. The challenge for the caregiver of the patient with chronic kidney disease. Nephrology Dialysis Transplantation. 2008;**23**:3749-3751. PMID: 19028759

[93] Tuncay FÖ, Mollaoğlu M, Fertelli TK. Care burden and social support of caregivers caring for patients with chronic diseases. LiteratürSempozyum Journal of Psychiatry Neurology Behavioral Sciences, October/November/December 2015, 2015;issue 8. http://www.literatursempozyum.com/pdf/m_1453712649.pdf

[94] Birol L. Nursing Process. 9th Ed, Izmir: Etki Publications, 2009: pp. 78-81

[95] GökÖzer F, TaşçıBeydağ KD, Cengiz Ş, Kiper S. Hopelessness levels of patients undergoing hemodialysis. Journal of the Fırat Health Services. 2009;**4**(10):123-136

[96] Karabulutlu Yılmaz E, Okanlı A. The evaluation of illness perceptions in hemodialysis patients. Journal of Anatolia Nursing and Health Sciences. 2011;**14**(4):25-30. ISSN: 1309-5471

[97] Özaltın G. Patients and patients' family in psychiatric nursing. Journal of Cumhuriyet University Nursing School, 1999;**3**(1):1-8

[98] Polat M. Home Care Rehabilitation. In: Konak, Ş. (Ed.) Social, Psychological and Medical Aspects of Home Care. First Edition, Kongre Bookstore. 2016; pp. 335-340. ISBN: 978-605-66925-1-2

[99] Zaybak A. Home Care for Patients with Invasive Procedures. Konak, Ş. (Ed.) Social, Psychological and Medical Aspects of Home Care. First Edition, Kongre Bookstore, 2016; pp. 269-293. ISBN: 978-605-66925-1-2

[100] Kılıçkesmez K, Ökçün B, Küçükoğlu S. Definition and Pathophysiology of Heart Failure. In Ö. Kozan and M. Zoghi (Eds.), A to Z Chronic Heart Failure 2010; (pp. 25-38). Ankara: Güneş Medicine Bookstores

[101] Ponikowski P, Voors AA, Anker SD, Bueno H, Cleland JG, Coats AJ, et al. 2016 ESC Guidelines For The Diagnosis And Treatment Of Acute And Chronic Heart Failure. European heart journal. 2015. ehw128. DOI: https://doi.org/10.1093/eurheartj/ehw128

[102] Molloy G, J Johnston DW, Witham MD. Family caregiving and congestive heart failure. Review and analysis. European Journal of Heart Failure, 2005;**7**(4):592-603. DOI: 10.1016/j.ejheart.2004.07.008

[103] Friedman MM, Bowden VR, Jones E. Family Nursing: Research, Theory & Practice. In: Friedman MM, Bowden VR, Jones E. (Eds.). Introduction to the family. Upper Saddle River: Prentice Hall. 2003: pp. 3-33

[104] Goldstein G, Kenet G. The impact of chronic disease on the family. haemophilia. 2002;**8**(3):461-465. DOI: 10.1046/j.1365-2516.2002.00642.x

[105] Williams LA. Theory of caregiving dynamics. In: Smith M, Liehr P (Eds.), Middle range theory for nursing 2008; pp. 261-276). New York: Springer Publishing Company

[106] Lloyd-Jones D, Adams RJ, Brown TM, Carnethon M, Dai S, De Simone G, et al. Heart disease and stroke statistics—2010 update. Circulation, 2010;**121**(7):e46–e215. DOI: 10.1161/CIRCULATIONAHA.109.19266

[107] Levy D, Kenchaiah S, Larson MG, Benjamin EJ, Kupka MJ, Ho KK, et al. Long-term trends In the incidence of and survival with heart failure. New England Journal of Medicine, 2002:**347**(18):1397-1402. DOI: 10.1056/NEJMoa020265

[108] McMurray J, Petrie M, Murdoch D, Davie A. Clinical epidemiology of heart failure: Public and private health burden. European Heart Journal. 1998;**19**:9-16. DOI: PMID:9886707

[109] Roger VL, Go AS, Lloyd-Jones DM, Adams RJ, Berry JD, Brown TM, et al. Heart disease and stroke statistics—2011 Update. A Report From the American Heart Association. Circulation, 2011;**123**(4):e18–e209. DOI: 10.1161/CIR.0b013e3182009701

[110] Heidenreich PA, Trogdon JG, Khavjou OA, Butler J, Dracup K, Ezekowitz MD, et al. Forecasting The future of cardiovascular disease in the united states. Circulatio. 2011;**123**(8):933-944. DOI: 10.1161/CIR.0b013e31820a55f5

[111] McMurray JJ, Adamopoulos S, Anker SD, Auricchio A, Böhm M, Dickstein K, . et al. Esc guidelines for the diagnosis and treatment of acute and chronic heart failure 2012. European Journal of Heart Failure. 2012;**14**(8):803-869. DOI: 10.1093/eurjhf/hfs105

[112] Johnson MJ. Management of end stage cardiac failure. Postgraduate Medical Journal. 2007;**83**(980):395-401. DOI: 10.1136/pgmj.2006.055723

[113] Stuart B. Palliative Care and hospice in advanced heart failure. Journal of Palliative Medicine. 2007;**10**(1):210-228. DOI: 10.1089/jpm.2006.9988

[114] Wingate S, Wiegand DLM. End-Of-Life care in the critical care unit for patients with heart failure. Critical Care Nurse, 2008;**28**(2):84-94

[115] Yancy CW, Jessup M, Bozkurt B, Butler J, Casey DE Jr, Drazner MH, et al. 2013 ACCF/AHA guideline for the management of heart failure: a report of theAmerican College of Cardiology Foundation/American Heart Association Task Force on Practice Guidelines. Journal of the American College of Cardiology 2013;**62**:147-239

[116] Dickstein K, Cohen-Solal A, Filippatos G, McMurray JJ, Ponikowski P, Poole-Wilson PA, et al. ESC guidelines for the diagnosis and treatment of acute and chronic heart failure 2008. European Journal of Heart Failure. 2008;**10**(10):933-989. DOI: 10.1016/j.ejheart.2008.08.005

[117] Demir M, Ünsar S. Heart failure and home care. Fırat Health Services Journal. 2008;**3**(8): 119-130

[118] Özer S, Sezgin ÖGD. Self-care in heart failure. Heart Failure Electronic Newsletter, 2015;**7**(4):1-3

[119] Özdemir Ü. Heart failure patient and family education. Heart Failure Electronic Newsletter. 2009;**1**:1-6. http://www.tdk.org.tr/KYBulteni/makale=66

[120] Riegel B, Jaarsma T, Strömberg A. A Middle-range theory of self-care of chronic illness. Advances in Nursing Science. 2012;**35**(3):194-204. DOI: 10.1097/ANS.0b013e318261b1ba

[121] Pinquart M, Sörensen S. Correlates of physical health of informal caregivers: A meta-analysis. Journals of Gerontology. Series B: Psychological Sciences and Social Sciences. 2007;**62**(2):126-137. DOI: 10.1093/geronb/62.2.P126

[122] Humphrey L, Kulich K, Deschaseaux C, Blackburn S, Maguire L, Strömberg A. The caregiver burden questionnaire for heart failure (CBQ-HF): Face and content validity. Health and quality of life outcomes. 2013;**11**(1):84. DOI: 10.1186/1477-7525-11-84

[123] Scott LD. Caregiving and care receiving among a technologically dependent heart failure population. Advances in Nursing Science. 2000;**23**(2):82-97. PMID: 11104326

[124] Strömberg A. The situation of caregivers in heart failure and their role in improving patient outcomes. Current Heart Failure Reports. 2013;**10**(3):270-275. DOI: 10.1007/s11897-013-0146-8

# 8

# Psychopathological Symptoms in Caregivers of Demented and Nondemented Patients

Fernando L. Vázquez, Patricia Otero,
Vanessa Blanco, Lara López and Ángela Torres

**Abstract**

Currently, more than 1 in 10 adults living in the Organization for Economic Co-operation and Development is involved in nonprofessional care of a dependent family member. The main causes of dependence are dementia, followed by other conditions such as cerebrovascular accidents, limb impairment, depression, and vision impairment. Although care provided by the caregiver is crucial to the well-being of the cared person, it can also have negative consequences on the caregiver's emotional state. This chapter aims to describe the psychopathological symptoms experienced by caregivers based on the condition of the person cared for. A bibliographic search was conducted to examine the effects of care on the emotional state of caregivers, distinguishing patients with dementia from those with other conditions. Depressive and anxiety symptoms were the most frequent psychopathological symptoms, both in caregivers of demented and nondemented patients, experienced by caregivers of patients with dementia, cerebrovascular accidents, traumatic brain injury, schizophrenia, cancer, amyotrophic lateral sclerosis, and autism spectrum disorder. In caregivers of patients with bipolar disorder and vision impairment, depressive symptoms were most prominent, whereas anxiety symptoms were common in caregivers of patients with spinal cord injuries. Sleep disturbances were found among caregivers of dementia and schizophrenia patients. Strategies for preventing psychopathological symptoms were provided and the importance of professional support when they occur was pointed out.

**Keywords:** caregiver, dementia, nondementia, psychopathology, symptoms

## 1. Introduction

Great discoveries and advances in hygiene, nutrition, medical technology, and social achievements have led to a decline in mortality and an increase in life expectancy [1]. In parallel with this increase in life expectancy, there has also been an increase in individuals dependent on caregivers, which is associated with both the aging of the population and the rising survival rates. In fact, it is estimated that there are around 349 million dependents around the world [2] and the proportion of disability-adjusted life years due to the number of years living with a disability increased globally to 31.2% in 2013 [3].

In addition, figures related to dependency are not limited to the person who suffers dependency. Individuals with a disability need the assistance and care of another person to carry out most of their daily activities. This responsibility usually falls on one of their relatives. Thus, currently more than one in 10 adults living in the Organization for Economic Co-operation and Development (OECD) countries is involved in the unpaid care of a dependent family member [4]. In the United States, an estimated 43.5 million adults have provided unpaid care to an adult or child with disability in the last 12 months [5]. In Europe, it is estimated that there are around 54.5 million nonprofessional caregivers [4]. **Figure 1** shows the percentages of caregivers by country.

The conditions that can lead a patient to require dependent care are varied, with up to 301 different diagnoses having been associated with different levels of dependency [3]. Among these, the main causes of dependence are, first, dementia, followed by other conditions such as cerebrovascular accidents, limb impairment, severe depression, and vision problems [6]. Typically, all these conditions require daily caregiver assistance [2].

Although the care provided by the caregiver is crucial to the well-being of the dependent person, it entails great costs and sacrifices for the caregiver in terms of leisure time, self-care, family life, money, work, and personal projects, all of which can affect their well-being. The impact of caregiving on the emotional state of caregivers is well documented [7]. Specifically, it has been found that 10.0% of caregivers have anxiety disorders [8] and between 8.9% and 32.0% have a major depressive episode [9, 10], being insomnia or hypersomnia, diminished ability to think or concentrate and depressed mood the most frequent symptoms (see **Table 1**) [10].

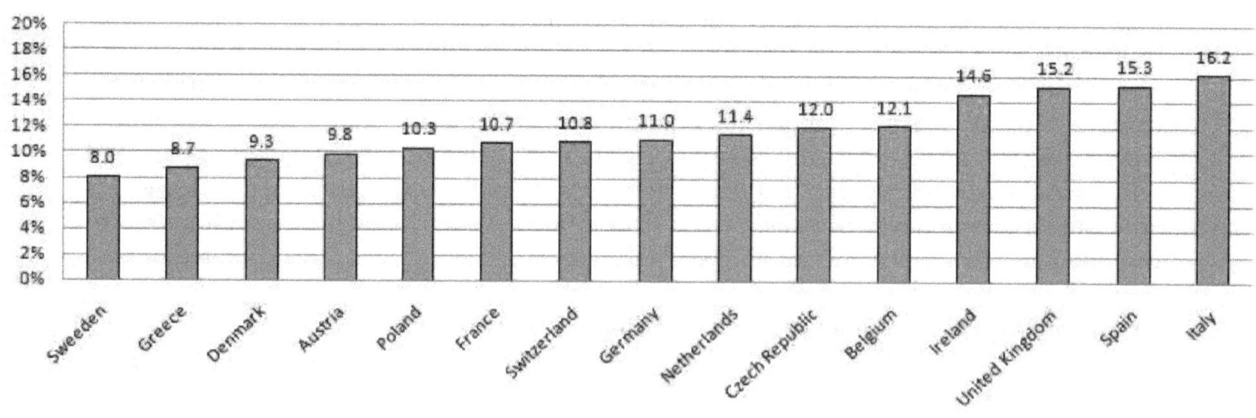


**Figure 1.** Percentage of the population reported to be nonprofessional caregivers. *Note*: Adapted from Colombo et al. [4]. Reproduced with permission.

| Symptom | Presence (%) | Absence (%) |
|---|---|---|
| 1. Depressed mood | 84.4 | 15.6 |
| 2. Diminished interest or pleasure | 75.6 | 24.4 |
| 3. Significant weight loss or gain | 80.0 | 20.0 |
| 4. Insomnia or hypersomnia | 93.3 | 6.7 |
| 5. Psychomotor agitation or retardation | 77.8 | 22.2 |
| 6. Fatigue or loss of energy | 71.1 | 28.9 |
| 7. Feelings of worthlessness or excessive or inappropriate guilt | 20.0 | 80.0 |
| 8. Diminished ability to think or concentrate or indecisiveness | 91.1 | 8.9 |
| 9. Recurrent thoughts of death, or a suicide attempt, or a specific plan for committing suicide | 77.8 | 22.2 |

**Table 1.** Clinical symptoms of major depressive episodes in nonprofessional caregivers.

It should be noted, however, that much of the information about the mental health of caregivers was obtained from studies of caregivers of people with dementia [11]; although more recently, there has been recognition that caregivers of patients who have other conditions also suffer from adverse effects [12, 13].

The aim of this chapter is to describe the psychopathological symptoms experienced by caregivers based on the condition of the person cared for and to compare the symptoms present in the caregivers of demented and nondemented patients.

## 2. Psychopathology of caregivers according to the diagnosis of the person being cared for

We reviewed the main psychopathological manifestations of the caregivers found in the scientific literature and organized them as a function of the diagnosis of their relatives (see **Table 2**). Specifically, we group them according to whether care is provided to a person with dementia or with other conditions.

### 2.1. Dementia

Dementia is a clinical syndrome that leads to a progressive deterioration of memory, intellect, personality, and physical abilities, and has serious consequences for individuals, their families, the health system, and the economy [14], affecting 24.3 million people worldwide [15]. Alzheimer's is the most prevalent form of dementia, with an average survival of 10 years,

| Dependent's diagnosis | Main psychopathological manifestations found in caregivers |
|---|---|
| Dementia | Depressive symptoms, major depressive disorder, anxiety symptoms, anxiety disorder, sleep disturbances, insomnia, anticipatory grief |
| Cerebrovascular accident | Depressive symptoms, anxiety symptoms |
| Traumatic brain injury | Depressive symptoms, anxiety symptoms |
| Bipolar disorder | Depressive symptoms |
| Schizophrenia | Depressive symptoms, anxiety symptoms, sleep disturbances, insomnia |
| Spinal cord injury | Anxiety symptoms, burden in the social role and adjustment to the ongoing recovery process, negative outcomes on the family system |
| Vision impairment and blindness | Depressive symptoms |
| Cancer | Depressive symptoms, anxiety symptoms, concerns about the future and fear of loss and loneliness |
| Amyotrophic lateral sclerosis | Depressive symptoms, anxiety symptoms, anticipatory grief |
| Autism spectrum disorder | Depressive symptoms, anxiety symptoms |

**Table 2.** Main psychopathological manifestations of caregivers according to the diagnosis of the person cared for.

though this varies depending on the age of onset [14]. As dementia progresses, the affected person requires an increasing amount of help [16] and time [17]. In this situation, caregivers are essential, and it is expected that the number of caregivers of people with dementia will increase significantly in the following decades, as it is estimated that the number of people with dementia will reach 75.6 million worldwide in the year 2030 [15].

It is well documented that caregivers of people with dementia experience mental health problems to a greater extent than noncaregivers [7]. Most of these caregivers present a high prevalence of elevated symptoms of depression and anxiety [7, 18].

Regarding depressive symptoms, previous research has found that between 27.9% and 55.0% of caregivers of patients with dementia have elevated depressive symptoms [11]. This is not a trivial fact; elevated depressive symptoms are one of the major predictors of the development of major depressive disorder [19] and have a mortality risk comparable to that of major depressive disorder [20]. In addition, previous research has found that between 15.0% and 32.0% of caregivers of patients with dementia meet the diagnostic criteria for a major depressive episode [21]. Risk factors related to depression in caregivers of people with dementia include loneliness, younger age (that the caregiver be under the age of 65), low income, being a wife, dedicating a greater number of daily hours to care, the patient presenting with behavioral disturbances (particularly angry or aggressive behavior), and the patient presenting a greater dependence for the basic activities of their daily life [22, 23].

In the context of anxiety, between 3.7% and 76.5% of caregivers present symptoms of anxiety [18] and between 10.0% and 16.0% suffer from an anxiety disorder [8, 24]. The severity of physical health consequences of the person with dementia and the caregiver's overload and their coping style (escape-avoidance and confrontation, especially) are factors associated with higher levels of anxiety [18].

In addition to these main psychopathological manifestations, it has also been found that two-thirds of these caregivers experience some form of sleep disturbance during the course of their caregiving career [25] and 41.0% suffer from insomnia [26]. Finally, and although it is not a pathological process, given the degenerative nature of dementia, many caregivers come to experience what is known as *anticipatory grief*,[1] which generates feelings of denial, anger, depression, and finally acceptance of reality. They progressively experience the loss of their loved one, even before he or she dies, with the consequent conflict of emotions and the feeling of being physically and emotionally exhausted.

## 2.2. Conditions other than dementia that lead to dependence

### *2.2.1. Cerebrovascular accident and traumatic brain injury*

#### *2.2.1.2. Cerebrovascular accident*

A cerebrovascular accident is a neurological condition attributed to acute focal damage of the brain cells due to a vascular cause (a significant decrease in blood flow in the brain or bleeding), also known as a stroke. In 2010 alone, 16.9 million people worldwide suffered a first stroke and 33 million people who have previously had a stroke were still alive [28].

In many cases, a cerebrovascular accident occurs in an instant and involves a permanent life change. Cognitive, behavioral, and personality changes can occur, and as a result, their autonomy can be limited or totally reduced. This can have a huge impact on the family, as it is likely they will be the main caregivers once the patient leaves the hospital [29].

Previous research has found that 55.0% of caregivers of people who have suffered a stroke have significant emotional distress [30], which manifests primarily as symptoms of depression and anxiety. In fact, between 18.8% and 33.0% of caregivers of people who suffered a cardiovascular accident were found to have clinically significant depressive symptoms [12, 31]. The depression of the caregiver was associated with the severity of the stroke, with the best predictor being the caregiver's depression in the acute phase of the illness and the patient's anxiety and depression [12, 31].

Furthermore, it was found that around 31.1% of stroke patient caregivers experienced elevated anxiety symptoms [31]. The predictors of anxiety among caregivers were anxiety, depression, and cognitive impairment of the patient [31].

[1] *Anticipatory grief*. This term refers to the mourning that takes place before the actual loss of a loved one. It occurs in those cases where the death of a loved one is an outcome that is already known (due, for example, to a terminal or degenerative disease). During this period of anticipation, the potential survivor begins the tasks of mourning and begins to experience different emotional responses before the death of the loved one [27].

#### 2.2.1.2. Traumatic brain injury

Traumatic brain injuries are another condition in which damage occurs in the brain, typically as a result of an external force (such as falls, vehicle collisions, or violence). The overall estimated incidence rate of traumatic brain injury is 262 per 100,000 populations in Europe [32], and in 2010, it was 824 per 100,000 populations in the United States [33]. It can result in an alteration of the individual's cognitive, physical, and/or emotional abilities. Thus, it can affect the emotional state of the caregiver.

It has been found that between 37.0% and 60.0% of caregivers of people with traumatic brain injury have clinically significant symptoms of depression [34, 35] and 39.0% of these caregivers experience elevated anxiety symptoms [35].

Two variables frequently studied in caregivers of people with traumatic brain injury are the behavioral and personality changes that occur in the patient and the effected family changes as a result of the caregiving situation. Regarding the behavioral and personality changes, relationships between the patient's disruptive behaviors and mental health indicators in caregivers have been found, but this relationship may be mediated by the caregiver's beliefs about these changes [36]. For example, believing that the behavior was under the control of the person with traumatic brain injury and/or was motivated by hostile intentions was associated with more depression, but less stress. This was because the perception that the other person is in control of their behavior gave the caregiver more confidence in their own ability to control the behavior through persuasion. Another affected variable is the family unit [35]. This is an important factor to bear in mind since it has been suggested that having family support may be one of the most effective variables in reducing depressive symptoms [37] and is related to improved well-being and general health [38].

### 2.2.2. Severe mental disorders

The importance of family in the care of people with severe mental illness has grown due to the deinstitutionalization of psychiatric patients [39]. However, providing care to a family member with a severe mental disorder is an overwhelming experience for the caregiver.

Caregivers of people with severe mental illness often exhibit depressive symptomatology, and care-related burden contributes significantly to such symptomatology [40]. Further aggravating the prevalence of depressive symptomatology, social support of the caregivers may decrease due to the social stigma associated with severe mental illness [40].

The two types of serious mental disorders that have received the most attention are bipolar disorder and schizophrenia. Severe depression is also considered a major cause of dependency and a condition requiring daily care [2, 6]. However, to the best of our knowledge, no studies have been done on the emotional consequences of caring for a family member with severe depression.

#### 2.2.2.1. Bipolar disorder

Bipolar disorder is characterized by unusual changes in mood (euphoria vs. depression), energy, activity level, and ability to perform daily tasks. The life prevalence of this disorder in caregivers is around 3.9% [41]. It can be especially stressful because of its chronic and cyclical nature. Caregivers may be concerned about future mood swings and about the likelihood of suicide [42].

Caregivers of patients with bipolar disorder experience more psychiatric symptoms, especially depression [42]. Specifically, it has been found that between 24.0% and 38.0% of caregivers of people with bipolar disorder present clinically significant depressive symptoms [43].

Given the variable course of the patient's illness, it is important to establish whether caregivers experience symptoms during subsyndromic phases and whether the severity of the patient's symptoms impacts the caregiver's symptoms [42]. However, some previous research has not found a significant association between the clinical state of the patient and the depressive symptoms of the caregiver [44]. In addition, the perceived stigma of the caregiver has been identified as significantly related to depression, which may reduce their coping effectiveness [44].

#### *2.2.2.2. Schizophrenia*

Schizophrenia is a severe mental disorder, characterized by profound disruptions in thinking, affecting language, perception, the sense of self, and the patient's ability to engage in day-to-day activities. It is estimated that schizophrenia affects 21 million people in the world [45]. Caregiving of a patient with schizophrenia involves assisting patients in daily tasks, which may disrupt caregiver behavior and their daily routine, among others [46].

Gupta et al. [13] conducted a study to examine the health status of caregivers of patients with schizophrenia compared to noncaregivers and caregivers of adults with other conditions. There were 398 schizophrenia caregivers, 158,989 noncaregivers, and 14,341 caregivers of other conditions from five European countries (France, Germany, Italy, Spain, and the United Kingdom); all were matched on baseline characteristics. Comparing the caregivers of people with schizophrenia and noncaregivers, it was found that caregivers presented a significantly higher proportion of difficulties sleeping (42.7% vs. 28.5%), insomnia (32.4% vs. 18.5%), anxiety (37.9% vs. 23.6%), and depression (29.4% vs. 19.4%). Comparing schizophrenia caregivers and other caregivers, schizophrenia caregivers were more likely to experience sleep difficulties (42.7% vs. 32.8%), insomnia (32.4% vs. 22.0%), and anxiety (37.9%).

### *2.2.3. Spinal cord injury*

A spinal cord injury is damage to the spinal cord; it causes changes in its function, either temporarily or permanently. These changes translate into loss of muscle function below the level of the lesion. Depending on the location and severity of damage along the spinal cord, the symptoms can vary widely, from pain or numbness to paralysis. The prognosis also ranges widely from full recovery to permanent tetraplegia (also called quadriplegia) in injuries at the level of the neck and paraplegia.

Caregivers of people with a spinal cord injury have to provide care in the basic daily life activities and as a result, the quality of their own life may be affected. However, research on psychopathological manifestations in caregivers of people with spinal cord injury is scarce though one study found caregivers of patients with a spinal cord injury to present more stress than noncaregivers [47]. Caregivers also experience significant burden, especially in the social role functioning and adjustment to the ongoing recovery process [48]. Likewise, in caregivers who are married to the patient when the spinal cord injury occurs, more negative outcomes on the family system have been reported [49].

#### 2.2.4. *Vision impairment and blindness*

Vision impairment is a decrease in the ability to see to the point where glasses cannot treat the impairment. It is often defined as the best corrected visual acuity worse than 20/40 or 20/60. The term blindness is used for the complete loss of vision. The most common causes of vision impairment are refractory errors, cataracts and glaucoma, macular degeneration, or diabetic retinopathy. It is estimated that in 2012, there were 285 million visually impaired people worldwide, with 246 million having low vision and 39 million being blind [50]. These problems can cause difficulties in daily activities, such as driving, reading, socializing, or walking. Thus, it is important to receive care and support from a loved one.

Despite their prevalence, little research has been conducted on the psychopathological manifestations of the caregivers of people with vision impairments. The only manifestation studied was depression, finding that between 3.8% and 16.0% of the caregivers of people with low vision and between 9.2% and 48.0% of the caregivers of totally blind people presented clinically significant depressive symptoms [51, 52].

Related variables for depression in caregivers were being a woman, daily hours required for close supervision of the patient, intensity of care-giving, low household income, being the parent of a blind adult child, and being caregivers of patients who have not completed vision rehabilitation programs [51, 52].

#### 2.2.5. *Cancer*

Cancer is characterized by the rapid creation of abnormal cells that grow beyond their usual boundaries and then invade adjoining parts of the body and spread to other organs. According to data from the World Health Organization [53], cancer is the second leading cause of death in the world, causing 1 in 6 deaths. In addition, its economic impact is $1.16 trillion per year and this is expected to continue increasing.

The diagnosis of cancer is a traumatic event that has a significant impact in the patients and their families [54, 55]. In addition, recent advances in the treatment of cancer have resulted in shorter periods of hospitalization and the dispensing of treatment using medical devices in their homes. As a result, patients have become more chronic patients who spend more time at home, resulting in more caregiving tasks being placed on caregivers [55].

Elevated levels of anxiety and depression have been found in caregivers of cancer patients [56], including higher levels of anxiety than depression. In the palliative phases, Grov et al. [57] found that anxiety levels were significantly higher in these caregivers than in noncaregiver normative pairs. In contrast, they found no significant differences in depression. The authors suggest that the elevated levels of anxiety may be related to concerns about the future and fear of loss and loneliness, issues of special relevance to impending death. However, the quality of life and anxiety do not differ significantly between caregivers in the palliative and curative stages of the disease, suggesting that both phases are equally stressful and challenging [58] and always include a concern about the future. However, in another study [59], clinically significant levels of depressive symptomatology were found, which did not change markedly over time of the disease.

### 2.2.6. *Amyotrophic lateral sclerosis (ALS)*

Amyotrophic lateral sclerosis (ALS) is a neuromuscular degenerative disease with a late-onset fatal prognosis, whose incidence rate is 2.16 per 100,000 person-years in Europe [60] and 5 per 100,000 for 2013 in the USA [61]. Life expectancy since diagnosis is usually about 3–5 years and the age of onset is between 50 and 65 years [62]. Patients with ALS need increasing attention in all daily life activities because as the disease progresses, their ability to write or speak decreases, as well as the ability to complete daily life tasks, and the demands for attention from their caregivers are progressively greater.

Depressive and anxiety symptoms have been found among caregivers of patients with ALS [63]. More specifically, it has been found that between 13.0% and 61.0% had moderate to severe levels of depression and about 16.0% take medication for depression [63–65]. However, caregivers may be actually experiencing anticipated grief and pain for the future loss than a typical situation of care, characterized by progressive but prolonged deterioration over time. In fact, in these cases, mutual support between patient and caregiver takes on an essential role, rather than a unilateral benefit that may exist in other care relationships [63].

In addition, between 16.0% and 75.6% demonstrated moderate to severe levels of anxiety [66, 67], with the anxiety traits of the caregiver being the best predictors of state anxiety [67].

### 2.2.7. *Autism and autism spectrum disorders*

Autism is a neurodevelopmental disorder characterized by difficulties in social interaction and communication and by repetitive behaviors [68]. It is estimated that 62 out of every 10,000 people in the world suffer from an autism spectrum disorder [69].

Due to the early age of onset of autism (i.e., early childhood), the main caregivers are usually the parents. The caregivers face the symptoms of the disorder and behavior problems [70] and other secondary difficulties such as social stigma and lack of understanding of the disease. In fact, anxiety and depression scores were higher in parents of children with autism spectrum disorders than in parents of children with normal development [68]. A meta-analysis found that mothers of children with developmental disorders, including autism spectrum disorder, had significantly more depressive symptoms than mothers with problem-free children, with an effect size of 0.39 [71]. When analyzing the long-term effects, Barker et al. [70] found that after 10 years of follow-up, there were no significant changes in depressive symptomatology, though anxiety did decrease.

Behavioral problems are one of the most important predictors of parental stress, along with obedience/tranquility and self-isolation/ritualism [72].

### 2.3. Comparison of psychopathological symptoms among caregivers of patients with dementia and without dementia

Previous research has suggested that caring for a person with dementia is more difficult and burdensome than caring for people with other conditions. There are several reasons why caregivers of people with dementia may be at increased risk for these adverse effects. On the one hand, they are exposed to difficult disruptive behaviors, cognitive impairment, and affective losses characteristic of the progression of dementia. On the other hand, patients with dementia require more supervision, express less gratitude for the help they receive, are more likely to be depressed, and may present with aggressiveness and personality changes [73, 74]. However, there are few studies that have compared the consequences on the emotional state of the caregivers of people with dementia with those of caregivers of dependent people without dementia, and the results have been contradictory.

Clipp and George [75] compared caregiver spouses of patients with dementia and cancer patients. They found that caregivers of patients with dementia had significantly greater stress, burden, and negative affect compared with caregivers of people with cancer. Furthermore, Ory et al. [76] found that caring for a person with dementia has more adverse effects than caring for a person with another condition, in terms of physical and emotional strain, physical and mental problems, time for leisure, and family conflict.

However, Crespo et al. [77] found no evidence that caregivers of people with dementia had a poorer emotional state (evaluated as depressive and anxiety symptoms) than those who cared for dependent relatives without dementia. Moreover, Papastavrou et al. [78] reported that caregivers of people with cancer were more depressed compared with caregivers of schizophrenia and of people with dementia, whereas caregivers of people with dementia reported the highest levels of burden. Finally, Loi et al. [79] found higher levels of depressive symptomatology and burden in caregivers of people with physical disabilities (fragility and vision difficulties) than in caregivers of people with dementia.

## 3. Strategies for preventing psychopathological symptoms

Regardless of the condition of the person cared for, caregivers may consider the following strategies to take care of their own well-being and prevent the onset of psychopathological symptoms [80, 81]

- *Finding information on the disease of the family member cared for.* It will allow the caregiver to better understand their behaviors and moods.
- *Asking for and accepting help.* It is important that caregivers do not wait until they feel overwhelmed to ask for help. They should try to get as many family members involved in caregiving as possible. The caregiver could prepare a list of simple tasks that others could help him/her with, and let the helper choose what he or she would like to do. For instance, one person might be willing to take the person cared for on a walk a couple of times a week, and someone else might offer to pick up groceries.

- *Maintaining personal relationships.* Caregivers should try to stay well connected with family and friends who can offer nonjudgmental emotional support. If it is difficult for them to leave home, they could invite a relative to visit them or phone some friend.
- *Setting realistic goals.* Caregivers can break large tasks into smaller steps that they can do one at a time. It is important to prioritize and focus on the things they can control.
- *Taking time for himself/herself.* Caregivers are encouraged to participate in pleasant activities that allow them to relax and have fun, such as reading a book, going to a movie, or taking a warm bath.
- *Reducing personal stress.* Caregivers can learn to recognize warning signs such as irritability or forgetfulness, identify sources of stress, distinguish what can and cannot change, and take some action to reduce stress. Stress reducers can be simple activities like gardening or having coffee with a friend. Relaxation and meditation can also help.
- *Staying positive.* Trying to look at the positive side of situations. Caregiving allows to make a difference in our loved one's life by making him/her feel more comfortable, safe, and loved. Caregiving might also have spiritual meaning. These deep, meaningful motivations can help sustain the caregivers through difficult times.
- *Taking care of personal health.* It is recommended that caregivers meet their own healthcare needs, which include establishing a good sleep routine and proper nutrition with healthy foods and plenty of water. Exercise regularly, for example, going for a walk twice a week.

## 4. Professional support when psychopathological symptoms occur

When the above is not enough and psychopathological symptoms occur, it is better to seek professional help from a psychologist or a psychiatrist. There are several psychological interventions that have demonstrated efficacy in decreasing depressive and anxiety symptoms [82, 83]. Cognitive-behavioral interventions are more effective in reducing depressive symptoms, group interventions are more effective in increasing social support and respite services are recommended for sleep problems [82, 83].

In addition, it is recommended to ask the professional as soon as possible, in order to act early, before mental illness develops, and thus avoid personal suffering. A few sessions might be enough. In fact, Otero et al. [84] found significant differences between a problem-solving intervention lasting only five sessions and a usual care control group in the reduction of depressive symptomatology ($d = 1.33$) and the onset of new cases of depression at 12-month follow-up (10.1% vs. 25.0%). In another study, Vázquez et al. [85] found significant differences between a five-session cognitive-behavioral intervention and a usual care control group in the reduction of depressive symptomatology ($d = 1.33$) and the incidence of depression (3.4% vs. 22.0%) at 12-month follow-up (see **Figure 2**). Both interventions were effective regardless of the condition of the person cared for [86, 87]; those changes in depressive symptomatology were also clinically significant [88] and homework tasks played a fundamental role in the reduction of depressive symptomatology [89].

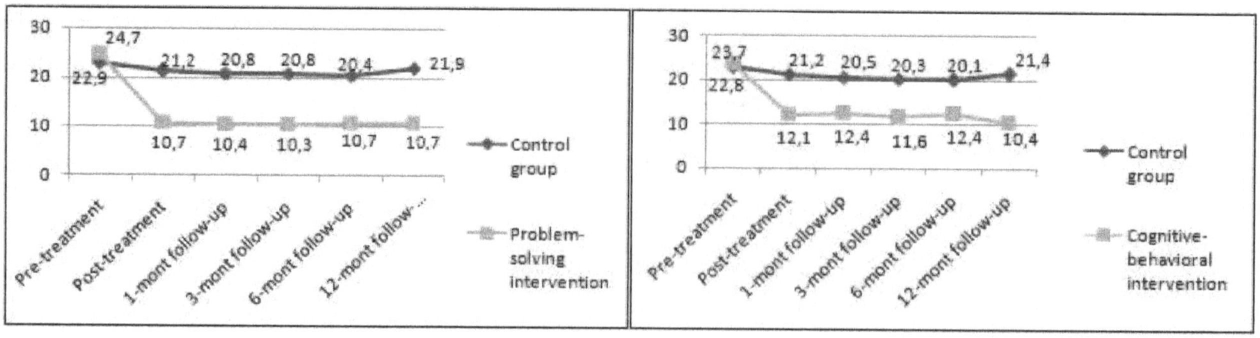


**Figure 2.** Depressive symptoms as a function of time in the two interventions from the studies by Otero et al. and Vázquez et al.

Caregivers may delay seeking professional health because of certain accessibility barriers including lack of time, not having someone to take over care during their absence, transportation problems, or stigma. For these cases, the efficacy of telephone-administered psychological interventions, that would allow caregivers to be treated for their psychopathological symptoms without the need to leave their home, is being studied. Thus, in a pilot study, Vázquez et al. [90] compared a cognitive-behavioral intervention via conference call, a behavioral activation intervention via conference call and a control group receiving usual care. They found that at post-treatment, depressive symptoms were significantly reduced in both intervention groups compared with the control group ($d$ = 2.18 and $d$ = 2.06) and there was a lower incidence of depression in the cognitive-behavioral group and the behavioral activation group when compared with the control group (0.0% for both interventions vs. 10.5% for the control group).

## 5. Conclusion

It is well documented that the burden of care assumed by nonprofessiona caregivers has negative consequences on their emotional well-being. Depressive and anxiety symptoms have been the most explored variables. Studies have found high levels of depressive and anxious symptomatology in all types of caregivers, regardless of the diagnosis of the dependent person (demented and nondemented patients). Depressive and anxiety symptoms were experienced by caregivers of patients with dementia, cerebrovascular accidents, traumatic brain injury, schizophrenia, cancer, ALS, autism, and autism spectrum disorder. Sleep disturbances were found in caregivers of dementia and schizophrenia patients. Only depressive symptoms were found in caregivers of bipolar disorder and vision impairment, while only anxiety symptoms were found in caregivers of spinal cord injury patients. Therefore, it is recommended that clinicians be prepared to evaluate and treat these symptoms in caregivers using psychological interventions with proven efficacy for the treatment of depressive and anxious symptoms in caregivers [84, 85].

There is no doubt that all the conditions that cause a situation of dependence result in stressors and demand that the caregiver must confront. However, the type of illness of the dependent person could be only one of the determining factors of the psychopathological manifestations in the caregivers. One possible explanation for these findings is that the effects of being a caregiver on mental health also depend on many other factors, both related to the care situation and the resources available to the caregiver (e.g., socioeconomic level) as well as the psychological resources available to the caregiver (e.g., coping style, the caregiver's beliefs about the problems of the dependent person, social support, or family conflict). Nonprofessional caregivers are a heterogeneous population with different profiles of psychopathological risk, as they vary in their exposure to the demands of care, in the style of coping with them, and in the resources they have at their disposal.

These findings must be interpreted taking into account certain limitations. Most of the work has focused on specific populations of caregivers and methodological limitations, and heterogeneity between studies makes comparisons difficult: the instruments used have been diverse; small samples make it difficult to generalize results; some studies have selected the participants according to different sociodemographic characteristics. There are few comparative studies among caregivers of people with dementia and without dementia. Finally, the cross-sectional nature of these studies prevents establishing cause-effect relationships.

Future research could analyze the specific contribution of each of the factors to the occurrence of depressive and anxiety symptoms in the caregiver population. The number of caregivers is expected to increase significantly in the coming decades, with as many as 613 million people needing care around the world by the year 2050 [2]. Thus, a better understanding of these variables would make it possible to ascertain the specific needs of caregivers and offer interventions that meet their needs. In fact, Zarit and Femia [91] recommended that psychological interventions not be applied to all caregivers indiscriminately, but that a selection of participants be made based on the risk factors to which they are exposed. Studies that have used this approach [80, 81] have achieved significant reductions in psychopathological symptoms such as depression and made strides in the prevention of the occurrence of mental disorders such as depression.

## Acknowledgements

This work was supported by the Ministry of Economy and Competitiveness of Spain [grant number 2012-PN162 (PSI2012-37396)] as well as the support received by the Ministry of Labor and Welfare (Xunta de Galicia).

## Author details

Fernando L. Vázquez[1]*, Patricia Otero[2], Vanessa Blanco[1], Lara López[1] and Ángela Torres[1]

*Address all correspondence to: fernandolino.vazquez@usc.es

1 University of Santiago de Compostela, Santiago de Compostela, Spain

2 University of A Coruña, A Coruña, Spain

## References


[1] World Health Organization, editor. The World Health Report 2002. Reducing Risks, Promoting Healthy Life. Geneva: World Health Organization; 2002

[2] Harwood RH, Sayer AA, Hirschfeld M. Current and future worldwide prevalence of dependency, its relationship to total population, and dependency ratios. Bulletin of the World Health Organization. 2004;**82**:251-258. DOI: 10.1590/S0042-96862004000400006

[3] Global Burden of Disease Study 2013 Collaborators. Global, regional, and national incidence, prevalence, and years lived with disability for 301 acute and chronic diseases and injuries in 188 countries, 1990-2013: A systematic analysis for the Global Burden of Disease Study 2013. Lancet. 2015;**386**:743-800. DOI: 10.1016/S0140-6736(15)60692-4

[4] Colombo F, Llena-Nozal A, Mercier J, Tjadens F. Help Wanted? Providing and Paying for Long-Term Care. Paris: OECD Publishing; 2011

[5] National Alliance for Caregiving and AARP Public Policy Institute. Caregiving in the U.S. 2015 [Internet]. 2015. Available from: http://www.caregiving.org/wp-content/uploads/2015/05/2015_CaregivingintheUS_Final-Report-June-4_WEB.pdf [Accessed February 10, 2017]

[6] Sousa RM, Ferri CP, Acosta D, Albanese E, Guerra M, Huang, Y, et al. Contribution of chronic diseases to disability in elderly people in countries with low and middle incomes: A 10/66 Dementia Research Group population-based survey. Lancet. 2009;**374**:1821-1830. DOI: 10.1016/S0140-6736(09)61829-8

[7] Pinquart M, Sörensen S. Differences between caregivers and noncaregivers in psychological health and physical health: A meta-analysis. Psychology and Aging. 2003;**18**:250-267. DOI: 10.1037/0882-7974.18.2.250

[8] Dura JR, Stukenberg KW, Kiecolt-Glaser JK. Anxiety and depressive disorders in adult children caring for demented parents. Psychology and Aging. 1991;**6**:467-473. DOI: 10.1037/0882-7974.6.3.467

[9] Livingston G, Manela M, Katona C. Depression and other psychiatric morbidity in carers of elderly people living at home. The British Medical Journal. 1996;**312**:153-156. DOI: 10.1136/bmj.312.7024.153

[10] Torres A, Blanco V, Vázquez FL, Díaz O, Otero P, Hermida E. Prevalence of major depressive episodes in non-professional caregivers. Psychiatry Research. 2015;**226**:333-339. DOI: 10.1016/j.psychres.2014.12.066

[11] Schulz R, O'Brien AT, Bookwala J, Fleissner K. Psychiatric and physical morbidity effects of dementia caregiving: Prevalence, correlates, and causes. Gerontologist. 1995;**35**:771-791. DOI: 10.1093/geront/35.6.771

[12] Berg A, Palomäki H, Lönnqvist J, Lehtihalmes M, Kaste M. Depression among caregivers of stroke survivors. Stroke. 2005;**36**:639-643. DOI: 10.1161/01.STR.0000155690.04697.c0

[13] Gupta S, Isherwood G, Jones K, Van Impe K. Assessing health status in informal schizophrenia caregivers compared with health status in non-caregivers and caregivers of other conditions. BMC Psychiatry. 2015;**15**:162. DOI: 10.1186/s12888-015-0547-1

[14] Hugo J, Ganguli M. Dementia and cognitive impairment: Epidemiology, diagnosis and treatment. Clinics in Geriatric Medicine. 2014;**30**:421-442. DOI: 10.1016/j.cger.2014.04.001

[15] World Health Organization (WHO). Dementia. Fact Sheet [Internet]. 2016. Available from: http://www.who.int/mediacentre/factsheets/fs362/en/ [Accessed: February 14, 2017]

[16] Ferrara M, Langiano E, Di Brango T, De Vito E, Di Cioccio L, Bauco C. Prevalence of stress, anxiety and depression in with Alzheimer caregivers. Health and Quality of Life Outcomes. 2008;**6**:93. DOI: 10.1186/1477-7525-6-93

[17] Langa KM, Chernew ME, Kabeto MU, Herzog AR, Ofstedal MB, Willis RJ, et al. National estimates of the quantity and cost of informal caregiving for the elderly with dementia. Journal of General Internal Medicine. 2001;**16**:770-778. DOI: 10.1111/j.1525-1497.2001.10123.x

[18] Cooper C, Balamurali T, Livingston G. A systematic review of the prevalence and associates of anxiety in caregivers of people with dementia. International Psychogeriatrics. 2007;**19**:175-195. DOI: 10.1017/S1041610206004297

[19] Joling KJ, van Marwijk HW, Veldhuijzen AE, van der Horst HE, Scheltens P, Smit F, et al. The two-year incidence of depression and anxiety disorders in spousal caregivers of persons with dementia: Who is at the greatest risk? The American Journal of Geriatric Psychiatry. 2015;**23**:293-303. DOI: 10.1016/j.jagp.2014.05.005

[20] Cuijpers P, Vogelzangs N, Twisk J, Kleiboer A, Li J, Penninx BW. Differential mortality rates in major and subthreshold depression: Meta-analysis of studies that measured both. British Journal of Psychiatry. 2013;**202**:22-27. DOI: 10.1192/bjp.bp.112.112169

[21] Cuijpers P. Depressive disorders in caregivers of dementia patients: A systematic review. Aging Ment Health. 2005;**9**:325-330. DOI: 10.1080/13607860500090078

[22] Beeson RA. Loneliness and depression in spousal caregivers of those with Alzheimer's disease versus non-caregiving spouses. Archives of Psychiatric Nursing. 2003;**17**:135-143. DOI: 10.1016/S0883-9417(03)00057-8

[23] Covinsky KE, Newcomer R, Fox P, Wood J, Sands L, Dane K, et al. Patient and caregiver characteristics associated with depression in caregivers of patients with dementia. Journal of General Internal Medicine. 2003;**18**:1006-1014. DOI: 10.1111/j.1525-1497.2003.30103.x

[24] Russo J, Vitaliano PP, Brewer DD, Katon W, Becker J. Psychiatric disorders in spouse caregivers of care recipients with Alzheimer's disease and matched controls: A diathesis-stress model of psychopathology. Journal of Abnormal Psychology. 1995;**104**:197-204. DOI: 10.1037/0021-843X.104.1.197

[25] McCurry SM, Logsdon RG, Teri L, Vitiello MV. Sleep disturbances in caregivers of persons with dementia: Contributing factors and treatment implications. Sleep Medicine Reviews. 2007;**11**:143-153. DOI: 10.1016/j.smrv.2006.09.002

[26] Simón MA, Bueno AM, Otero P, Blanco V, Vázquez FL. Insomnia in female family caregivers of totally dependent patients with dementia: An exploratory study. Women Health. Forthcoming

[27] Worden JW. Grief Counselling and Grief Therapy. A Handbook for the Mental Health Practitioner. New York: Springer Publishing Company; 1997

[28] Feigin VL, Forouzanfar MH, Krishnamurthi R, Mensah GA, Connor M, Bennett DA, et al. Global and regional burden of stroke during 1990-2010: Findings from the Global Burden of Disease Study 2010. Lancet. 2014;**383**:245-255. DOI: 10.1016/S01406736(13)61953-4

[29] Kreutzer JS, Gervasio AH, Camplair PS. Primary caregivers' psychological status and family functioning after traumatic brain injury. Brain Injury. 1994;**8**:197-210. DOI: 10.3109/02699059409150973

[30] Anderson C, Linto J, Stewart-Wynne EG. A population-based assessment of the impact and burden of caregiving for long-term stroke survivors. Stroke. 1995;**26**:843-849. DOI: 10.1161/01.STR.26.5.843

[31] Atteih S, Mellon L, Hall P, Brewer L, Horgan F, Williams D, et al. Implications of stroke for caregiver outcomes: Findings from the ASPIRE-S study. International Journal of Stroke. 2015;**10**:918-923. DOI: 10.1111/ijs.12535

[32] Peeters W, van den Brande R, Polinder S, Brazinova A, Steyerberg EW, Lingsma HF, et al. Epidemiology of traumatic brain injury in Europe. Acta Neurochirurgica. 2015;**157**:1683-1696. DOI: 10.1007/s00701-015-2512-7

[33] Centers for Disease Control and Prevention. Rates of TBI-related Emergency Department Visits, hospitalizations, and deaths – United States, 2001-2010 [Internet]. Available from: https://www.cdc.gov/traumaticbraininjury/data/rates.html [Accessed: March 19, 2017]

[34] Douglas JM, Spellacy FJ. Correlates of depression in adults with severe traumatic brain injury and their carers. Brain Injury. 2000;**14**:71-88. DOI: 10.1080/026990500120943

[35] Marsh NV, Kersel DA, Havill JH, Sleigh JW. Caregiver burden at 6 months following severe traumatic brain injury. Brain Injury. 1998;**12**:225-238. DOI: 10.1080/026990598122700

[36] Riley GA. Stress and depression in family carers following traumatic brain injury: The influence of beliefs about difficult behaviours. Clinical Rehabilitation. 2007;**21**:82-88. DOI: 10.1177/0269215506071279

[37] Wells R, Dywan J, Dumas J. Life satisfaction and distress in family caregivers as related to specific behavioural changes after traumatic brain injury. Brain Injury. 2005;**19**:1105-1115. DOI: 10.1080/02699050500150062

[38] Grant JS, Elliott TR, Weaver M, Glandon GL, Raper JL, Giger JN. Social support, social problem-solving abilities, and adjustment of family caregivers of stroke survivors. Archives of Physical Medicine and Rehabilitation. 2006;**87**:343-350. DOI: 10.1016/j.apmr.2005.09.019

[39] Ohaeri, JU. The burden of caregiving in families with a mental illness: A review of 2002. Current Opinion in Psychiatry. 2003;**16**:457-465. DOI: 10.1097/01.yco.0000079212.36371.c0

[40] Song LY, Biegel DE, Milligan SE. Predictors of depressive symptomatology among lower social class caregivers of persons with chronic mental illness. Community Mental Health Journal. 1997;**33**:269-286. DOI: 10.1023/A:1025090906696

[41] Kessler RC, Berglund PA, Demler O, Jin R, Merikangas KR, Walters EE. Lifetime prevalence and age-of-onset distributions of DSM-IV disorders in the National Comorbidity Survey Replication (NCS-R). Archives of General Psychiatry. 2005;**62**:593-602. DOI: 10.1001/archpsyc.62.6.593

[42] Steele A, Maruyama N, Galynker I. Psychiatric symptoms in caregivers of patients with bipolar disorder: A review. Journal of Affective Disorders. 2010;**121**:10-21. DOI: 10.1016/j.jad.2009.04.020

[43] Perlick DA, Rosenheck RA, Miklowitz DJ, Chessick C, Wolff N, Kaczynski R, et al. Prevalence and correlates of burden among caregivers of patients with bipolar disorder enrolled in the Systematic Treatment Enhance Program for Bipolar Disorder. Bipolar Disorders. 2007;**9**:262-273. DOI: 10.1111/j.1399-5618.2007.00365.x

[44] Perlick DA, Miklowitz DJ, Link BG, Struening E, Kaczynski R, Gonzalez J, et al. Perceived stigma and depression among caregivers of patients with bipolar disorder. British Journal of Psychiatry. 2007;**190**:535-536. DOI: 10.1192/bjp.bp.105.020826

[45] World Health Organization (WHO). Schizophrenia [Internet]. Available from: http://www.who.int/mental_health/management/schizophrenia/en/ [Accessed: March 20, 2017]

[46] Ochoa S, Vilaplana M, Haro JM, Villalta-Gil V, Martinez F, Negredo MC, et al. Do needs, symptoms or disability of outpatients with schizophrenia influence family burden? Social Psychiatry and Psychiatric Epidemiology. 2008;**43**:612-618. DOI: 10.1007/s00127-008-0337-x

[47] Weitzencamp DA, Gerhart KA, Charlifue SW, Whiteneck GG, Savic G. Spouses of spinal cord injury survivors: The added impact of caregiving. Archives of Physical Medicine and Rehabilitation. 1997;**78**:822-827. DOI: 10.1016/S0003-9993(97)90194-5

[48] Stambrook M, MacBeath S, Moore AD, Peters LC, Zubek E, Friesen IC. Social role functioning following spinal cord injury. Paraplegia. 1991;**29**:318-323. DOI: 10.1038/sc.1991.46

[49] Crewe NM, Krause JS. Marital relationships and spinal cord injury. Archives of Physical Medicine and Rehabilitation. 1988;**69**:435-438

[50] World Health Organization (WHO). Visual Impairment and Blindness. Fact Sheet No. 282 [Internet]. [Updated: 2014]. Available from: http://www.who.int/mediacentre/factsheets/fs282/en/ [Accessed: March 20, 2017]

[51] Braich PS, Lal V, Hollands S, Almeida DR. Burden and depression in the caregivers of blind patients in India. Ophthalmology. 2012;**119**:221-226. DOI: 10.1016/j.ophtha.2011.07.038

[52] Khan Z, Braich PS, Rahim K, Rayat JS, Xing L, Iqbal M, et al. Burden and depression among caregivers of visually impaired patients in a Canadian population. Advances in Medicine. 2016;**2016**:4683427. DOI: 10.1155/2016/4683427

[53] World Health Organization (WHO). Cancer. Fact Sheet [Internet]. 2017.Available from: http://www.who.int/mediacentre/factsheets/fs297/en/ [Accessed: February 8, 2017]

[54] Kurtz ME, Kurtz JC, Given CW, Given B. Relationship of caregiver reactions and depression to cancer patients' symptoms, functional states and depression – A longitudinal view. Social Science & Medicine. 1995;**40**:837-846. DOI: 10.1016/0277-9536(94)00249-S

[55] Nijboer C, Tempelaar R, Sanderman R, Triemstra M, Spruijt RJ, van den Bos, GA. Cancer and caregiving: The impact on the caregiver's health. Psycho-oncology. 1998;**7**:3-13. DOI: 10.1002/(SICI)1099-1611(199801/02)7:1<3::AID-PON320>3.0.CO;2-5

[56] Sklenarova H, Krümpelmann A, Haun MW, Friederich HC, Huber J, Thomas M, et al. When do we need to care about the caregiver? Supportive care needs, anxiety, and depression among informal caregivers of patients with cancer and cancer survivors. Cancer. 2015;**121**:1513-1519. DOI: 10.1002/cncr.29223

[57] Grov EK, Dahl AA, Moum T, Fosså SD. Anxiety, depression, and quality of life in caregivers of patients with cancer in late palliative phase. Annals of Oncology. 2005;**16**:1185-1191. DOI: 10.1093/annonc/mdi210

[58] Valeberg BT, Grov EK. Symptoms in the cancer patient: Of importance for their caregivers' quality of life and mental health? European Journal of Oncology Nursing. 2013;**17**:46-51. DOI: 10.1016/j.ejon.2012.01.009

[59] Given B, Wyatt G, Given C, Gift A, Sherwood P, DeVoss D, et al. Burden and depression among caregivers of patients with cancer at the end of life. Oncology Nursing Forum. 2004;**31**:1105-1117. DOI: 10.1188/04.ONF.1105-1117

[60] Logroscino G, Traynor BJ, Hardiman O, Chió A, Mitchell D, Swingler RJ, et al. Incidence of amyotrophic lateral sclerosis in Europe. Journal of Neurology Neurosurgery and Psychiatry. 2010;**81**:385-390. DOI: 101136/jnnp.2009.183525

[61] Centers for Disease Control and Prevention. Prevalence of amyotrophic lateral sclerosis – United States, 2012-2013. Morbidity and Mortality Weekly Report. 2016;**65**:1-12

[62] Zarei S, Carr K, Reiley L, Diaz K, Guerra O, Altamirano PF, et al. A comprehensive review of amyotrophic lateral sclerosis. Surgical Neurology International. 2015;**6**:171. DOI: 10.4103/2152-7806.169561

[63] Rabkin JG, Albert SM, Rowland LP, Mitsumoto H. How common is depression among ALS caregivers? A longitudinal study. Amyotrophic Lateral Sclerosis. 2009;**10**:448-455. DOI: 10.3109/17482960802459889

[64] Miyashita M, Narita Y, Sakamoto A, Kawada N, Akiyama M, Kayama M, et al. Care burden and depression in caregivers caring for patients with intractable neurological diseases at home in Japan. Journal of the Neurological Sciences. 2009;**276**:148-152. DOI: 10.1016/j.jns.2008.09.022

[65] Trail M, Nelson ND, Van JN, Appel SH, Lai EC. A study comparing patients with amyotrophic lateral sclerosis and their caregivers on measures of quality of life, depression, and their attitudes toward treatment options. Journal of the Neurological Sciences. 2003;**209**:79-85. DOI: 10.1016/S0022-510X(03)00003-0

[66] Lillo P, Mioshi E, Hodges JR. Caregiver burden in amyotrophic lateral sclerosis is more dependent on patients' behavioural changes than physical disability: A comparative study. BMC Neurology. 2012;**12**:156. DOI: 10.1186/1471-2377-12-156

[67] Vignola A, Guzzo A, Calvo A, Moglia C, Pessia A, Cavallo E, et al. Anxiety undermines quality of life in ALS patients and caregivers. European Journal of Neurology. 2008;**15**:1231-1236. DOI: 10.1111/j.1468-1331.2008.02303.x

[68] Almansour MA, Alateeq MA, Alzahrani MK, Algeffari MA, Alhomaidan HT. Depression and anxiety among parents and caregivers of autistic spectral disorder children. Neurosciences. 2013;**18**:58-63

[69] Elsabbagh M, Divan G, Koh YJ, Kim YS, Kauchali S, Marcín C, et al. Global prevalence of autism and other pervasive developmental disorders. Autism Research. 2012;**5**:160-179. DOI: 10.1002/aur.239

[70] Barker ET, Hartley SL, Seltzer MM, Floyd FJ, Greenberg JS, Orsmond GI. Trajectories of emotional well-being in mothers of adolescents and adults with autism. Developmental Psychology. 2011;**47**:551-561. DOI: 10.1037/a0021268

[71] Singer GH. Meta-analysis of comparative studies of depression in mothers of children with and without developmental disabilities. American Journal of Mental Retardation. 2006;**111**:155-169. DOI: 10.1352/0895-8017(2006)111[155:MOCSOD]2.0.CO;2

[72] Levacalier L, Leone S, Wiltz J. The impact of behaviour problems on caregiver stress in young people with autism spectrum disorders. Journal of Intellectual Disability Research. 2006;**50**:172-182. DOI: 10.1111/j.1365-2788.2005.00732.x

[73] Müller-Spahn F. Behavioral disturbances in dementia. Dialogues in Clinical Neuroscience. 2003;**5**:49-59

[74] Rabins PV. Behavioral disturbances of dementia: Practical and conceptual issues. International Psychogeriatrics. 1996;**8**:281-283. DOI: 10.1017/S1041610297003487

[75] Clipp EC, George LK. Dementia and cancer: A comparison of spouse caregivers. Gerontologist. 1993;**33**:534-541. DOI: 10.1093/geront/33.4.534

[76] Ory MG, Hoffman RR, Yee JL, Tennstedt S, Schulz R. Prevalence and impact of caregiving: A detailed comparison between dementia and nondementia caregivers. Gerontologist. 1999;**39**:177-185. DOI: 10.1093/geront/39.2.177

[77] Crespo M, López J, Zarit SH. Depression and anxiety in primary caregivers: A comparative study of caregivers of demented and nondemented older persons. International Journal of Geriatric Psychiatry. 2005;**20**:591-592. DOI: 10.1002/gps.1321

[78] Papastavrou E, Charalambous A, Tsangari H, Karayiannis G. The burdensome and depressive experience of caring: what cancer, schizophrenia, and Alzheimer's disease caregivers have in common. Cancer Nursing. 2012;**35**:187-194. DOI: 10.1097/NCC.0b013e31822cb4a0

[79] Loi SM, Dow B, Moore K, Hill K, Russell M, Cyarto E. The adverse mental health of carers: Does the patient diagnosis play a role? Maturitas. 2015;**82**:134-138. DOI: 10.1016/j.maturitas.2015.06.034

[80] Family Caregiver Alliance. Take Care of You: Self Care for Family Caregivers [Internet]. Available at https://www.caregiver.org/taking-care-you-self-care-family-caregivers [Accessed: April 18, 2017]

[81] Family Caregiver Alliance. Depression and Caregiving [Internet]. Available at https://www.caregiver.org/depression-and-caregiving [Accessed: April 19, 2017]

[82] Pinquart M, Sörensen S. Helping caregivers of persons with dementia: Which interventions work and how large are their effects? International Psychogeriatrics. 2006;**18**:577-595. DOI: 10.1017/S1041610206003462

[83] Sörensen S, Duberstein P, Gill D, Pinquart M. Dementia care: Mental health effects, intervention strategies, and clinical implications. The Lancet Neurology. 2006;**5**:961-973. DOI: 10.1016/S1474-4422(06)70599-3

[84] Otero P, Smit F, Cuijpers P, Torres A, Blanco V, Vázquez FL. Long-term efficacy of indicated prevention of depression in non-professional caregivers: Randomized controlled trial. Psychological Medicine. 2015;**45**:1401-1412. DOI: 10.1017/S0033291714002505

[85] Vázquez FL, Torres A, Blanco V, Otero P, Díaz O, Ferraces MJ. Long-term follow-up of a randomized clinical trial assessing the efficacy of a brief cognitive-behavioral depression prevention intervention for caregivers with elevated depressive symptoms. The American Journal of Geriatric Psychiatry. 2016;**24**:421-432. DOI: 10.1016/j.jagp.2016.02.050

[86] Blanco V, Rohde P, Vázquez FL, Torres A. Identification of caregivers at greatest risk of major depression in two prevention studies. Psychotherapy Research. 2014;**24**:578-593. DOI: 10.1080/10503307.2013.847989

[87] Otero P, Smit F, Cuijpers P, DeRubeis RJ, Torres A, Vázquez FL. Differential response to depression prevention among a sample of informal caregivers: Moderator analysis of longer-term follow-up trial data. Psychiatry Research. 2015;**230**:271-278. DOI: 10.1016/j.psychres.2015.09.005

[88] Blanco V, Otero P, López L, Torres A, Vázquez FL. Predictores del cambio clínicamente significativo en una intervención de prevención de la depresión [Clinically significant predictors of change in an intervention for the prevention of depression]. Revista Iberoamericana de Psicología y Salud. 2017;**8**:9-20. DOI: 10.23923/j.rips.2017.08.002

[89] Otero P, Vázquez FL, Hermida E, Díaz O, Torres A. Relationship of cognitive behavioral therapy effects and homework in an indicated prevention of depression intervention for non-professional caregivers. Psychological Reports. 2015;**116**:841-854. DOI: 10.2466/02.PR0.116k22w7

[90] Vázquez FL, Torres A, Otero P, Blanco V, Díaz O, Estévez LE. Analysis of the components of a cognitive-behavioral intervention administered via conference call for preventing depression among non-professional caregivers: A pilot study. Aging and Mental Health. Advanced online. DOI: 10.1080/13607863.2016.1181714

[91] Zarit S, Femia E. Behavioral and psychosocial interventions for family caregivers. American Journal of Nursing. 2008;**108**:47-53. DOI: 10.1097/01.NAJ.0000336415.60495.34

9

# Overburden in Alzheimer's Patient Caregivers

María del Carmen Pérez-Fuentes,
María del Mar Molero Jurado and
José Jesús Gázquez Linares

**Abstract**

The figure of the caregiver of dependent elderly people is presently the subject of a large volume of scientific publications. In various disciplines of health and social sciences, an analysis of the terminology referring to these caregivers, specifically those who are untrained and unpaid for such care, in recent scientific publications, is considered necessary. This chapter makes a comprehensive analysis of the characteristics and needs of caregivers of elderly dependents with Alzheimer's disease. From a realistic and practical point of view, it is the impact of research on improving the quality of life of caregivers which is important. In addition, this analysis attempts to complete a process addressing theoretical and methodological aspects, in which various problems are detected, for their effective application in the field of care of dependency.

**Keywords:** overburden, Alzheimer's patients, caregivers, intervention, quality of life

## 1. Introduction

Sometimes, living longer involves dependence on care in which the needs become more and more obvious. One of the most frequent causes of such dependency in the elderly population is Alzheimer's disease. Over 35 million people were suffering from some type of dementia in 2010 and world forecasts for 2030 and 2050 double and triple this figure, respectively [1]. In this urgent scope of action, the World Health Organization [2] takes a stand by identifying dementia as one of today's priority public health problems.

Even though there are a multitude of care models and resources placed at the service of these patients [3, 4], a large part of this population receives care within their own family setting [5]. This is why the volume of research analyzing the profile of the family caregiver, skills for their patient's care, and improving their relationship with the patient has intensified [6]. In this field, the concept of caregiver overburden [7] and its repercussion on their physical and mental health, social relations, mood, etc., as well as their quality of life [8], is of special interest.

This chapter provides a complete analysis of the characteristics and needs of the caregivers of the elderly who have become dependent because of Alzheimer's disease. All of this is from a realistic and practical viewpoint that what is important is the repercussion of research on the improvement of the quality of life of the caregiver. Furthermore, this analysis attempts to make a complete review covering all the theoretical and methodological where problems are found in their effective application in the area of care of dependency.

First, the terminology used to refer to the different caregiver profiles is reviewed, and the problem which could arise in research on the subject as a consequence is analyzed. Once the specific profile to be studied has been identified, the needs that should be considered in an intervention for this specific caregiver typology are discussed. At this point, having set the basis for intervention, we propose an inventory for evaluating caregiver overburden in Alzheimer's patient family caregivers who have no specialized training.

## 2. Conceptual approach to the concept of caregiver

The term "care" is widely used and has been studied from different approaches, especially in the areas of study which refer to overburden of the caregiver [9–11], associated factors [12–15], or instruments for its measure [16–18].

On a conceptual level, the contributions of Heidegger [19] in developing the phenomenological concepts of care and cure are significant. From this perspective, care becomes the way in which human beings exert control over themselves, or, in other words, feel that they are in possession of their own existence or not. In this phenomenological discourse, the relationship established between lifestyle and state of health-illness is important to the extent that they are closely related to care. It is precisely through care behavior that daily structure is formed, where man is positioned between satisfaction of his needs and health.

As inferred from Heidegger's theoretical proposal, although the action of caring for someone is inherent in human nature, the concept as such is relatively new. This novel character of the terminology related to care reveals difficulties in its operationalization and its limits for use in the concept of caregiver, especially in research [20].

The traditional definitions of caregiver have been characterized by elements related directly to the tasks typical of caregiving [21]. Nevertheless, sometimes emotional aspects are included, which, according to authors such as Pearlin et al. [22], are inevitably present in the caregiving relationship. These authors define caregiving as "the behavior expression of commitment to the wellbeing or protection of another person" (p. 583).

## 2.1. Types of "family" caregivers

In spite of the surge in the concept of the caregiver since the 1970s, to date, there is a wide diversity in the terms used synonymously in the literature, making this a concept vulnerable to lack of specificity [23].

In the study of the concept of the caregiver, attention has been given to the skills necessary to perform the work [24], the consequences or impact it has on their well-being [25], and even the profile itself [26]. But in any case, it deals with a word that maintains a close bond with the family.

Family care models, in which one member undertakes care of another who has become dependent, make family dynamics a variable of interest [27]. Such is the bond created between the caregiver and his relative that in fact studies have revealed that even after the patient has been admitted to an institution, the relatives still keep acting as caregivers [28].

Starting out from the family context as the source of care, different questions may be asked which lead to different senses of the term. The most basic would be the answer to the question, who is providing the care? In this case, there are two specific possibilities, a relative or someone in the immediate social circle, such as neighbors, family friends, etc. In any case, it is someone significant to the person receiving the care.

Some of the terms identified in the literature include the concept "informal caregiver," and characterize them as those who perform the work of caring for dependent persons in their home, without being associated to any health care and/or service entity [29].

When full responsibility for care falls on a single person, normally someone in the immediate social circle, without training in the tasks of caregiving and for which no payment is received, some authors [30] use the term "primary informal caregiver."

Although they sound similar, and their meanings are as well, the use of the terms "primary" and "main" caregiver is differentiated.

"Primary caregiver" is discussed in the literature with regard to attention to the most immediate and basic needs (physical and emotional), with affective involvement, and therefore an important figure for the person receiving care [31–33]. Other studies have chosen the term "main caregiver," but with the same characteristics as the first. That is, again, a person who is close to the recipient and gives priority attention to their physical and emotional needs in a commitment to continuous assistance [34, 35].

Another question that could be derived from the use of different terms is with regard to the type of work done by the caregiver [36]. For example, while some caregiving work may need to be meticulous, other tasks deal with protection or help. The view of the patient is also different depending on the term applied. Assistance is directed at a necessarily vulnerable individual and/or who is unprotected, whereas the term attention is oriented toward a goal of intervention, more toward action than covering primary needs. Thus, the particular use of concepts, such as help, care, assistance, or attention, becomes the basis of the ambiguity in which the caregiver works.

### 2.2. The main caregiver of elderly dependents

Caregivers form a social class in itself [37]. From this perspective, different models are proposed for analyzing the figure of the main caregiver, with direct involvement in intervention and help strategies.

The caregiver-resource model defines the main caregiver as an instrument for optimizing attention given to the dependent, so their well-being falls onto a second plane. In this case, the purpose of intervention is to maintain or increase informal help as much as possible. Thus, caregivers are trained in patient needs and how to care for them, that is, provide them with the skills necessary to perform caregiving work adequately. Professional caregivers may often include family members who give care as a resource collaborating in the dependent person's care [38].

In the caregiver-client model, the recipient is understood as a secondary receiver of formal services. Therefore, the need argued is for the main caregiver to have recourse to services during intervention that improve their quality of life and decrease the negative impact of caregiving on their own well-being. From this perspective, interventions would include the main caregiver as a vulnerable agent, and therefore with important needs that have to be covered by help and/or relief services, alternative service resources, and training in strategies to lessen overburden [39].

To start with, the care of a family member in one's own home is something conceived of as natural, to the extent that it is a responsibility expected from the family. However, if the caregivers do not have social help or do not have access to the resources necessary for it, they are going to be compelled to develop "home" remedies for their care and to transform/adapt their homes [40], which are then no longer natural contexts for the family to live together in, and become a substitute for a service center.

Since the beginning of the century, there has been exponential growth in the population over 65 years of age and a noticeable increase in those over 80 [41]. Demographic reports show the prevalence and incidence of illnesses that are plainly higher in the more advanced age groups, as well as chronicity, disability, and dependency rates. Neurological pathologies are one of the most costly groups of diseases for the health-care system and for the society as a whole, since in addition to the process of the illness itself, there is a psychological impact, diminishing quality of life, disability for work, loss of social skills, and the burden of caregivers and dependency (p. 175) [42].

### 2.3. Review of the terminology used to refer to the caregiver in scientific publications

At the present time, the figure of the caregiver of elderly dependents is the subject of a large volume of scientific publications [43]. In various health-care and social science disciplines, the terminology used to refer to caregivers is often confusing [44]. Some of the difficulties identified on a conceptual level of care are related to the lack of operative definitions and terminology incoherent with its multidimensional character [45] and the concept of overburden [46]. From a more operative approach to the design of effective intervention with caregivers, it may be said that the existence of problems for its conceptual delimitation leads to trouble differentiating case-specific care typologies [47]. This specificity in data processing is precisely a characteristic which should be present from the moment a study is proposed, directed toward a specific type of care, instead of a generic typology which is only theoretically common to all caregivers [48].

From this viewpoint, the terminology referring to the caregiver, especially for those who have no technical training and are unpaid for their caregiving labor, must be analyzed in recent scientific publications. Therefore, a review of the terminology used in scientific publications on the subject was done to provide data on the current state of the problem described [49].

The study methodology consisted of systematically reviewing scientific literature on the subject. Publications in several different international databases were reviewed for this, comparing two production periods, 1996–2005 and 2006–2016.

Given the characteristics and scope of database coverage, the descriptors in Spanish and/or English ("family caregivers," "informal caregivers," and "non-professional caregivers") are presented. For all cases, it is limited to the search in the title of the document. In addition, the results were filtered by the document type "journal article," and were limited to the search at the time interval. As for the language of the publication, the options "Spanish" and "English" were selected in the databases that have this filter, and they were manually revised in the cases for which they did not have this function. On the other hand, for the selection of publications, the inclusion criteria are established, which were applied in the manual review of the titles, in each of the databases. The established inclusion criteria were as follows: (1) journal articles, (2) papers published in Spanish or English, and (3) containing the title of the descriptors used. On the other hand, for the exclusion criteria, the following were applied: (1) work that deals with the care of a relative, but does not include the terminology analyzed in the title, and (2) works published in a language other than Spanish or English.

The preliminary results suggest a more frequent use of the term "family caregiver" in publications, both in English and in Spanish. At the same time, differences were detected in the use of terminology, with attention to variables such as production period, subject matter, and type of journal. The Z-statistic was applied for comparative analysis to check for significant differences in percentages.

First, examining the scientific production periods (**Table 1**), it is observed that in general, the volume of publications including the descriptors (both in Spanish and in English) in the title was higher in 2006–2016. However, when the percentages of the two periods are compared, the term "family caregivers" (in Spanish) is significantly more representative ($Z = 3.91$; $p < 0.001$) in 1996–2005 than in 2006–2016. The same thing occurred for the English descriptor ("family caregivers"), which was significantly higher ($Z = 4.48$; $p < 0.001$) than in 2006–2016.

The percentage use of the descriptor "non-professional caregivers" (in Spanish) was also significantly higher ($Z = -2.02$; $p < 0.05$) in 2006–2016. It was also in this second period when a significantly higher percentage ($Z = 6.84$; $p < 0.001$) of the descriptor "informal caregivers" appeared in the titles.

| Descriptors | 1996–2005 | | 2006–2016 | |
|---|---|---|---|---|
| | *N* | % | *N* | % |
| "family caregivers" (in Spanish) | 65 | 3.66 | 104 | 2 |
| "non-professional caregivers" (in Spanish) | 0 | 0 | 12 | 0.23 |
| "informal caregivers" (in Spanish) | 39 | 2.19 | 124 | 2.39 |
| "family caregivers" | 1430 | 80.60 | 3907 | 75.39 |
| "non-professional caregivers" | 1 | 0.05 | 17 | 0.32 |
| "informal caregivers" | 239 | 13.47 | 1018 | 19.64 |
| **Total** | 1774 | 100 | 5182 | 100 |

**Table 1.** Number of publications containing descriptors in the title by production period.

No significant differences in the total percentages of the number of publications that included each of the descriptors in the title by subject (Health Sciences and Social Sciences) were found for any of them in 2006–2016. However, the descriptor which appeared the most in the title was "family caregivers" (in Spanish) in both Health Sciences and Social Sciences (**Table 2**).

In Health Sciences, the descriptor most used in nursing publications was "family caregivers" (in Spanish) ($n$ = 34), followed by "informal caregivers" (in Spanish) ($n$ = 21). In Geriatrics, "informal caregivers" (in Spanish) was in first place ($n$ = 6) followed by "informal caregivers" ($n$ = 3) in second.

The secondary subject matter Generalities stressed more frequent use by publications that included the descriptor "family caregivers" (in Spanish) ($n$ = 10) in the title, followed by "informal caregivers" (in Spanish) ($n$ = 3).

On the other hand, in the Social Sciences, in Psychology, the term most frequently used was "family caregivers" (in Spanish) ($n$ = 16) and second "informal caregivers" (in Spanish) ($n$ = 8).

| Descriptors | Health Sciences | | Social Sciences | |
|---|---|---|---|---|
| | *N* | % | *N* | % |
| "cuidadores familiares" (in Spanish) | 48 | 44.85 | 17 | 44.73 |
| "cuidadores no profesionales" (in Spanish) | 2 | 1.86 | 3 | 7.89 |
| "cuidadores informales" (in Spanish) | 35 | 32.71 | 15 | 39.47 |
| "family caregivers" | 19 | 17.75 | 3 | 7.89 |
| "non-professional caregivers" | 0 | 0 | 0 | 0 |
| "informal caregivers" | 3 | 2.80 | 0 | 0 |
| **Total** | 107 | | 38 | |

By authors. Source: Dialnet database (2006/2016).

**Table 2.** Number of publications containing the descriptors in the title by subject.

This one "informal caregivers" (in Spanish) was also in first place ($n = 7$) in Sociology/Social Work, followed by the term "non-professional caregivers" (in Spanish) ($n = 2$).

Finally, the number of articles that contain each of the descriptors in the title, classified by journal (**Table 3**), shows a trend toward the preferential use of the term "family caregivers" (in Spanish) in nursing journals (Aquichan, International Nursing Review, and Index de Enfermería), Geriatrics (Gerokomos and Revista Española de Geriatría y Gerontología), and psychology/education/multidisciplinary (Anales de Psicología and European Journal of Investigation in Health, Psychology and Education).

| Descriptors | Journals | No. of titles |
|---|---|---|
| "cuidadores familiares" (in Spanish) | Aquichan | 6 |
| | Gerokomos: Revista de la Sociedad Española de Enfermería Geriátrica y Gerontológica | 3 |
| | International Nursing Review | 3 |
| | Index de Enfermería | 2 |
| | Revista Española de Geriatría y Gerontología | 2 |
| | Revista Ciencia y Cuidado | 2 |
| | Anales de Psicología | 2 |
| | European Journal of Investigation in Health, Psychology and Education | 2 |
| | Investigación y Educación en Enfermería | 1 |
| | Evidentia: Revista de Enfermería basada en la Evidencia | 1 |
| | Respuestas | 1 |
| | Enfermería Global | 1 |
| | Metas de Enfermería | 1 |
| | Cultura de los Cuidados | 1 |
| | Clínica y Salud | 1 |
| | Duazary | 1 |
| | Facultad Nacional de Salud Pública | 1 |
| | Revista de Psicología | 1 |
| | Revista de Calidad Asistencial | 1 |
| "cuidadores no profesionales" (in Spanish) | Revista Española de Geriatría y Gerontología | 1 |
| | Metas de Enfermería | 1 |
| | Clínica y Salud | 1 |
| | Estudios Financieros: Revista de trabajo y seguridad social | 1 |
| | Humanismo y Trabajo Social | 1 |
| | Revista de Derecho Social | 1 |
| | Revista del Ministerio de Trabajo e Inmigración | 1 |

| Descriptors | Journals | No. of titles |
|---|---|---|
| "cuidadores informales" (in Spanish) | Enfermería Clínica | 2 |
| | Revista ROL de Enfermería | 2 |
| | Enfermería Global | 2 |
| | Trabajo Social y Salud | 2 |
| | Gerokomos: Revista de la Sociedad Española de Enfermería Geriátrica y Gerontológica | 1 |
| | Revista Española de Geriatría y Gerontología | 1 |
| | Revista Multidisciplinar de Gerontología | 1 |
| | International Journal of Developmental and Educational Psychology | 1 |
| | Aquichan | 1 |
| | Hygia de Enfermería | 1 |
| | Actas Españolas de Psiquiatría | 1 |
| | International Nursing Review | 1 |
| | Metas de Enfermería | 1 |
| | Neurología | 1 |
| "family caregivers" | Research in Nursing and Health | 4 |
| | Cancer Nursing an International Journal for Cancer Care | 4 |
| | Revista de Pesquisa: Cuidado é Fundamental online | 4 |
| | Investigación y Educación en Enfermería | 3 |
| | Journal of the American Geriatrics Society | 2 |
| | Nursing Research, an AJN Company Publication | 2 |
| | Aquichan | 1 |
| | American Journal of Occupational Therapy | 1 |
| | Sociology of Health & Illness | 1 |
| "informal caregivers" | Journal of the American Geriatrics Society | 3 |
| | Documentos de Trabajo (FEDEA) | 1 |
| | Cancer Nursing an International Journal for Cancer Care | 1 |

By author. Source: Dialnet database (2006/2016).

**Table 3.** Number of publications with the descriptors in the title by journal.

In addition to representative journals in the disciplines mentioned above, the descriptor "family caregivers" (in Spanish) was found in titles in journals in other disciplines, such as law (Revista de Derecho Social) and social work (Estudios Financieros, Humanismo y Trabajo Social, and Revista del Ministerio de Trabajo e Inmigración).

The term "informal caregivers" (in Spanish) was used the most as part of the titles published in nursing journals (Enfermería Clínica, Rol de Enfermería, and Enfermería Global) and social work (Trabajo Social y Salud).

Of the two English descriptors, more titles were found with "family caregivers," most of them in nursing journals (Research in Nursing and Health, Cancer Nursing and International Journal for Cancer Care, and Revista de Pesquisa Cuidado è Fundamental Online).

When the descriptor "informal caregivers" was entered, the most frequent presence was found in publications in geriatrics journals (Journal of the American Geriatrics Society). Finally, no journals with publications that included the term "non-professional caregivers" in the title were found in the database searched dated in the last decade.

These data suggest that, in spite of a generalized trend toward the use of the expression "family caregivers" (in Spanish) (and "family caregivers" in English), it would be necessary to review the characteristics of each of the caregiver profiles in each concrete case.

One of the reasons for these differences in the use of terminology could be related to the desire to differentiate this type of caregiver from the assistance provided by health-care professionals [50]. Another of the questions inherent in this diversity of terms is the volume of publications generated in a certain discipline. Since, as seen in the data found by subject matter (and secondary subjects), even though not significant, differences were observed in the use of terms such as "non-professional caregivers" (in Spanish), more frequent in the social sciences (especially sociology and social work). This diverse use of the terminology also occurs in journals published in different scientific disciplines and/or professional fields.

In brief, the trend in the use of terminology associated with caregivers without technical training who are unpaid for their work has been identified and described. The need for updating terms and a proposal for alternatives sufficiently operative to overcome the difficulties in comparing the results of different studies where concepts related to caregiving are dealt with are justified.

## 3. Needs for intervention in the family caregiver without specialized training: variables related to overburden levels

Alzheimer's disease continues at present to be the most frequent type of dementia and one of the main causes of dependency in the population over 65 years of age [51]. It affects all the dimensions of life (emotional, cognitive, and social) of the patients, and in turn leads to a series of consequences which make it extensive to their closest family setting [52]. Therefore, it is of interest to analyze the patient-caregiver relationship to find out the feelings present in the caregiver, as a result of interaction with the patient [53]. Caron and Caron [54] found that the family response to the impact of the diagnosis may vary from negation to overprotection and even aggressiveness in care. According to the authors, all this would be to reduce the anxiety which incoherencies in interaction with the patient can cause.

Information on the diagnosis of Alzheimer's disease is currently under debate, with no unanimity yet arrived at. The details that surround the communication of the diagnosis are complicated, and affect both the patient and caregivers [55]. Scientific literature on the subject has found advantages in making and communicating the diagnosis to the person affected [56, 57]. Some of these advantages are ending the feeling of uncertainty by knowing the changes they are undergoing better, having information on the course and evolution of the disease, its treatment and the options for care available, as well as taking part in planning short-term goals, and participating in decision-making on care to be received in the more advanced stages.

Some authors believe that communicating Alzheimer's diagnosis to the patient involves more negative effects than positive. Some of the arguments from this perspective refer to the moderate effect of available treatments, lack of understanding as cognitive deterioration progresses, in addition to a diagnosis based on probability, so knowledge of the diagnosis could have negative effects on the health of the person affected [58].

It is usually thought that a timely, precise explanation of the diagnosis and its implications is basic to better planning and management of the disease [59]. In the study Who cares? [60], in which caregivers were asked what type of information they received in the diagnosis, half of them provided information on the disease and the medication available. However, few of them received any information on the resources and help available to the caregiver.

After the critical moment of the diagnosis, the caregiver is left in a situation of uncertainty and uneasiness. This is due in part to ignorance of the disease and the care it requires. In this situation, prior beliefs the caregiver has about the disease may positively or negatively influence the feeling of burden. Along this line, some authors [61] affirm that the more negative beliefs of the caregiver are, the more likely intense feelings of overburden, thereby making the caregiver more vulnerable to stress and anxiety.

In the case of family caregivers, the responsibility for providing quality care and the anxiety of not having technical preparation for it can lead to risk to their mental health [62, 63]. These and other concerns about ignorance of the disease and the care it requires arise at the critical moment of diagnosis of the disease [64], moment at which the caregiver is the most vulnerable to the feeling of burden. Situations such as these become more evident in the case of Alzheimer's patient caregivers, since they have the added difficulty of not having an early diagnosis and the consequent negative impact on emotional responses of the caregiver which usually affect the quality of care. Situations such as these, which become more evident in caregivers of Alzheimer's patients, must have already dealt with the added difficulty of not having an early diagnosis, with the consequent negative impact on the emotional responses of the caregiver, and which usually affect the quality of care. Therefore, training of family caregivers in symptomatology and evolution of the disease, or in the management of daily situations, could reduce the level of overburden and even largely avoid its appearance [65]. It is therefore a matter of providing the caregiver with tools that assist in approaching stressful situations that take place during care and interaction with the patient.

The care of a dependent person is often associated with significant risk to the health and well-being of the caregiver [66]. The burden perceived by the caregiver is related to the functional state of the patient, the time devoted to care, social support, and perception of their own health condition [67]. In a sample of non-professional caregivers, it was observed that almost 50% evaluated their health as poor or very poor [68].

In other cases, more somatic complaints [69], more frequent demand for and use of health-care services and drugs have been found in caregivers [70]. Depression is often a problem in non-professional caregivers; however, the proposals for intervention continue to be mostly palliative [71]. Thus, there are proposals for intervention programs based on solving the problems to prevent clinical depression in family caregivers [72].

Another problem that arises up for caregivers of Alzheimer's patients is variability and evolution of their psychiatric symptoms and behavior, making them more dependent. In this respect, some authors [73] positively correlate this symptomatology with the feeling of burnout in caregivers of this type of patient. The European survey [60] showed that carers found that difficulties in performing daily activities, such as washing, and behavioral symptoms are the most problematic to cope with, and they were the reason for seeking help in just as many cases as cognitive problems. Behavioral symptoms such as aggression and personality changes, which often cause a familiar to behave completely out of normative, are especially distressing for carers.

Given the impact of neurodegenerative diseases such as Alzheimer's, it becomes necessary to give attention to the variables that can deteriorate the main caregiver's well-being, but also to the extent that it is going to have a direct or an indirect repercussion on the quality of care being given, from a psychosocial adjustment approach [74]. Most of the initiatives along this line concentrate on recovering physical health and reestablishing support networks and the personal and social well-being of the caregiver, who after several years of dedication to such care has developed a considerable burden [75].

In short, knowing the specific needs of the caregivers and the real situation of their care is the first step in defining adequate support, not to reduce overburden as much as to avoid its appearance by finding out what the critical needs are from the beginning.

## 4. Evaluation of overburden in caregivers without specialized training in Alzheimer's patients

The above review of both terminology and needs of a specific caregiver profile suggests the necessity for taking another step further and materializing these contributions in the proposal of a burden evaluation instrument that enables approach to the difficulties with which caregivers are faced before they develop into a certain degree of overburden [76].

Although a wide variety of resources for the evaluation of the caregiver's burden is available [17], a stable preference since the decade of the 1990s for the reiterative use of generic scales such as the Zarit has been observed [7].

The Zarit Caregiver Burden Interview (ZBI) was originally an interview for evaluating primary caregivers of patients with dementia. This interview, with items found based on the most frequent areas mentioned by caregivers (according to the experience of the authors themselves), caretaker health, psychological well-being, finances, social life, and social relations, was administered to a sample of caregivers. It consists of 29 items which the caregiver answers with the best choice from "not at all" to "extremely" [77].

The Revised Memory and Behavior Problems Checklist is an instrument designed to evaluate the behavior problems of patients with dementia, although in the original study, the sample was composed of patients and their caregivers. As described by the authors, the instrument may be used for medical, cognitive, or psychological evaluation in any older person. It contains two subscales, one of them concentrating on observable behavior of the patient and the other on the reactions of the caregiver. The test is a 24-item self-report which the caregiver answers on a five-point Likert-type scale. It is reliable and validated, with an alpha of 0.84 for the patient behavior subscale and 0.90 for caregiver burden [78].

The Caregiver Appraisal Inventory (CAI) was derived from two different projects, one in which a relief program for caregivers of persons with dementia was carried out, and another called "institutionalization study," in which they followed the process of caregiving in the time elapsed between the application of the family for admission in an institution and the first month after admission. It is made up of 21 items (two for evaluation of the caregiving domain, 10 for the subjective burden, five for satisfaction or positive aspects of care, and four on impact). Concerning psychometric properties, internal consistency is acceptable on all the subscales [79].

Finally, for construction of the Caregiver Burden Inventory, a sample of caregivers of persons with senile dementia, Alzheimer's, or organic syndrome was used. The CBI establishes a multidimensional five-factor model of burden (related to the restrictions on caregiver time, feelings of being "left out" with respect to their peers, psychological well-being, social, and emotional burden). It is made up of 24 items which the caregiver answers on a four-point Likert-type scale. The psychometric properties found by the authors were a Cronbach's alpha of 0.85 for the time and developmental burden factors, 0.86 on the factor psychological burden, 0.73 on social burden, and 0.77 on emotional burden [80].

In line with the contributions described above, a model is proposed that argues for the development of an instrument to evaluate the specific needs of the family caregiver of Alzheimer's patients [45]. Therefore, the following factors should be considered for early detection of burnout in this concrete profile of caregivers (**Figure 1**). On one hand, the authors propose factors related to the caregiver, such as reaction (feelings) to the diagnosis, physical health, and knowledge of the illness. On the other, attention is given to the factors related to the patient, such as level of dependence. Finally, special attention should be given to the symptomatology,

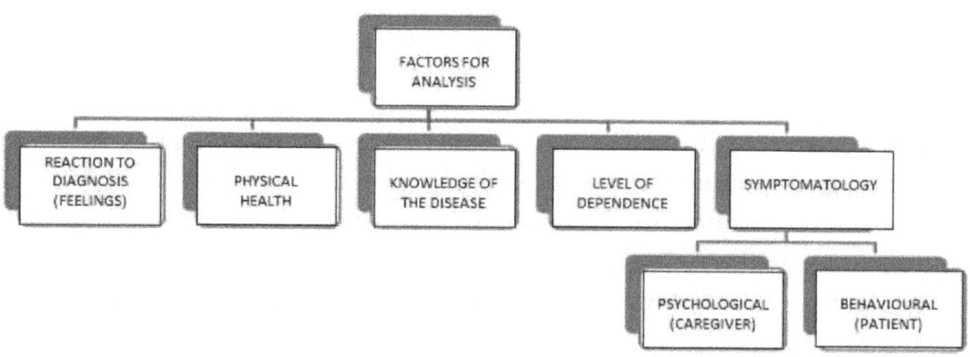


**Figure 1.** Factors of necessary for analysis of the family caregiver.

which in this case is presented as a two-dimensional factor, caretaker psychological symptomatology, and patient-behavioral symptomatology.

From this perspective and for the purpose of validating an instrument for early detection of the needs of family caregivers of Alzheimer-type dementia patients enabling the design of early intervention to avoid overburden syndrome in the caregiver, the Inventario de predictores de sobrecarga en cuidadores familiares sin formación especializada de enfermos de Alzheimer (Overburden Predictor Inventory for Alzheimer's patient family caregivers without specialized training) (IPSO-CA24) was developed. It is an evaluation instrument with a multidimensional approach to overburden in line with the current trend of considering the characteristics of patient and caregiver needs together. The psychometric properties are analyzed based on a descriptive study with a sample of caregivers. Starting from the results of the first implementation of the instrument, it is possible to identify six dimensions which function as overburden predictors [81]. Both the questionnaire and scales are available at the following link: www.grupocuidadores.com/ipso.

## Author details

María del Carmen Pérez-Fuentes, María del Mar Molero Jurado* and
José Jesús Gázquez Linares

*Address all correspondence to: mmj130@ual.es

University of Almeria, Almeria, Spain

## References

[1] Prince M, Bryce R, Albanese E, Wimo A, Ribeiro W, Ferri CP. The global prevalence of dementia: A systematic review and meta-analysis. Alzheimer's & Dementia. 2013;**9**(1): 63-75

[2] World Health Organization and Alzheimer's Disease International. Dementia: A Public Health Priority. Geneva: World Health Organization; 2012

[3] Herrera E, Muñoz I, Martín V, Cid M. Experiencias españolas en la promoción de la autonomía personal en las personas mayores. Gaceta Sanitaria. 2011;**25**(8):147-157

[4] Rodríguez G. Políticas sociales de atención a la dependencia en los regímenes de bienestar de la Unión Europea. Cuadernos de Relaciones Laborales. 2011;**29**(1):13-42

[5] Abellán A, Esparza C. Solidaridad familiar y dependencia entre las personas mayores. Madrid, Informes Portal Mayores, IMSERSO; 2010. p.99

[6] Gázquez JJ, Pérez-Fuentes MC, Molero MM, Mercader I. Inteligencia emocional y calidad de vida del cuidador familiar de pacientes con demencia. Revista de Comunicación y Salud. 2015;**5**:1-15

[7] Martos A, Cardila F, Barragán A, Pérez-Fuentes MC, Molero MM, Gázquez JJ. Instrumentos para la evaluación de la sobrecarga del cuidador familiar de personas con demencia. European Journal of Investigation in Health, Psychology and Education. 2015;**5**(2): 281-292

[8] Molero MM, Pérez-Fuentes MC, Gázquez JJ, Mercader I, Abad T. Evaluación de la calidad de vida relacionada con la salud en población mayor: Revisión de instrumentos específicos. In: Gázquez JJ, Pérez-Fuentes MC, Molero MM, Mercader I, editors. Calidad de vida, Cuidadores e intervención para la mejora de la salud en el envejecimiento. Granada: Editorial GEU; 2013. pp. 93-100

[9] Seidmann S, Stefani D, Pano CO, Acrich L, Pupko VB. Sentimiento de sobrecarga y apoyo social en cuidadores familiares de enfermos crónicos. Revista de Psicología. 2013;**22**(1): 45-62

[10] Caqueo-Urízar A, Miranda-Castillo C, Lemos S, Lee S, Ramírez M, Mascayano F. An updated review on burden on caregivers of schizophrenia patients. Psicothema. 2014;**26**(2):235-243. DOI: 10.7334/psicothema2013.86

[11] Fernández de Larrinoa P, Martínez S, Ortiz N, Carrasco M, Solabarrieta J, Gómez I. Autopercepción del estado de salud en familiares cuidadores y su relación con el nivel de sobrecarga. Psicothema. 2011;**23**(3):388-393

[12] Delgado E, Suárez O, de Dios R, Valdespino I, Sousa Y, Braña G. Características y factores relacionados con sobrecarga en una muestra de cuidadores principales de pacientes ancianos con demencia. Medicina de Familia. 2014;**40**(2):57-64. DOI: 10.1016/j.semerg.2013.04.006

[13] Flores N, Jenaro C, Moro L, Tomsa R. Salud y calidad de vida de cuidadores familiares y profesionales de personas mayores dependientes: Estudio comparativo. European Journal of Investigation in Health, Psychology and Education. 2014;**4**(2):79-88. DOI: 10.1989/ejihpe.v4i2.55

[14] Kang HS, Myung W, Na DL, Kim SY, Lee JH, Han SH, Choi SH, Kim SY, Kim S, Kim DK. Factors associated with caregiver burden in patients with Alzheimer's disease. Psychiatry Investigation. 2014;**11**(2):152-159. DOI: 10.4306/pi.2014.11.2.152

[15] Lanzón T, Díaz A. Papel predictor de las variables tipo de cuidador, nivel de dependencia y tiempo dedicado al cuidado en el impacto del estresor: Cuidar a un familiar dependiente. European Journal of Investigation in Health, Psychology and Education. 2015;**4**(3):193-202. DOI: 10.1989/ejihpe.v4i3.66

[16] Graessel E, Berth H, Lichte T, Grau H. Subjective caregiver burden: Validity of the 10-item short version of the Burden Scale for Family Caregivers BSFC-s. BMC Geriatrics. 2014;**14**:23. DOI: 10.1186/1471-2318-14-23

[17] Crespo M, Rivas MT. La evaluación de la carga del cuidador: Una revisión más allá de la escala de Zarit. Clínica y Salud. 2015;**26**(1):9-16. DOI: 10.1016/j.clysa.2014.07.002

[18] Martín-Carrasco M, Domínguez-Panchón AI, Muñoz-Hermoso P, González-Fraile E, Ballesteros-Rodríguez J. Instrumentos para medir la sobrecarga en el cuidador informal del paciente con demencia. Revista Española de Geriatría y Gerontología. 2013;**48**(6):276-284. DOI: 10.1016/j.regg.2013.06.002

[19] Heidegger M. El Ser y el Tiempo. Madrid: Fondo de Cultura Económica; 2000

[20] Hermanns M, Mastel-Smith B. Caregiving: A qualitative concept analysis. The Qualitative Report. 2012;**17**(75):1-18

[21] Swanson EA, Jensen DP, Specht J, Johnson ML, Maas M, Saylor D. Caregiving: Concept analysis and outcomes. Scholarly Inquiry for Nursing Practice. 1997;**11**(1):65-76

[22] Pearlin LK, Mullan JT, Semple SJ, Skaff MM. Caregiving and the stress process: An overview of concepts and their measures. The Gerontologist. 1990;**30**(5):583-594

[23] Rivas JC, Ostiguín, RM. Cuidador: ¿concepto operativo o preludio teórico?. Enfermería Universitaria. 2011;**8**(1):49-54

[24] Eterovic CA, Mendoza SE, Sáez KL. Habilidad de cuidado y nivel de sobrecarga en cuidadoras/es informales de personas dependientes. Enfermería Global. 2015;**14**(2):235-248. DOI: http://dx.doi.org/10.6018/eglobal.14.2.198121

[25] Northouse LL, Katapodi MC, Schafenacker AM, Weiss D. The impact of caregiving on the psychological well-being of family caregivers and cancer patients. Oncology Family Caregivers. 2012;**28**(4):236-245. DOI: http://dx.doi.org/10.1016/j.soncn.2012.09.006

[26] Mendoza RM, Hernández EL, Medina M, Company MC, Gómez ML, Estrada L, Navarro FJ, Fiuza MD. Perfil del cuidador principal en el área de salud de Gran Canaria. Ene Revista de Enfermería. 2014;**8**(2): 0-0. DOI: http://dx.doi.org/10.4321/S1988-348X2014000200002

[27] Moreno A, Ortega M, Gamero C. Los modelos familiares en España: Reflexionando sobre la ambivalencia familiar desde una aproximación teórica. Revista Española de Sociología. 2017;**26**(1):1-19

[28] Kong EH. Family caregivers of older people in nursing homes. Asian Nursing Research. 2008;**2**(4):195-207

[29] Zwaanswijk M, Peeters JM, van Beek AP, Meerveld JH, Francke AL. Informal caregivers of people with dementia: Problems, needs and help in the initial stage and in subsequent stages of dementia: A questionnaire survey. The Open Nursing Journal. 2013;**7**:6-13. DOI: 10.2174/1874434601307010006

[30] Islas NL, Ramos B, Aguilar MG, García ML. Perfil psicosocial del cuidador primario informal del paciente con EPOC. Revista del Instituto Nacional de Enfermedades Respiratorias. 2006;**19**(4):266-271

[31] Seguí JD, Ortiz-Tallo M. Factores asociados al estrés del cuidador primario de niños con autismo: Sobrecarga, psicopatología y estado de salud. Anales de Psicología. 2008; **24**(1):100-105

[32] Caqueo-Urízar A, Segovia-Lagos P, Urrutia-Urrutia U, Castillo CM, Lechuga EN. Impacto de la relación de ayuda de cuidadores primarios en la calidad de vida de pacientes con cáncer avanzado. Psicooncología. 2013;**10**(1):95-108

[33] Vázquez OG, Castillo ER, Huertas LA, García AM, Ponce JLA, Manzanilla EO. Aguilar SA. Guía de práctica clínica para la atención psico-oncológica del cuidador primario informal de pacientes con cáncer. Psicooncología. 2015;**12**(1):87-104

[34] Calero-García MJ, Ortega AR, Jiménez C. El impacto del cuidador principal en el deterioro funcional y cognitivo del anciano hospitalizado. European Journal of Investigation in Health, Psychology and Education. 2012;**2**(2):41-52. DOI: 10.1989/ejihpe.v2i2.13

[35] Martínez T, Serrano P, Del Rincón C, Martino R. Repercusiones en el cuidador principal del niño hospitalizado a domicilio en cuidados paliativos pediátricos. Medicina Paliativa. 2016;**23**(2):79-92. DOI: 10.1016/j.medipa.2013.12.004

[36] Biurrun A. La asistencia de los familiares cuidadores en la enfermedad de Alzheimer. Revista Española de Geriatría y Gerontología. 2001;**36**(6):325-330. DOI: 10.1016/S0211-139X(01)74751-8

[37] Twigg J. Cuidadores de los ancianos: Modelos para un análisis. In: Jamieson A, Illsley R, editors. Comparación de las políticas europeas de atención a las personas ancianas. Barcelona: SG Editores y Fundación Caja Madrid; 1993. pp. 35-51

[38] Delicado MV, Candel E, Alfaro A, López M, García C. Interacción de enfermería y cuidadoras informales de personas dependientes. Atención Primaria. 2004;**33**(4):193-199

[39] Tirado G, López-Saez A, Capilla C, Correa A, Geidel B. La Valoración en el Síndrome del Cuidador. Desarrollo Cientif Enferm. 2011;**19**(3):102-106

[40] De la Cuesta C, Sandelowski M. The material world and craft of caregiving for relatives with dementia. Journal of Transcultural Nursing. 2005;**16**(3):218-225

[41] Imserso. Informe 2014: Las Personas Mayores en España Datos Estadísticos Estatales y por Comunidades Autónomas. Madrid: Imserso; 2015

[42] Domingo EP, Sierra MG, Valero MM, Castiñeira MPO. El Libro Blanco del Parkinson en España—Aproximación, análisis y propuesta de futuro. Madrid: Real Patronato sobre Discapacidad (Ministerio de Sanidad, Servicios Sociales e Igualdad) y Federación Española de Parkinson; 2015

[43] García-Pereira S, Quevedo-Blasco R. Análisis de las revistas iberoamericanas de Psicología y de Educación indexadas en el Journal Citation Reports del 2013. European Journal of Education and Psychology. 2015;**8**(2):85-96. DOI: 10.1016/j.ejeps.2015.09.003

[44] Ruiz-Robledillo N, Moya-Albiol L. El cuidado informal: Una visión actual. Revista de Motivación y Emoción. 2012;**1**:22-30

[45] Pérez-Fuentes MC, Molero MM, Gázquez JJ, Mercader I, Soler F, Núñez A. Factores a tener en cuenta en la detección precoz del burnout en cuidadores familiares de enfermos

de Alzheimer. In: Gázquez JJ, Pérez-Fuentes MC, Molero MM, Mercader I, Soler F, editors. Calidad de vida, cuidadores e intervención para la mejora de la salud en el envejecimiento Volumen II. Almería: ASUNIVEP; 2014. pp. 155-160

[46] Van der Lee J, Bakker TJEM, Duivenvoorden HJ, Dröes RM. Multivariate models of subjective caregiver burden in dementia: A systematic review. Ageing Research Reviews. 2014;**15**:76-93. DOI: 10.1016/j.arr.2014.03.003

[47] Papastavrou E, Tsangari H, Karayiannis G, Papacostas S, Efstathiou G, Sourtzi P. Caring and coping: the dementia caregivers. Aging and Mental Health. 2011;**15**(6):702-711. DOI: 10.1080/13607863.2011.562178

[48] Zarit SH, Femia EE, Kim K, Whitlatch CJ. The structure of risk factors and outcomes for family caregivers: Implications for assessment and treatment. Aging & Mental Health. 2010;**14**(2):220-231. DOI: 10.1080/13607860903167861

[49] Molero MM, Pérez-Fuentes MC, Gázquez JJ. Cuidadores familiars, no profesionales o informales: Revisión de la terminología en publicaciones científicas. Revista Facultad de Ciencias de la Salud UDES. 2016;**3**(1):59-67. DOI: 10.20320/rfcsudes.v3i1.107

[50] Vives M, Orte C, Sánchez L. Identificación de competencias y habilidades del buen profesional que trabaja con personas mayores a través de la técnica Delphi. European Journal of Investigation in Health, Psychology and Education. 2016;**6**(1):37-46

[51] Organización Mundial de la Salud. Demencia: Una prioridad de Salud Pública. Washington, DC: OMS; 2013

[52] Armayor AC, Vivar C, Durán CN. Dependencia y familia cuidadora: reflexiones para un abordaje familiar. Anales del Sistema Sanitario de Navarra. 2012;**34**(3):463-469

[53] Hooker SA, Grigsby ME, Riegel B, Bekelman DB. The impact of relationship quality on health-related outcomes in heart failure patients and informal family caregivers: An integrative review. The Journal of Cardiovascular Nursing. 2015;**30**(4):S52-S63. DOI: 10.1097/JCN.0000000000000270

[54] Caron R, Caron L. The mental stress of the accompaniment in Alzheimer's disease. Encephale. 2011;**37**(6):439-447

[55] Robles MJ, Cucurella E, Formiga F, Fort I, Rodríguez D, Barranco E, Catena J, Cubí D. La información del diagnóstico en la demencia. Revista Española de Geriatría y Gerontología. 2011;**46**(3):163-169

[56] Drickamer MA, Lachs MS. Should patients with Alzheimer's disease be told their diagnosis? The New England Journal of Medicine. 1992;**326**:947-951. DOI: 10.1056/NEJM199204023261410

[57] Smith A, King E, Hindley N, Barnetson L, Barton J, Jobst KA. The experience of research participation and the value of diagnosis in dementia: Implications for practice. Journal of Mental Health. 1998;**7**:309-321. DOI: http://dx.doi.org/10.1080/09638239818120

[58] Carpenter B, Dave J. Disclosing a dementia diagnosis: A review of opinion and practice, and a proposed research agenda. The Gerontologist. 2004;**44**(2):149-158

[59] Pinner G, Bouman WP. Attitudes of patients with mild dementia and their carers towards disclosure of the diagnosis. International Psychogeriatrics. 2003;**15**(3):279-288

[60] Alzheimer Europe. Who Cares? The State of Dementia Care in Europe. 2006. Available from: http://www.alzheimer-europe.org/./Alzheimer-Europe./Whocares-The-state-of-dementia-care-in-Europe

[61] Feldberg C, Tartaglini MF, Clemente MA, Petracca G, Cáceres F, Stefani D. Vulnerabilidad psicosocial del cuidador familiar. Creencias acerca del estado de salud del paciente neurológico y el sentimiento de sobrecarga. Neurología. 2011;**3**(1):11-16

[62] De Valle-Alonso MJ, Hernández-López IE, Zúñiga-Vargas ML, Martínez-Aguilera P. Sobrecarga y Burnout en cuidadores informales del adulto mayor. Enfermería Universitaria. 2015;**12**(1):19-27. DOI: 10.1016/j.reu.2015.05.004

[63] Vázquez FL, Blanco V, Hermida E, Otero P, Torres A, Díaz-Fernández O. Eficacia de las intervenciones psicológicas breves para reducir los síntomas depresivos en cuidadores: Revisión sistemática y meta-análisis. Revista de Psicopatología y Psicología Clínica. 2015;**20**(3):173-188. DOI: 10.5944/rppc.vol.20.num.3.2015.15891

[64] Rosa E, Lussignoli G, Sabbatini F, Chiappa A, Di Cesare S, Lamanna L, Zanetti O. Needs of caregivers of the patients with dementia. Archives of Gerontology and Geriatrics. 2010;**51**(1):54-58. DOI: 10.1016/j.archger.2009.07.008

[65] Saavedra FJ, Bascón MJ, Sánchez SA, Calderón MG, Moreno DM. Cuidadoras de familiares dependientes y salud: Influencia de la participación en un taller de control de estrés. Clínica y Salud. 2013;**24**(2):85-93

[66] Brown RM, Brown SL. Informal caregiving: A reappraisal of effects on caregivers. Social Issues and Policy Review. 2014;**8**(1):74-102. DOI: 10.1111/sipr.12002

[67] Richardson TJ, Lee SJ, Berg-Weger M, Grossberg GT. Caregiver health: Health of caregivers of Alzheimer's and other dementia patients. Current Psychiatry Reports. 2013;**15**(7):1-7. DOI: 10.1007/s11920-013-0367-2

[68] Gila MJ, Sánchez RO, Gómez-Caro S, Oropesa AS, Morena JC, Moreno FJ. El rol de cuidador de personas dependientes y sus repercusiones sobre su calidad de vida y su salud. Revista Clínica de Medicina Familiar. 2009;**2**(7):332-334

[69] Manso ME, Sánchez MDP, Flores IC. Salud y sobrecarga percibida en personas cuidadoras familiares de una zona rural. Clínica y Salud. 2013;**24**(1):37-45. DOI: http://dx.doi.org/10.5093/cl2013a5

[70] Urdaneta E, Etxeberria I, Galdona N, Yanguas JJ, García A, Buiza C. Perceived social help, psychosomatic complaints and burden: The relationship with negative affect in Alzheimer caregivers. Alzheimer's & Dementia. 2008;**44**:660

[71] Cardila F, Martos A, Barragán AB, Pérez-Fuentes MC, Molero MM, Gázquez JJ. Prevalencia de la depresión en España: Análisis de los últimos 15 años. European Journal of Investigation in Health, Psychology and Education. 2015;**5**(2):267-279

[72] Vázquez FL, Otero P, Torres A, Hermida E, Blanco V, Díaz O. Una intervención breve de solución de problemas para la prevención indicada de la depresión en cuidadoras. Psicothema. 2013;**25**(1):87-92

[73] Corazza DI, Pedroso RV, Andreatto CA, Scarpari L, Garuffi M, Costa JL, Santos-Galduróz RF. Los predictores psiconeuroinmunológicos de la sobrecarga de cuidado en ancianos cuidadores de pacientes con enfermedad de Alzheimer. Revista Española de Geriatría y Gerontología. 2014;**49**(4):173-178. DOI: 10.1016/j.regg.2014.03.007

[74] Rodríguez-Fernández A, Ramos-Díaz E, Madariaga JM, Arrivillaga A, Galende N. Steps in the construction and verification of an explanatory model of psychosocial adjustment. European Journal of Education and Psychology. 2016;**9**(1):20-28. DOI: 10.1016/j.ejeps.2015.11.002

[75] Sánchez R, Molina E, Gómez-Ortega O. Intervenciones de enfermería para disminuir la sobrecarga en cuidadores: Un estudio piloto. Revista Cuidarte. 2016;**7**(1):1171-1184. DOI: http://dx.doi.org/10.15649/cuidarte.v7i1.251

[76] Garand L, Rinaldo DE, Alberth MM, Delany J, Beasock SL, Lopez OL, Dew MA. Effects of problem a solving therapy on mental health outcomes in family caregivers of persons with a new diagnosis of mild cognitive impairment or early dementia: A randomized controlled trial. The American Journal of Geriatric Psychiatry. 2013;**22**(8):771-781

[77] Zarit SH, Reever KE, Bach-Peterson J. Relatives of the impaired elderly. Correlates of feelings of burden. The Gerontologist. 1980;**20**:649-654

[78] Teri L, Truax P, Logsdon R, Uomoto J, Zarit S, Vitaliano PP. Assessment of behavioral problems in dementia: The Revised Memory and Behavior Problems Checklist (RMBPC). Psychology and Aging. 1992;**7**(4):622-631

[79] Lawton MP, Kleban M, Moss M, Rovine M, Glicksman A. Measuring caregiving appraisal. Journal of Gerontology. 1989;**44**:61-71

[80] Novak M, Guest CI. Application of a multidimensional caregiver burden inventory. The Gerontologist. 1989;**29**:798-803

[81] Pérez-Fuentes MC, Gázquez JJ, Ruiz MD, Molero MM. Inventory of overburden in Alzheimer's patient family caregivers with no specialized training. International Journal of Clinical and Health Psychology. 2017;**17**:56-64. DOI: http://dx.doi.org/10.1016/j.ijchp.2016.09.004

# 10

# Caregiving and Experiences of Health, Illness and Coping in the Context of Paediatric and Adolescent HIV and Poverty

Antonio G. Lentoor

**Abstract**

The contextual challenges in the context of HIV negatively impact the social ecology of the families. The consequences of this are that it adversely impacts the psychosocial functioning of caregivers and health and well-being of the children. The findings showed that caregiving is performed, not only in the context of maternal HIV infection, but also in the context of inadequate material and financial resources and single-head households where women assume the primary caregiving role. Caregiving is also complicated by the issue of maternal death and abandonment, where relatives (i.e. mainly grandparents) assume the role of the primary caregivers of children infected with HIV. On the other hand, emerging studies that started to focus on enhancing resilience in children whose caregiver is HIV positive holds promise to the fact that adequate interventions can have long-lasting benefits on the developmental and psychological trajectory of HIV-positive children and their HIV-positive caregivers. Consequently, the link between poverty and HIV/AIDS has been established, and its impact on perinatal, infancy and early-childhood development outcomes is clearly documented.

**Keywords:** HIV, paediatric HIV, maternal HIV, poverty, caregiving

## 1. Introduction

The role of caregiving for a child in many cultures is the primary responsibility of the mother. Young children, especially, are more dependent on their caregivers and, as a result, are vulnerable to declines in the quality of caregiving [39]. Given the multigenerational nature of HIV infection, it is worthwhile, from a research perspective, to explore what impact the disease is having on this role, more so given the fact that 98% of children infected with HIV results from mother-to-child transmission [59]. Furthermore, with more and more perinatally infected infants progressing into childhood and adolescence, the need for empirical data to demonstrate and help understand the impact this pandemic is having on the surviving children and their family structures is underscored. This is especially so given that some surviving children are raised by mothers infected with HIV as well as many being orphans living in abject poverty [15, 43]. For example, it has been shown that South Africa has more than 60% of double orphans being raised by grandmothers or relatives other than the biological parent [53] and are living in poverty, which poses additional challenges in caregiving. It has been argued that poverty exposes perinatally HIV-positive children to various psychosocial risk factors, which often co-occur and impact negatively on the child's neurodevelopment, thereby contributing to poor health, lack of readiness for school, poor academic performance and psycho-emotional problems in childhood and adolescence [29]. This chapter presents a systematic and critical review of the literature on caregiving in the context of HIV/AIDS and poverty associated with perinatally HIV (PHIV) infection in children.

## 2. Body

### 2.1. Methodology

Literature searches were carried out using PubMed, PsycINFO and Google Scholar. A combination of words with the subject terms was used to identify relevant articles. The search terms included 'HIV&rsquo, 'HIV infection', 'Child and Adolescent HIV', 'Paediatric HIV', 'Maternal HIV', 'Biological and Non-Biological Caregivers and HIV', 'HIV and Poverty', 'Stress and HIV Illness', 'Nutrition and HIV', 'Caregiving and HIV', 'HIV Orphans', 'Attachment and HIV' and 'Extended Relatives and HIV'. Appropriate journal articles were identified, while in addition to this, the author also used the references cited in the identified articles to find other publications. The search and appropriateness of the articles were guided by the following broad objective to be addressed in the chapter which was

- To understand the challenges associated with caregiving in the context of child and adolescent HIV.

In order to meet the objective, the following questions were guiding the literature search:

- What are the experiences of being HIV positive (caregiver health status) and a caregiver of an HIV-positive child (child health status)?
- How does HIV influence the caregiving capacity of the primary caregiver of an HIV-positive child?
- How does poverty impact the experience of an HIV-positive caregiver to care for an HIV-positive child?
- Does having to live in an impoverished context have any impact on the overall physical, psychological and social health of the caregiver and the child living with HIV?

- What network of support system is in place for assistance in caregiving of the HIV-positive child, and how does this impact on coping with having to care for an HIV-positive child?

Procedure for the inclusion of relevant articles:

All online abstracts of the selected studies were reviewed, and eligible studies were obtained and reviewed by the author. Studies were included in the review if they met following criteria:

- focus was on HIV/AIDS,
- children younger than 16 years (account for paediatric and adolescence) and were perinatally infected by their mothers,
- HIV, poverty, child and caregiver's physical and/or psychological health outcomes were focus of the study,
- raised by either biological mother or extended relative, and
- both qualitative and quantitative studies were included.

### 2.2. Findings

#### *2.2.1. Poverty, psychosocial risk factors and caregiving*

Despite the shift in South Africa's political dispensation from apartheid to democracy, it should be noted that a large number of South African citizens still live in abject poverty [52] as is the case in many Sub-Saharan countries. It is estimated that the South African child population accounts for approximately 18.7 million, with 2.3 million of them still being forced to live in shacks or some form of informal dwelling [27]. Moreover, from this population, approximately 30% under the age of five live in over-crowded conditions. In a study conducted in 2007 by the Housing Development Agency, it was found that approximately 6000 households are still headed by children under the age of 18 [41].

Living conditions for a large number of people are still characterised by a lack of access to quality basic services, including adequate housing, electricity, safe and clean running water, toilet facilities and refuse removal services [51]. A study conducted by Iversen et al. found that nearly 7 million children in the country still do not have access to clean, safe, drinking water in their households [27]. According to StatsSA, about 25.2% of households in the Eastern Cape had no access to flush toilets as compared to the Western Cape which had more than 50% accessibility [51]. In terms of access to piped water, the Eastern Cape is considered the worst, remaining below the national average. While it can be argued that some improvement did occur since the new political dispensation assumed power, a large number of children are still exposed to harsh socioeconomic living conditions [27, 41, 51]. These conditions create an environment that fuels vulnerability to mental and physical illness and easily spreads diseases.

The capacity to care for children usually suffers as the impaired mental state of a parent living with a primary chronic life-threatening illness like HIV does not only disrupt parenting ability but also adversely influence the attachment between parent and child [30]. The disruption is further exacerbated by the fact that HIV often co-exists with poverty, which means the infected mother and child will probably live in socioeconomically disadvantaged contexts that pose additional challenges [13, 18, 23]. Research has established a link between the negative effects of poverty on parental roles and child development [16, 35–38]. Poverty has also been associated with negative parental health, which independently and jointly impacts the child's cognitive and social-emotional well-being in an adverse manner [15, 32]. Furthermore, economic deprivation creates a catalyst for psychological stress and vulnerability among caregivers, which further predisposes them to depression [28]. Hence, a caregiver confronting impoverishment on a daily basis is more likely to be stressed, which in turn may impede the quality and quantity of her parenting [9, 31]. The implication of this dynamic has an overwhelmingly negative effect on the child's developmental outcome. Low socioeconomic status (SES) has also proven to be associated with a variety of obstacles hindering effective rearing, such as inadequate nutritional provision, lack of time for cognitively stimulating activities in the parent-child dyad and poor parent-child relationships owing to associated stress [23]. The association between SES and home environment therefore suggests that children infected with HIV and who are living in poverty also live in less stimulating and less supportive home environments. This is certainly plausible given the reciprocal nature of the child-parent dyad and their environment. Additionally, maternal infection may affect the quality of caregiving which, when combined with poverty, may further frustrate the attachment relationship, resulting in poor child-development outcomes that is even observable in late adolescence [15, 30]. Studies focusing on healthy, pre-term, disabled and chronically ill children also support the premise that poverty serves as a risk factor for poor cognitive and socio-emotional functioning outcomes [32]. Some researchers argue that poverty is the single factor most associated with HIV/AIDS vulnerability, physical and mental ill health, impaired parent-child dyads and child development outcomes [15, 20–22, 28, 29].

#### 2.2.2. *Parental health and relationship to caregiving*

Until recently, most research focused exclusively on parenting interactions with healthy children and those children confronting chronic illness and disabilities [55, 57]. While there is a growing number of studies on the plight of caregivers infected and affected by HIV/AIDS in developed countries, there are still very few from developing countries [39]. Not only do HIV-positive mothers have to battle their own illness and witness the deaths of others in the same predicament, they also have to deal with the knowledge that their children are infected with the disease and still raise them [22, 24]. As a result, they are often burdened with the inability to confront their own mortality as well as that of their children. It is documented that childhood chronic illness brings about significant strain on the family system, including high rates of maternal depression and anxiety, marital distress and adjustment problems [5, 6, 55, 56]. Likewise, parental illness has been shown to impact caregiving capacity and to increase the risk of psychological problems in affected children [19, 42].

The caregiving behaviour of a parent and the quality of the early parent-child relationship are two factors that have been identified as influencing and promoting development outcomes in children [3, 45, 46]. As stated by Sameroff et al. '...development, particularly in the earlier years, is a function of ongoing cycles of child-caregiver transaction that weave together the fabric of psychological functions, including the mental health of the young child' [49].

Based on this premise, the caregiver's health and overall well-being is thus of critical importance in relation to exploring the child's health and well-being. Mothers infected with HIV commonly live as single parents, in economically disadvantaged environments with not much social support and their children may therefore be at risk of ill health [9]. When a caregiver confronts a chronic illness, the children usually suffer as the caregiver's capacity to care for them becomes interrupted [45]. The consequences of such a disruption can have multiple adverse effects on the psychological functioning, neurodevelopment, physical health and well-being of the affected children [46, 47]. In addition to this, poor child-health adds even greater demands to a caregiver's already strained load [45]. Consequently, in situations where a caregiver is infected with HIV, she is now confronted with the dual challenge of being a patient and a caregiver [22].

The multiple stressors associated with being HIV positive and caring for HIV-positive children are most likely to place these women at an increased risk of mental health problems, which in turn will exacerbate the stress associated with parenting. This may result in a vicious cycle impacting the caregiver-child dyad negatively. Positive caregivers may be unable to cope with the stressful reality of their HIV illness and may also be overburdened by carrying the sole responsibility of caring for their infected children [9]. Being HIV positive is also associated with the increased risk of having mental disorders (see [8] for review). For example, one of the most commonly associated mental illnesses is depression, which is rooted in life circumstance, illness, poor support networking structures and daily life stress [8]. The emotional toll of parenting can be high, partly because parents are relatively socially isolated and do not always get support from the community and their extended family [9]. Many HIV-positive mothers must deal with their illness in isolation owing to the stigma associated with the disease, as well as prevalence of HIV-related discrimination remaining rife in communities, and their fear of rejection and abandonment by relatives and close associates [25, 26]. These experiences further compound the stress experienced by mothers as caregivers, thus complicating the problems inherent in parenting. Literature on research investigating the impact of maternal stress and depression is in consensus, in that it has been associated with adverse outcomes on both parenting and childhood neurocognitive and socio-emotional development (see [20–22, 28, 30]). With regard to the impact of parental depression on the parenting role, research suggests that there is a breakdown in attachment between the caregiver and child, and as a result, the caregiver-child relationship suffers. Furthermore, due to the debilitating nature of parental depression, parents are less likely to carry out their functioning role as parents and as a result are less likely to engage in behaviour repertoires consistent with enhancing a child's neurocognitive, social and emotional development and well-being [20–22, 30].

Caring for a child is a time-consuming and emotionally taxing activity that becomes exponentially more burdensome if the caregiver is ill and has a child suffering from a chronic illness; hence, their increased vulnerability to developing depression, especially in the absence of poor social and financial support structures [54]. The caregiver may be overwhelmed with constant concerns over the child's health and worries about the future and as a result may be flooded with feelings of inadequacy. These concerns may create heightened levels of distress and in turn these caregivers may experience a lack of confidence in their ability to parent as they are unable to meet their children's needs. In a study conducted by McLearn and colleagues, the parenting practices of depressed mothers were investigated, and the researchers concluded that depressed mothers engaged in parenting practices were most likely to impact negatively on the children's overall development [34]. Parenting practices showed no clear structure and routine, and parents were less likely to engage in play behaviour with the child, breastfeed, talk to, read books to, or respond to the child's non-verbal cues [34]. The consequent effect on the child's developmental outcome can be devastating and may even have long-lasting implications. As indicated by Knitzer et al. [30], depressed caregivers are more likely to expose their children to health risks and less likely to adhere to health advice for themselves and their children. Depressed caregivers will also find it more difficult to respond to and manage chronic illness in their children [30]. As a result, children parented by depressed caregivers are known to display a spectrum of cognitive and socio-emotional problems [20–22], including strong associated behavioural problems such as attention-deficit/hyperactivity disorder, conduct problems, anger and violent behaviour, depression and anxiety [29, 30]. Moreover, cognitive deficits observed in children who are exposed to depressed caregivers have shown to negatively affect school readiness and the success of these children [30], and they have even exhibited deficits in social competencies [28]. Consequently, these children who have a greater tendency to engage in negative social behaviours are at greater risk of peer pressure and have a low social concept. Finally, children parented by depressed caregivers have a high risk for developing antisocial behaviour [20–22]. As indicated by Forsyth [19], children born to mothers infected with HIV have shown to present more psycho-developmental problems, which is likely to be a consequence of the disruption in the parenting and caring capacity of the mother as a result of the HIV infection and the associated stress that is accompanied by the illness.

#### 2.2.3. *Impact of HIV on parental interaction*

The strain of caring for a sick child while managing one's own illness and bearing responsibility for children is a tremendous burden on many mothers infected with HIV [6]. As is the case of rearing children with other chronic illnesses, maternally HIV-infected children tend to make unique and often greater demands on their caregivers. Therefore, it is plausible to assume parenting for caregivers of children infected with HIV is marked by increased worry, emotional pain and other concerns when compared to caregivers of children without illness [11]. Coscia et al. [15], in their study exploring the relationship between home environment and HIV-infected children's cognitive functioning, found an association between parental interaction and disease severity. As the child's disease progressed, the caregiver's interaction became less stimulating and supportive, thus creating a higher vulnerability for poor cognitive development and socio-emotional functioning. These researchers suggest that as the HIV-positive child becomes more ill, perhaps the caregivers' relationship with the child weakens. One hypothesis is that the HIV-positive caregiver does not expect the HIV-infected child to survive beyond early childhood and this influences the caregiver's capacity to bond with the child. Another hypothesis is that the sheer burden of caring for a chronically ill child, particularly under harsh conditions, may cause resentment. Equally, HIV can be argued to cause a breakdown in the quality and quantity of the critical early relationship between the caregiver and child. Poor bonding, for example, may in turn impact on developmental outcomes.

As shown in studies of pre-term babies, environmental factors such as effective parenting characterised by warmth, sensitivity, consistency and connectedness have a positive relationship with cognitive and social-emotional competence [50, 55].

Effective parenting has been shown to facilitate healthy caregiver-child dyads and is associated with greater optimal development outcomes in children [48]. This premise is located within the theoretical perspective of secure attachment coined by John Bowlby [10]. Bowlby was the first of many theorists who described the importance of caregiver-child relationship and its effect on children's development outcomes [10, 45]. According to Bowlby, securely attached children have an internal representation of the caregiver as stable, responsive and caring that serve to provide the child with a secure basis from which they can explore their environment, grow and develop [10]. Subsequent research related to parenting has successfully demonstrated the relevance of attachment models. Treyvaud and colleagues, in a study of pre-term infants, found a positive relationship between cognitive development and sensitive caregiving [55]. Therefore, children whose caregivers interacted with them in a warm and positive manner showed particularly positive outcomes in cognitive development [55]. Similar results were echoed in a study conducted by Richter and Grieve [46], where the relationships between home environment and cognitive functioning were explored among a sample of South Africans. Consensus from these studies was that facilitative, warm, positive and sensitive caregiving contributed to positive cognitive development and healthy psychological functioning in these ill-health children. Thus, the results illustrate that the quality of a caregiver's interactions and his/her ability to create an environment conducive of learning and development is positively associated with cognitive development in children and operates as a protective factor against the adverse effects of poverty. Richter [48] recommended that such effective parenting is important and should be encouraged as it can mediate the effects of poverty and promote development in children. Consequently, the findings of these particular studies are encouraging as they demonstrate the importance of enhancing caregiver-child interaction, which in turn can promote optimal outcomes in children.

### *2.2.4. Role of extended relatives*

On the other hand, the increasing HIV pandemic in South Africa poses a substantial threat with a detrimental impact on the provision of care for children. As biological parents become ill or even die and are unable to care for their children, the responsibility of caring for these children is often transferred to grandmothers, aunts, other children and relatives [1, 7, 12, 13, 43, 44]. As a consequence of the impact of HIV, the family structure may change. Due to the incapacitating nature of HIV/AIDS or even deaths of parents, the need to provide some form of guardianship for the affected and infected children must be prioritised [14]. As indicated by Richter [48], it is not uncommon in the African context for relatives to assume a caretaking role of HIV orphans. However, the assumption of caretaking responsibility often occurs in the context of other factors such as having to raise other grandchildren and cousins. These relatives are often still in the process of grieving for multiple family members who died of HIV and are even confronted with continued stigmatisation from the community [1, 2, 43]. This often places additional stress on relatives caring for HIV-infected children.

Furthermore, the above-mentioned caregivers may experience heightened levels of psychological distress as a result of the increased stress associated with their situation and may require social and health support too [4, 44]. Literature, on grandparents as caregivers of HIV-infected orphans, shows for example, that caregivers' personal ill health may prevent them from adequately responding to the needs of the child [40]. In the context of limited capacity, foster caregivers, particularly grandparents, may prioritise the physical well-being of children over the learning, intellectual and emotional needs of said children. Correspondingly, the coexistence of HIV with poverty further limits caring capacity as caregivers frequently have difficulty accessing health services, they have to deal with complex medical treatment and struggle to acquire financial assistance to meet the health and nutritional needs of the children [13, 35–38].

#### *2.2.5. Enhancing resilience as a protective coping mechanism*

Research has shown that parental illness impacts negatively on positive parenting as it increases parental stress and disrupts the parent-child relationship. This has stimulated interventions that can enhance positive parenting in HIV-positive caregivers in low-and middle-income countries. While evidence suggests that maternal illness is considered a risk for poor outcome in their children, where HIV-positive mothers were given the opportunity to enhance their capacity to deal with their illness and to strengthen parent-child relationship, the outcomes proved to benefit both the mental health of the caregiver and the child [33, 39]. A few studies that emerged have started looking at the resilience in young children whose mothers are living with HIV in an attempt to improve developmental and psychosocial outcomes for both the HIV-infected mother and the child [17, 33, 39, 47, 58]. In the study with HIV-positive mothers from South Africa, there were also HIV-positive mothers who were able to express their own desires to live positively, for themselves and their children; they were also able to recognise how their own behaviour was affecting their children, and this had a positive impact on their ability to parent and communicate effectively with their children [58]. This suggests that there are caregivers who show resilience and work very hard to care for their children. Interventions directed at the mother-child relationship were able to further enhance HIV-positive mothers' capacity to cope better with their own illness and, as a result, be able to build psychological resilience in their children [58]. It is well demonstrated that resilience has the capacity to affect the long-term trajectory of a child's emotional, cognitive and adaptive functioning. In another large study conducted in Tswane, South Africa, among 390 mother-child pairs, an intervention that focused on mother-child dyads was not only able to enhance the parent-child relationship, but it also resulted in significant reduction in children's externalising behaviours, while improving the children's adaptive functioning [17], for at least a year following the intervention. Evidently, also in the study was a significant reduction in depression among children. Importantly, benefits were not only noticeable for the children but also for the HIV-positive caregivers who engaged in less-frequent avoidant coping behaviour [17]. A similar finding was found in Murphey and Marelich, who established that HIV-positive mothers in their study were able to better cope, and this translated into better adaptive potential in their children [39]. The benefit of interventions focusing on caregiver-child dyads has the potential to have a long-lasting resilient effect on both children and their HIV-positive caregivers. Recently, the first large study that examined the relationship between HIV/AIDS and positive parenting, using a sample of 2477 caregiver-child dyads, was conducted in KwaZulu-Natal [31]. Findings from the study indicated that HIV-positive caregivers and those caring for AIDS-orphaned children engaged in less positive parenting in comparison to non-affected families. However, non-HIV sick caregivers or those caring for orphans with other chronic illnesses were not associated with any positive parenting. The findings were mediated by psychosocial risk factors such as poverty, caregiver's depression, etc. However, the study does suggest that a parenting programme that is aimed at improving caregiver psychological health and encouraging positive parenting has the potential to safeguard against risks of poor child psychological and physical health outcomes in HIV-affected families living in poverty. This finding is promising that HIV-exposed caregivers have the ability to engage positively with their children, albeit, as the finding suggests, the effect size was small [31]. This nevertheless suggests, if adequately tailored interventions are implemented to look at strengthening the child-caregiver relationship, that it can ameliorate the children's response to the exposed adversities. This, in turn, has the potential to have a lasting impact on children's developmental and psychological outcome. The findings from these studies are promising as it indicates that while many children are at risk for various negative psychosocial outcomes, mothers living with HIV and those caring for AIDS orphans can be resilient and are able to take adequate care of their children, despite the challenges.

### 2.3. Conclusion

In conclusion, the findings from this systematic review show that HIV-positive caregivers and those caring for HIV-orphaned children also often live in poverty-stricken contextual realities which pose additional challenges to the caregiving context. The consequences of this are that it has adverse effects on psychosocial, health, and well-being of both the children and the caregivers. However, on the other hand, some intervention studies with HIV caregivers and/or HIV-positive children, albeit limited, do hold the promise to ameliorate the adverse impact of both HIV and poverty on caregiving.

## Acknowledgements

This chapter results from research performed as part of a doctoral study on the 'The relationship between psychosocial factors and poor neurocognitive and socio-emotional development in children perinatally infected with HIV in South Africa' at the University of KwaZulu Natal, South Africa. This publication is based on research that has been supported in part by the University of Cape Town's Research Committee (URC).

## Author details

Antonio G. Lentoor

Address all correspondence to: antonio.lentoor@westerncape.gov.za

UCT Department of Psychiatry and Mental Health, Valkenberg Hospital, Cape Town, South Africa

## References

[1] Akintola A. Towards Equal Sharing of AIDS Caring Responsibilities: Learning from Africa. Geneva: United Nations [Internet]. 2008. Available from: http:www.un.org/womanwatch/daw [Accessed: 13 December 2010]

[2] Akintola O. Defying all odds: Coping with the challenges of volunteer caregiving for patients with AIDS in South Africa. Journal of Advanced Nursing. 2008;**63**(4):357-365

[3] Anderson P, Doyle LW, Victorian Infant Collaborative Study Group. Neurobehavioral outcomes of school-age children born extremely low birth weight or very preterm in the 1990s. JAMA. 2003;**289**(24):3264-3272

[4] Asante KO. Social support and the psychological wellbeing of people living with HIV/AIDS in Ghana. African Journal of Psychiatry. 2012;**15**(5):340-345

[5] Bachanas PJ, Kullgren KA, Schwartz KS, McDaniel JS, Smith J, Nesheim S. Psychological adjustment in caregivers of school-age children infected with HIV: Stress, coping, and family factors. Journal of Pediatric Psychology. 2001;**26**(6):331-342

[6] Bachanas PJ, Kullgren KA, Schwartz KS, Lanier B, McDaniel JS, Smith J, Nesheim S. Predictors of psychological adjustment in school-age children infected with HIV. Journal of Pediatric Psychology. 2001;**26**(6):343-352

[7] Bauman LJ, Foster G, Johnson Silver E, Berman R, Gamble I, Muchaneta L. Children caring for their ill parents with HIV/AIDS. Vulnerable Children and Youth Studies. 2006;**1**(1):56-70

[8] Brandt R. The mental health of people living with HIV/AIDS in Africa: A systematic review. African Journal of AIDS Research. 2009;**8**(2):123-133

[9] Brandt R, Dawes A, Bray R. Women coping with AIDS in Africa: Contributions of a contextually grounded research methodology. Psychology, Health & Medicine. 2006;**11**(4):522-527

[10] Bretherton I. The origins of attachment theory: John Bowlby and Mary Ainsworth. Developmental Psychology. 1992;**28**(5):759

[11] Button S, Pianta R, Marvin R. Partner support and maternal stress in families raising young children with cerebral palsy. Journal of Developmental and Physical Disabilities. 2001;**13**(1):61-81

[12] Cluver L, Gardner F, Operario D. Psychological distress amongst AIDS-orphaned children in urban South Africa. Journal of Child Psychology and Psychiatry. 2007;**48**(8):755-763

[13] Cluver L, Gardner F, Operario D. Poverty and psychological health among AIDS-orphaned children in Cape Town, South Africa. AIDS Care. 2009;**21**(6):732-741

[14] Cluver LD, Orkin M, Boyes ME, Gardner F, Nikelo J. AIDS-orphanhood and caregiver HIV/AIDS sickness status: Effects on psychological symptoms in South African youth. Journal of Pediatric Psychology. 2012;**37**(8):857-867

[15] Coscia JM, Christensen BK, Henry RR, Wallston K, Radcliffe J, Rutstein R. Effects of home environment, socioeconomic status, and health status on cognitive functioning in children with HIV-1 infection. Journal of Pediatric Psychology. 2001;**26**(6):321-329

[16] Costello EJ, Compton SN, Keeler G, Angold A. Relationships between poverty and psychopathology: A natural experiment. JAMA. 2003;**290**(15):2023-2029

[17] Eloff I, Finestone M, Makin JD, Boeving-Allen A, Visser M, Ebersöhn L, Ferreira R, Sikkema KJ, Briggs-Gowan MJ, Forsyth BWC. A randomized clinical trial of an intervention to promote resilience in young children of HIV-positive mothers in South Africa. AIDS. 2014;**28**(0 3):S347-S357. DOI:10.1097/QAD.0000000000000335

[18] Engle PL, Black MM. The effect of poverty on child development and educational outcomes. Annals of the New York Academy of Sciences. 2008;**1136**(1):243-256

[19] Forsyth BW. Psychological aspects of HIV infection in children. Child and Adolescent. Psychiatric Clinics of North America. 2003;**12**(3):423-437

[20] Gagliardi A, Honigfeld L. Addressing Maternal Depression: Opportunities in the Pediatric Setting. Farmington, CT: Child Health and Development Institute of Connecticut; 2008

[21] George D, Mallery M. Using SPSS for Windows Step by Step: A Simple Guide and Reference. Boston, MA: Allyn Bacon

[22] Hacle K, Somlai A, Kelly J, Kalichman S. Woman living with HIV/AIDS: The dual challenge of being a patient and a caregiver. Health and Social Work. 1997;**22**(1):53-62

[23] Hochhauser CJ, Gaur S, Marone R, Lewis M. The impact of environmental risk factors on HIV-associated cognitive decline in children. AIDS Care; 2008;**20**(6):692-699

[24] Hughes C, Caliandro G. Effects of social support, stress, and level of illness on caregiving of children with AIDS. Journal of Pediatric Nursing. 1996;**11**:347-358

[25] Ingram D, Hutchinson SA. Defensive mothering in HIV-positive mothers. Qualitative Health Research. 1999;**9**(2):243-258

[26] Ingram D, Hutchinson SA. Double binds and the reproductive and mothering experiences of HIV-positive women. Qualitative Health Research. 2000;**10**(1):117-132

[27] Iversen PO, Du Plessis L, Marais D, Morseth M, Herselman M. Nutritional health of young children in South Africa over the first 16 years of democracy. South African Journal of Child Health. 2011;**5**(3):72-77

[28] Kiernan KE, Huerta MC. Economic deprivation, maternal depression, parenting and children's cognitive and emotional development in early childhood1. The British Journal of Sociology. 2008;**59**(4):783-806

[29] Kiernan KE, Mensah FK. Poverty, maternal depression, family status and children's cognitive and behavioural development in early childhood: A longitudinal study. Journal of Social Policy. 2009;**38**(04):569-588

[30] Knitzer J, Theberge S, Johnson K. Reducing Maternal Depression and Its Impact on Young Children: Toward a Responsive Early Childhood Policy Framework. Policy Roundtable. New York: National Center for Children in Poverty; 2008

[31] Lachman JM, Cluver LD, Boyes ME, Kuo C, Casale M. Positive parenting for positive parents: HIV/AIDS, poverty, caregiver depression, child behavior, and parenting in South Africa. AIDS Care. 2014;**26**(3):304-313

[32] Mani A, Mullainathan S, Shafir E, Zhao J. Poverty impedes cognitive function. Science. 2013;**341**(6149):976-980

[33] Mavhu W, Berwick J, Chirawu P, Makamba M, Copas A, Dirawo J, Willis N, Araya R, Abas MA, Corbett EL, Mungofa S, Laver SM, Cowan FM. Enhancing psychosocial support for HIV positive adolescents in Harare, Zimbabwe. PLoS One. 2013;**8**(7):e70254

[34] McLearn KT, Minkovitz CS, Strobino DM, Marks E, Hou W. The timing of maternal depressive symptoms and mothers' parenting practices with young children: Implications for pediatric practice. Pediatrics. 2006;**118**(1):e174-e182

[35] McLeod JD, Shanahan MJ. Poverty, parenting, and children's mental health. American Sociological Review. 1993;**58**(3):351-366

[36] McLeod JD, Shanahan MJ. Trajectories of poverty and children's mental health. Journal of Health and Social Behavior. 1996;**37**(3):207-220.

[37] McLoyd VC. The impact of economic hardship on black families and children: Psychological distress, parenting, and socioemotional development. Child Development. 1990;**61**(2):311-346

[38] McLoyd VC. Socioeconomic disadvantage and child development. American Psychologist. 1998;**53**(2):185

[39] Murphy DA, Marelich WD. Resiliency in young children whose mothers are living with HIV/AIDS. AIDS Care. 2008;**20**(3):284-291

[40] Musile C. Health, Stress, Coping and Social Support in grandmothers as caregivers. Health Care Woman International. 1998;**19**:441-455

[41] National Department of Human Settlement 2009/2010 Informal Settlement Atlas, provided by the HAD. Retrieved from htt://www.thehda.co.za/uploads/images/HDA_Eastern_Cape_Report_lr.pdf 2012.07.15

[42] Patcher L, Auinger P, Palmer R, Weitzman M. Do parenting and the home environment, maternal depression, neighborhood, and chronic poverty affect child behavioral problems differently in different racial-ethnic. Groups. Pediatrics. 2006;**117**:1329-1338

[43] Petersen I, Bhana A, Myeza N, Alicea S, John S, Holst H, McKay M, Mellins C. Psychosocial challenges and protective influences for socio-emotional coping of HIV+ adolescents in South Africa: A qualitative investigation. AIDS Care. 2010;1-9. **22**(8):970-978

[44] Petersen I, Swartz L, Bhana A, Flisher AJ. Mental health promotion initiatives for children and youth in contexts of poverty: The case of South Africa. Health Promotion International. 2010.daq026. **25**(3):331-341

[45] Richter L. The impact of HIV/AIDS on the development of children. A generation at risk. 2004;9-31

[46] Richter LM, Grieve KW. Home environment and cognitive development of black infants in impoverished South African families. Infant Mental Health Journal. 1991;**12**(2):88-102

[47] Richter L, Dawes A, de Kadt J. Early childhood. In: Petersen I, Bhana A, Flisher A, Swartz L & Richter L, editors. Promoting Mental Health in Scarce-Resource Context: Emerging Evidence and Practice. Cape Town: HSRC Press; 2010. pp. 99-123

[48] Richter LM. The Importance of Caregiver-Child Interactions for the Survival and Healthy Development of Young Children: A Review. Geneva: World Health Organization; 2004

[49] Sameroff A. A unified theory of development: A dialectic integration of nature and nurture. Child Development. 2010;**81**(1):6-22

[50] Smith K, Landry S, Swank P. The influence of early paterns of positive parenting on children's preschool outcomes. Early Education and Development. 2000;**11**(2):387-403

[51] Statistics South Africa. Community Survey. Pretoria: Statistics South Africa; 2007

[52] Statistics South Africa. Quarterly Labour Force Survey, 31 July. Pretoria: Stats SA, 2012

[53] Statistics South Africa General Household Survey. Pretoria: Stats SA, 2004. Available from: www.statssa.gov.za/publications/P0318/P03182014.pdf

[54] Tompkins TL, Henker B, Whalen CK, Axelrod J, Comer LK. Motherhood in the context of HIV infection: Reading between the numbers. Cultural Diversity and Ethnic Minority Psychology. 1999;**5**(3):197

[55] Treyvaud K, Anderson VA, Howard K, Bear M, Hunt RW, Doyle LW, *Inder TE, Woodward L*, Anderson PJ. Parenting behavior is associated with the early neurobehavioral development of very preterm children. Pediatrics. 2009;**123**(2):555-561

[56] Treyvaud K, Anderson VA, Lee KJ, Woodward LJ, Newnham C, Inder TE, Doyle LW, Anderson PJ. Parental mental health and early social-emotional development of children born very preterm. Journal of Pediatric Psychology. 2010;**35**(7):768-777

[57] Treyvaud K, Anderson VA, Lee KJ, Woodward LJ, Newnham C, Inder TE, Doyle LW, Anderson PJ. Parental mental health and early social-emotional development of children born very preterm. Journal of Pediatric Psychology. 2009;**35**(7):768-777

[58] Visser M, Finestone M, Sikkema K, Boeving-Allen A, Ferreira R, Eloff I, Forsyth B. Development and piloting of a mother and child intervention to promote resilience in young children of HIV-infected mothers in South Africa. Evaluation and Program Planning. 2012;**35**(4):491-500

[59] WHO/UNAIDS/UNICEF. Towards Universal Access. Scaling Up Priority HIV/AIDS Interventions in the Health Sector. Progress Report. Geneva: WHO. 2010; Retrieved from: http://www.who.int/hiv/pub/towards_universal_access_report_2010.pdf

# 11

# The Role of Educational Technology in Caregiving

Maria José Lumini, Fátima Araújo and Teresa Martins

**Abstract**

Huge demographic and socio-economic changes are part of the experience of present societies. One consequence is the aging of the population and increasingly more people without the capacity for self-care. The provision of intergenerational care, namely caring for the older individuals, is a focus of attention for health professionals, but is also part of the political and social agenda. There is a need to regulate, support, and facilitate the daily life of families who have a dependent aged member. In contemporary societies, the use of information and communication technologies (ICT) is an important driver of innovation, responsible for a large transformation of living standards and new social behaviors. Within the scope of the provision of informal care, ICT can provide a great support, representing a primordial tool for updating the organizations in order to improve their efficiency, incorporating and making available services, and anticipating needs. Thus, the development of equipment, electronic applications, and websites for the elderly or their family caregivers should be conceptualized and customized to the profile of these users. A major challenge faced by healthcare institutions is to focus their services by organizing them around citizens' needs.

**Keywords:** technologies, caregiving, self-care, impairment, nursing

## 1. Introduction

The human being is by nature a gregarious being and the family is a primordial system to ensure the continuity and development of its members throughout the whole life cycle. The family is a systemic and dynamic unit and it influences and receives influences not only from each of its members, but also from the context in which it is inserted.

Throughout history, despite the structural and functional changes that took place in families, societies recognize them an important social role, not only toward the socialization and protection of their members, but also due to its supportive and helping function in the events during the different developmental stages as well as by assisting family members when they experience health/disease processes [1, 2].

The double population aging process (both in the base and top of the pyramid) observed in a large majority of current societies and particularly in developed countries, is accompanied by a successive decrease in the number of people who are able to respond to the challenges of caring for someone who may be unable to perform daily life activities (basic and instrumental), contrasting with an increasing number of elderly/very old people, often presenting chronic diseases associated with high levels of dependency. In fact, concomitantly with this demographic aging, the populations portray an epidemiological profile showing a prevalence of chronic and degenerative diseases that are potentially incapacitating. In the group of the elderly, along with these chronic problems that may progress gradually or with frequent acute episodes, with recurrent hospitalizations, there are other events that generate dependence that may abruptly present themselves, such as cerebrovascular accident (CVA) and fall events, whether they are associated or not with hip fractures.

These transitions (demographic and epidemiological) have prompted a (re-)emergence of an interest for informal systems on the political agenda, not only as a source of welfare provision, but also as an important resource for the continuity of care in situations of disease, particularly regarding society's older members. In fact, structural changes require new policies that ensure the sustainability of health systems and social support.

Whether the situation of dependency sets in unexpectedly or gradually, it requires the family to change its family dynamics in order not only to respond to the needs of the family member with Daily Life Activities (DLA) impairment, but also to regain their stability. The chronic illness and the functional compromise of the person with dependence have repercussions not only on the individual with a health problem, but also on the family, forcing constant adaptations in the family system. Compared to developmental transitions, health/illness transitions constitute an accidental crisis in the family, presenting a more disastrous character due to the unexpected way they are installed, and the need for rapid decision-making, creating situations that the family did not have time, neither knowledge nor maturity to face [3, 4].

After a period marked by the intrahospital occurrence of birth, death, and illness, the recent austerity policies have emphasized the role of the family in social protection and provision of well-being to its members, transferring to them a growing responsibility regarding the continuity of care when one of its members is affected by a health/illness process associated with different levels of functional disability [5].

Across the world, aggressive austerity policies have been implemented, especially in the health and social areas. These policies, in order to overcome the deficiencies, transfer to the caregiver an increased responsibility for the support and provision of care [1], even if the responses provided by the health services/teams are insufficient and inadequate when confronted with the physical, cognitive, and emotional needs expressed by the families/family caregivers [6, 7].

The experience of caring for a dependent person always implies a family (re-)adaptation, namely in terms of its functional dimension, by the need to redefine roles among the different elements of the system, in order to respond to the needs of the dependent person [6].

The scientific literature has identified multiple variables that can interfere in the way each individual and family adapt and manage the disease/dependence situation, finding favorable responses to the continuity of care. Among these variables are the resources the family has, as well as the capacity to mobilize and manage them, the stage of the life cycle in which the family finds itself, the cohesion among its members, the coping strategies that it is able to mobilize [3, 8] as well as the experience of previous similar experiences [4, 7]. There are also variables related to the type and beginning of the disease, expected results, and the level of dependence of the person who receives care [9].

The worsening of the functional level and the poor quality of life of the patient have a great impact on the family caregiver (FC) overload, not only because they require more time and requirements (physical, psychological, emotional, and economic) and also because family carers tend to have more concerns regarding meeting the needs and expectations of their sick relatives at the expense of their own needs, thus "forgetting themselves" [10].

In the face of a health-care transition experienced by a family member, care is usually provided by an informal support system (family or significant person), in which an individual assumes the unpaid responsibility of care with occasional support (instrumental, financial, and emotional) from other elements of the family [11, 12]. The literature presents several denominations for the family individual assuming these roles: informal caregiver; family caregiver, and primary caregiver. The first designation (informal caregiver) essentially aims to differentiate them from formal care, given by paid health professionals (e.g., nurses, doctors, and physiotherapists), both in public and private services. The designation of family caregiver refers to relationship of kinship, ties of consanguinity and affections with the person cared for. The term primary caregiver seeks to distinguish the person from the group of family members who participate in care, assuming the role of coordination and greater responsibility.

But irrespective of the designation, it is desirable that in the family, there is intergenerational collaboration among several members in the care for the dependent person, because it enriches the approach and care provided, also contributing to prevent and attenuate the caregiver's overload [11].

The selection of the person who usually takes care of the elderly person with self-care dependence essentially reflects four major criteria: gender (woman), kinship (spouse, daughters), physical proximity (living together), and affective proximity (conjugal). Although informal support has particular roots in the family system and/or affective bonds, the way a family member becomes FC does not always result from a willing decision, but from a "moral and social obligation" aggravated by a growing tendency by the aggressive and austerity policies (health and social security) to delegate to the family the responsibility of caring for their elderly dependent relatives [13].

In a sociological research on the role of the family and social networks in the production of well-being, it can be seen that in present societies, and particularly in the countries of southern Europe, intergenerational aid is processed essentially in a descending direction (from parents to children) and has still great relevance in domestic work, in the health care of children and the elderly. However, care for the elderly is a supportive area where aid clearly flows in an inverse flow (from children to parents) and the activated links are fundamentally feminine, showing that "what is mobilized is not properly the family, but rather women in the family" [1]. In fact, despite the many socio-political transformations and consequent changes in the family system in situations of illness and incapacity of one of its members, the female member continues to emerge as the main caretaker [1, 6, 10, 14, 15] because presently this duty is socially expected from women.

In countries where aging has been more significant, especially in southern Europe, where the number of families composed by very old couples has become expressive, it is increasingly frequent that continuity of care within the family is given by elderly caregivers, particularly women who care for their husbands, in fragile health and themselves having some type of handicap [6, 16, 17].

In several cultures and in particular for the Portuguese population in a situation of dependence, the family is the dependents' first choice. Institutionalization has a negative connotation and is only accepted when there is no alternative. In fact, in cases of illness and disability affecting the elderly, the family and home are the first choice for a large number of elderlies in order to receive the care they need, implying a greater family support [18].

The transition to this new role not only involves changes in the individual's life and family organization, but also requires the acquisition of new knowledge and skills, in order to be able to respond safely to the (increasingly complex) needs of family members returning home after a critical event that generates dependency or after a worsening of their chronic illness.

As observed in [5], in 2000, health policies lead to increasingly early hospital discharges, with patients leaving hospitals in a very fragile state, making it difficult for the FC and the family to be adequately prepared for the new role in a short space of time. At the global level, this home services provision has been strengthened as an important measure for the sustainability of health services, and under these circumstances, most FCs do not feel prepared to provide the care their family member needs when the patient returns home [7].

Although in some contexts, health services at community level develop programs aimed at providing some continuity in the preparation and support of FC, usually more directed towards the instrumental care of dependent persons, literature has shown that families often perceive it as falling short of their needs [6, 7]. In fact, more and more families take responsibility for the care of their families, but support policies and (health and social) services do not provide them with the necessary support and help [7, 10].

At the beginning of this century, the scientific community has reinforced the importance given to the problem of caring families, and particularly regarding the members responsible for managing and caring for their loved ones that are not to able to care for themselves. The research results show that their difficulties (physical, psychic, social, and economic), have a negative impact on their well-being and health, hindering or impeding an adequate transition to the role of caregiver [8, 18–20].

Using an advanced nursing perspective, the process of breaking away from the biomedical model that still characterizes health care in several countries as well as incorporating the evidence produced on a caregiving family approach, health professionals, and specifically nurses should direct their practices to the family member caregiver who is considered as a care client and an authentic care partner and not just as a resource to ensure continuity of care for its dependent members [21]. In this context, the preparation to return home should be a central concern both in the hospital and in the community context [22]. Home-based care is the proximity care preferable of the population; so, nurses should help families in the transition process experienced when one of their members is afflicted with chronic illness/dependency, accompanying the family/family caregivers wherever they live in order to develop this new role, giving support and managing the resources (internal and external to the family) according to the identified needs (both for the person cared and for the family), facilitating them to make a healthy transition and consequently to rediscover a new balance.

The preparation of the family caregiver at the level of the cognitive knowledge, skills, and competences associated with the caring process is one of the strategies identified to reduce the overload. The most recent literature has echoed some implemented programs (in an anticipatory care approach) to respond to the needs of the family/FC, aiming at preventing overload in the person who is most involved in the provision of care. Although studies have reported some benefits associated with interventions (care training, education and counseling, problem solving, psycho-educational support, coping strategies, information, and help groups), studies are very heterogeneous and reveal methodological weaknesses lowering their level of evidence [18, 21, 23]. The scientific community faces the challenge of developing clinical trials of high methodological quality to produce evidence with transferability potential for decision-making in clinical practice.

Taking into account that the elderly of the next decade are the current adults, with experience in the use of new technologies, it is pertinent that health services can optimize this resource as a complementary intervention, both for the elderly and for family caregivers. Although the research on this subject is still very incipient, the results obtained in a quasi-experimental study (pre and post test) using the conceptual framework from Meleis's theory of transitions [8, 24], show that tele-health care associated with a structured plan for the preparation of hospital discharge presented promising results in reducing FC overload and improved the mastery level with which FC in the intervention group were able to manage stress [25].

## 2. New technologies: a path to the future

In recent years, as a result of demographic evolution and the global aging of the population, changes in policies paradigms have taken place, namely the privatization of some services that provide care, the reinforcement of home support services, and the use of Information and Communication Technologies (ICT) [26, 27].

The use of ICTs for health organizations is today one of the most important resources. The value of technology comes from the capacity to use it, resulting not only from the information provided, but also mainly from its interpretation. It is necessary for health professionals to value the flow of information they access and to derive benefits from them to add value to the care they provide. On the other hand, the technology has an important utility represented by the remote connection when the groups or individuals geographically disperse [28].

In contemporary societies, the use of ICT is a relevant engine of innovation. Information Technologies have become a key tool for updating administration, making it possible to improve efficiency, incorporating and making available services and anticipating needs [29]. Its relevance stands out for both the handling of information and document management, as well as the provision of services to the citizen (even when they are face-to-face).

Society is facing enormous socio-economic changes. These include the great changes in living standards and new social behaviors, with the subsequent competitiveness of organizations as a result of the recent strategic resources of the twenty-first century, namely the development of ICT.

The major challenge that continues challenging the healthcare institutions relate to how to focus the provision of services on the citizens, structuring these services around their needs [30].

The scientific background points to a growing use of educational platforms for citizens' health education. The Internet is considered a privileged means of communication and information used to interact with the population in need of health care.

The great Internet revolution arrived through the Internet of Things (IoT), defined as the technological revolution of everyday objects interconnected via the Internet. The main purpose is to connect through sensors means of transport, clothing and watches, among other things, without human intervention. This means that the IoT will allow the interconnection of real-world objects with the virtual world through wireless (RFID) sensors. With IoT, the equipment is controlled and monitored remotely and is usually wireless. These sensors are capable of connecting household appliances, transport facilities, clothing and everything else, running without batteries. According to the report of the International Data Corporation (IDC), it is estimated that the quantities of these sensors will reach 30 billion in 2020. By IDC predictions, the IoT will be included in 212 billion things globally by the end of 2020 [31]. The main objective is to provide intercommunication of objects among them, exchanging information about status, location, functionalities, problems, etc. Algorithms will be responsible for processing this information, generating a large amount of data that will be stored on powerful servers in the cloud. The IoT is considered a global concept that will evolve from Machine to Machine (M2M) and other technologies.[1]

In future, several sectors will use Machine to Machine (M2M) applied, in particular in the health sector. Its application includes electronic health, m-health, telemedicine and assisted

[1]Machine-to-Machine is where "machines" use network resources to communicate with the remote applications' infrastructure for monitoring and control purposes, either of the "machine" itself or the surrounding environment. The potential interconnection of intelligent objects and the way we interact with the environment is how the Internet of Things is imagined, where the physical world will merge with the digital world.

living. Clients with non-critical health conditions can be monitored with sensors (e.g., blood pressure or blood sugar levels), sent home and supervised remotely by medical staff, and clients can often be instructed on how to interpret the data by themselves. It is important to emphasize the importance of these mechanisms in situations of remote surveillance of elderly people. Both scientific evidence and organizations such as the WHO and the EU have been urging member states to implement information and communication technologies in health care units. It is important to highlight the importance of introducing the new information technologies in health, not only in instruments for health organizations and professionals, but also in individual health plans, in particular in diagnostic and prevention instruments (e.g., blood pressure monitors), health care treatment and management devices and programs (e.g., smartphone devices).

The contribution in Ref. [32] regarding the development of a conceptual framework of information quality of a health platform defines quality dimensions and associated drivers specified for the education of an adult population. The five dimensions of health information quality were identified: completeness of information, understanding of information, relevance of information, depth of information, and accuracy of information; and the main driver themes: content, design, links, consumer resources, search functionality, supporting references, user focus, content FAQ, open access, policy statements and website performance.

It is now evident that technological developments keep pace with the aging of the population and provide important opportunities. For example, the Internet may allow for continuous connection between family members despite distance, access to information that can guide an older person's self-care or support caregivers. Support resources are more functional and accessible than in the past and handheld devices provide new opportunities for personalized health care and monitoring [33]. Thus, these social and technological changes lead to the need of redefining policies in order to benefit from the new opportunities that innovative approaches provide.

### 2.1. The paths of technological innovation

Political, economic, and social actors increasingly recognize innovation as a means for the sustainable development of organizations, thrusting their access to international markets. Innovating means creating new things, but in the opinion of [34], the innovations correspond to new creations with economic or social significance, mostly made by companies. They are the result of interactive processes among the multiple actors that are part of the innovation system, namely innovation in products, services, companies, public administration or society. Thus, innovation in organizations is related to the implementation of new ideas, whether related to new products or new business opportunities [35]. Innovation must be part of the DNA of winning organizations [35].

According to the OECD [36], innovation is already an important factor of economic growth in countries such as Sweden, Finland, or the United States of America. According to the calculations of this organization, in these countries, the investment in intangible assets (R&D, software, databases, patents) is already equal to or greater than the investment in physical assets (machinery, equipment or infrastructures).

Two of the great theories driving innovation are Technological Push and Demand Pull. The first theory, defends the idea that economic development is driven by innovation, where, through a dynamic process, new technologies, new skills, and new industries replace those that once dominated the market. This method wastermed "creative destruction" [37]. In this theory, the ideas that precede the creation of an innovation result from scientific research and the accumulation of the knowledge generated by it, and these ideas are not necessarily associated with a market need. The technology push theory is thus well identified with the linear model of innovation (pipeline) where, in a unidirectional sense and in a phase continuum, innovation starts in scientific research, advancing then to development, production and finally diffusion, with no feedback at any of these phases [34].

Based on the economic theory of market failures, governments have been promoting innovation by directly and indirectly supporting scientific research and the development of its results, in line with the idea that increasing the number of laboratories, researchers or registered patents should lead to an increase in the number of innovations and, hence, in sales, resulting in economic growth and job creation.

Examples of public policies for technology push include research and development (R&D) support, investment in infrastructure (laboratories), tax benefits for companies investing in R&D and support for education/training of researchers.

From the point of view of the demand-pull (or demand-side) innovation theory, it is argued that the capacity to generate innovation is dispersed throughout society and all its "actors" often require market demand for these innovations. For the demand-pull theory, demand is the main gravitational force that attracts resources and skills to innovation in order to meet social or market needs. Thus, a demand-side public policy seeks to increase demand and stimulate companies to respond to the needs of end users (market). It should also seek to reduce (legal, regulatory, and procedural) barriers to innovation, to stimulate end-users to adopt innovations, and to promote the emergence of new markets [37]. The process of innovation is thus achieved by numerous and complex factors. The enterprises rarely innovate sole, but through interaction with other organizations/institutions, they learn and transfer knowledge. These interactions between actors acting in different institutional contexts are therefore crucial to the process of development and diffusion of innovations [38].

In recent years, interest in holistic innovation policies (including the entire innovation cycle) has increased, recognizing the importance of interaction between the different elements of this process [34].

Demand-side innovation policies have an influence on the market; the main foundations for their use according to [39] are to overcome system and market failures and solve key societal challenges.

In Ref. [37], a study presents some examples where the effect of demand and lead users was decisive for the emergence of a new technology/innovation, among these, the Internet. Initially, the work that led to the development of the internet was done to meet the special needs of the US Department of Defense. After the development of the technology, a group of scientific researchers who had worked on that solution used it to establish communications between research laboratories.

Thus, it is essential to introduce the definition of Public Procurement of Innovation (PPI) referring to the public purchase of innovative products or services. It occurs when a public institution places a purchase order to satisfy certain needs (or functions of public responsibility) of a product or service that, although it does not exist at the moment, can be developed in a reasonable period of time. The primary objective of the PPI is to respond to problems in society. It is proposed that it may contribute to the development of knowledge about the user's personal experience, based on the available results [40].

Innovative situations, including ICT, have the potential to contribute to the provision of high quality and personalized healthcare while simultaneously increasing the efficiency of our care systems. Due to research studies that emphasize the need to include strategies that integrate interactive educational technologies in the training of people in the organizational contexts [41–44], it becomes a challenge to implement and highlight health policies that include the training and application of educational technologies and their dominance in the educational processes of users and families.

The World Health Organization's World Health Report on Aging states that between the years 2000 and 2050, the number of people aged 60 and over will double; and that by 2050, more than one in five people will be over 60 years [33]. Against this backdrop, the report addresses these challenges, recommending equally profound changes in the way health policies should be formulated and health services delivered to aging populations. Some of the important recommendations to be considered include the need to make an individual assessment taking into account that the factors influencing the health of the elderly are in equal proportion individual (behaviors, age-related changes, genetic factors, and diseases) and also related to the environment in which they live (housing, support technologies, transport and services, and social and health support). Promoting healthy aging involves changing attitudes about aging and the elderly, creating environmentally friendly environments for all ages, adapting health systems to people's needs, and developing long-term care systems [27, 33].

WHO defines active aging as the process of optimizing health, social participation, and safety opportunities in order to improve quality of life as people age [45]. Europe is known for its capacity for innovation and its future involves the development of actionable initiatives, among which the "Innovation Union" is highlighted. Part of this strategy is the production of smart, sustainable, and inclusive growth that translates into tertiary quality care for the elderly [46, 47].

One of the initiatives carried out by the Innovation Union was the creation of the European Innovation Partnership on Active Healthy Aging, (EIP-AHA)[2] [48]. Under this EIP-AHA [48] partnership, innovative ICT-based solutions should play an important role in achieving the objectives. Its strategic implementation plan sets out the priorities for accelerating and

---

[2]EIP-AHA access: http://ec.europa.eu/research/innovation-union/index_en.cfm?section=active-healthy-ageing&pg=about

intensifying innovation in the field of active and healthy aging across the EU in three areas: disease prevention and health promotion, health care and treatment, autonomous living and social inclusion. Thus, the objectives of the innovation partnership by 2020 are to allow citizens to live longer with good health, to increase their average number of healthy years by two years (number of years a person of 65 can expect to live without limitations), and achieve this goal by improving the sustainability and efficiency of our social and health systems, creating a market both in the EU and globally for innovative products and services with new business opportunities [49].

In Portugal, there are institutions and researchers that are part of this European Partnership, seeking to carry out initiatives, scientific research, and technological applications that promote general well-being and healthy aging, namely Ageing@Coimbra which is a consortium aimed at enhancing the role of the elderly in society and the application of good practices for general well-being and active and healthy aging. It is considered by the EU as European Reference Region for Active and Healthy Aging, a unique status within the Portuguese territory. It acts through the following action groups: adherence to therapy; prevention of falls; prevention of frailness; remote health monitoring; and elder-friendly services [50].

Simultaneously, in order to respond to this challenge, the concept of Ambient Assisted Living (AAL), which aims at the application of ICTs in the health field, results from the fusion of areas such as science, technology, health, and engineering. In this way, the AAL concept aims to increase the time the elderlies can live in their preferred environment, with autonomy and independence, through assistance in their daily activities [51]. In practical terms, AAL systems help prevent and classify situations such as falls, physical immobility, day-to-day activities, health parameter monitoring, and behavioral analysis. In general, the following objectives can be defined to respond to the concept of AAL: (1) to extend the time that people can live in their preferred environment, increasing their autonomy, self-confidence and mobility; support the maintenance of the health status and functional capacities of the elderly; (2) promote a healthier lifestyle for individuals at risk; (3) increase security, prevent social isolation and support the maintenance of a multifunctional network around the individual; (4) support caregivers, family members and care organizations; and (5) increase the efficiency and productivity of resources used in aging societies [52]. Some examples of home care projects will be presented considering the abovementioned background.

Thus, the project AAL4ALL[3] presents an idea by developing an ecosystem of products and services for Ambient Assisted Living (AAL) associated with a business model and validated through a large-scale pilot study. The project aims to bring together key stakeholders (public institutions, industry, user organizations, and R&D institutions) to discuss the definition of a basic set of AAL services of general interest. Analysis of standards, as well as other existing international activities, is the key principle of the project to avoid reinventing the wheel, focusing all efforts on implementing solutions to identified gaps. The definition of reference models for different environments will serve to reduce the risk of investment and to shorten the time-to-market of products and services developed in the future. The project is broken

[3]Project AAL4AAL link: http://www.aal4all.org/?lang=Pt

down into a number of areas that respond to the challenges and market segments for products (home and mobile users, ICT and logistics services, and users of care providers) in an integrated way.

The *European Joint Action*[4] is a project aimed at the prevention of chronic diseases, in particular cardiovascular diseases and type-2 diabetes. One of the fundamental objectives is the development of a platform for the exchange of knowledge, providing a more advanced updated repository and best practices on chronic diseases.

The project *Valorisation of Innovative Technologies for Aging in Europe* (VInTAgE)[5] was born in response to the i2010 European Initiative on Inclusion. The project aimed to propose innovative solutions to make information and communication technologies more accessible and attractive for the elderly, promoting benefits for their quality of life and independence in respect of them.

*The Fall Prevention Project*: For an active aging in community, two European cities (FP-FAAC:2EC)[6] aim to contribute to active aging through the prevention of falls and associated injuries. It is being developed with national and international partners. At a national level, they partner with a group of Health Centers of Porto and at international level, the University of Cordoba. The orientation of the project is based on a methodological approach of action-research, focusing on the process centered on praxis, seeking to change the practices in use, together with the actors of the contexts.

The project *Interactive Educational Technologies for Family Carers* (INTENT-CARE)[7] is a platform aimed at family caregivers who care for dependent people. Innovative solution is selected to be a part of the platform: Innovation Procurement Platform—AHA Innovative Solutions of the European Commission. It is proposed to contribute to the development of knowledge about the personal experience of the user, based on the available results. In addition, this knowledge is intended to help meeting user needs in order to increase the use of technologies. This project aims to develop and validate an interactive tool that allows specific information to be provided to family caregivers of people with dependency that complements their orientation and promotes their autonomy. The main innovative element will be the interactive design of the platform allowing a quick response to the needs of the user, aiding in the decision process and the selection of the most relevant information. The contents will be constructed focusing on the basic needs of daily life, in order to overcome difficulties regardless of the clinical diagnosis of the patients. This platform will be supported by demonstration videos of procedures and audio documents. Family caregivers already supporting dependent family members will enact videos to be produced to this end. Through the reliable information that the platform provides, adapted to the needs of family caregivers, this technological tool is an important facilitator to improve the care provided to dependent people. The current socio-professional context advocates the adoption of multiple resources and health policies that promote the

[4]European Joint Action link: http://www.chrodis.eu/

[5]VInTAgE link: http://www.vintageproject.eu/index.php/pt/pthome/7-general/67-itthevintageproject-2

[6]Project developed for professors from ESEP. FPFAAC link: http://www.esenf.pt/pt/i-d/projetos-internacionais/fp-faac/

[7]Project developed for professors from ESEP. Intent-Care link: http://www.esenf.pt/pt/i-d/projetos-internacionais/intent-care/

training of family caregivers, contributing to the sustainability of the National Health Service. This research suggests new educational strategies aimed at the family caregivers, using information and communication technologies [53].

One of the platforms developed within the framework of active aging is the "Aging well academy,"[8] a new online platform that aims to be a reliable source of information and counseling for seniors and caregivers on health prevention for the senior population promoting active and healthy aging. Developed by Porto4Ageing, the Center for Excellence in Active and Healthy Aging coordinated and promoted by the University of Porto and Porto City Council, this project aims to fill the gap in Portugal regarding the lack of reliable tools on health for the elderly, providing information on issues such as vaccination, healthy living habits, and adequate use of antibiotics.

The Porto4Ageing[9] was also responsible for selecting the Porto Metropolitan Area as one of the 74 reference sites in Active and Healthy Aging throughout Europe since 2016. The Porto4Ageing consortium has the specific objective of being an aggregating center and a forum for the discussion of issues related to active and healthy aging in the Porto metropolitan area, bringing together the various regional actors who work and who have an interest in this area, already comprising more than 90 partner institutions from four different profiles (universities and research centers, policy makers, users and industry). This quadruple-helix partnership, which involves different stakeholders (decision makers/caregivers, business/industry, academia/research and civil society/users), who are well placed to drive structural change, is far beyond the scope reachable by one organization on its own, in order to innovate and test in real-world contexts.

The HEARTEN project[10]—the HF collaborative tool for HF management, a project developed for people with heart failure. The HEARTEN project is designed to give heart failure patients extra support in everyday tasks and routine. According to an agent from the European Heart Network, this contributes to improving patients' overall quality of life.

The eWALL[11] is the outcome of a EC-funded project that contributes to the prolongation of independent living of various patient types and senior citizens. Unlike traditional eHealth/eCare solutions, eWALL offers a new experience to the users by creating Caring Home Environments based on advanced sensing and reasoning in an unobtrusive way.

The "Active Ageing at Home"[12] (AA@H) project delivers services to improve quality of life for elderly people by means of ICT solutions based on AAL paradigms, building a comprehensive platform. The proposed scenario includes a set of AAL solutions available to the seniors. It means to improve the sense of safety and comfort perceived by self-sufficient elderly people, and to foster active aging behaviors in their home environment. The key concepts of AA@H

[8]Aging well academy link: http://24.sapo.pt/tecnologia/artigos/academia-do-bem-envelhecer-a-plataforma-que-promove-a-saude-e-vacinacao-na-terceira-idade
[9]Porto4Ageing link: https://noticias.up.pt/porto4ageing-participa-em-tres-projetos-de-promocao-do-envelhecimento-saudavel/
[10]HEARTEN project link: www.hearten.eu
[11]eWALL project link: http://ewallproject.eu/
[12]Active Ageing at Home project link: http://activeageingathome.eresult.it/

are adaptability (seniors' needs change in time and the system adapts to variable requirements) and personalization (seniors can choose among a set of services and design their own support platform).

In addition to these programs, we list some proposals for ongoing activities, initiatives focusing on physical exercise (Portuguese National Walking and Running Program) and nutrition (*Health Ageing with Innovative Functional Foods/Needs for degenerative and metabolic diseases /INOVAFUNAGEING and Bioactive Natural Food Ingredients for aging-people functional diet/ NutriBioFun)* [54].

It is important to use examples of experiences from different countries to illustrate how specific situations can be addressed through innovative solutions. These solutions range from comprehensive care strategies focused on older people to health policies that enable older people to live with wellness and safety.

New technologies must be designed to allow interaction and meeting people's needs [45]. They do not replace face-to-face education with distance education; they are rather intended to move into a situation of interaction with other alternative forms of learning where professionals, patients, caregivers, and organizations are considered potential learning subjects [32, 55–57]. Technology has the potential to help patients and caregivers to become more autonomous in managing their own health and care [53, 55]. The Internet can be used as a complement to the provision of information through a helpline associated with a broad program of health promotion strategies [58]. In these studies, the use of educational technologies as a caring activity can be an innovative way of experiencing, in a healthy way, the transitions of the dependent person and the family caregiver. Thus, it is necessary to advance in more evidence-based ways, recommended to be used in the health area. Its use is a valuable resource in the educational strategies adopted by health professionals in the training of dependent people as well as family caregivers.

## 3. Recommendations for the development of new technologies for the elderly and their caregivers

ICT and the Web are resources with a strong impact on people's lives and well-being. The computer, the mobile phone, and the tablet are today's examples of essential work equipment, which are also used in leisure activities. Many of us cannot imagine our day to day life without these devices. The older population and those caring for them (usually with a close demographic profile) have had a more modest use of these resources due to the limitations associated with aging and the fact that they have not had prior used these technologies.

However, the use of ICT and an accessible Web can directly or indirectly support (through caregivers) social participation and independence at more advanced ages. There is a need to create more inclusive and facilitating measures for older people and their caregivers to also have access to information technologies and other electronic devices that facilitate a better quality of life. Some studies emphasize that the elderly have an interest and possibility of achieving good interaction and mastery in the use of technologies, improving their social interaction and mental stimulation [59, 60].

Physiological changes, associated with the aging process, determine a wide range of functionality and disabilities in the elderly, which may limit the use of new technologies. However, elderlies could get more value in the use of computer technologies and their role in communicating with others, their usefulness in risk management as well as functionalities that provide more well-being. Hence, the need to rethink and devise strategies promotes the inclusion of older people in this process.

Thus, there is a need to look at the process of aging and the physical, emotional, and social changes associated with it. We will only address the most relevant and which may become obstacles in the use of technologies. These include sensory decline as well as reduced attention and working memory.

Vision and hearing are two senses that undergo significant changes during the aging process. From the age of 40, humans begin to have more difficulties in reading a text with small print at a short distance. The eye loses the ability to detect fine details, loses contrast sensitivity, and the ability to distinguish similar colors. Between 40 and 80 years, contrast sensitivity may decrease to less than 83%. It is easier to see red and yellow compared to blue and green, and it is difficult to distinguish darker blue from black. There is pupil shrinkage, resulting in a greater need for light, and a decreased ability to adjust for changing light levels. For example, at age 60, the retina receives only 40% of the usual light (compared with the retina at age 20) and, at 80 years, it receives only 15% of the usual light [61]. There is also a progressive reduction in visual field with loss of peripheral vision.

At the hearing level, there is also a gradual impairment with age, with an increasing inability to hear high-pitched sounds.

Also mental and motor skills, namely dexterity, decrease with age. The presence of incapacitating pathologies such as arthritis and Parkinson's disease, hinder or even inhibit the use of technological equipment, such as the mouse, pointing devices and even the use of the keyboard [61].

Aging changes the way we think. The ability to simultaneously recall and process new information, perform complex cognitive tasks, and understand text can be hampered, making it difficult to use computers and other electronic equipment. Some people may have a clear thinking process in their 80s, while others already have severe cognitive impairment at 60. Despite this variability, three areas are particularly relevant in the development of technologies for the elderly: memory, attention, and decision-making [62].

There are different types of memory. These are differently affected by the aging process. For example, procedural memory (that is, remembering how it is done) is usually not affected. People can learn new skills and reproduce them over time. But other types of memory are affected as we age. Short-term memory and episodic memory are the most vulnerable. Older people often find it difficult to handle the content of their working memory. This means that they may have trouble understanding how to combine complex new concepts into a product or interface. Prospective memory (remembering to do something in the future) is also affected. This is particularly relevant to the usual tasks, such as remembering to take medications on time every day. Older people use paper records or calendars as memory aids to remember appointments, tests, and other future events, while younger people turn to electronic calendars and synchronize a set of applications that automatically update [62].

The pace of task execution is substantially slower with age. The elderly require more time to complete the tasks. Older people are less capable of dividing attention among multiple tasks. Regarding the design and development of technology products, the option for solutions that help people focus on one thing at a time may have benefits for all age groups.

Young people tend to weigh many options before choosing one. Older people base their decisions using other mental schemes, choosing in particular what enhances their prior knowledge and also pay attention to the opinions of experts (for example, their personal doctor for health decisions).

However, aging does not only have to be associated with negative aspects, but it is a stage of life in which it is necessary to invest in the full potential to carry out actions that allow the inclusion, participation and experience in a family and social context giving the maximum quality of life.

Older people are usually alert, persistent, and dedicated to learning what they recognize as interesting and accessible to their abilities [62]. Pickering [62] uses a funny expression regarding the attention of older people compared with young people, noting that the average person's attention has fallen below the level of a goldfish. The author notes that older people interact differently with the world and often find meaning and pay attention to things that younger people ignore.

Most creators of electronics, applications, and websites are young people who design interfaces based on commonly known concepts and features. The technological industry places its bets mainly on products for young people since they are their main clients. Most young people grew up playing, studying, and making use of a large number of equipment and applications. But many of the older ones lived without computers and may have never had contact with interface elements that we consider mundane. In the development of equipment, app and websites, there is usually little sensitivity to the physical and psychological problems of the elderly. However, it is important to pay attention to the detail that in the next decade, the number of elderly people with technological illiteracy will decrease substantially.

Accessibility and usability are two central concepts in the design and development of materials and technological equipment. Accessibility refers to the ease of accessing a given resource, even if architectural barriers, communication availability, physical access, adequate equipment and programs, content and presentation of information in alternative formats are created. Usability is defined by the International Organization for Standardization – ISO 9241, "The extent to which a user can use a product to achieve specific goals with effectiveness, efficiency and satisfaction in a specified context" [63]. The greater the ease of learning and memorizing, the faster the tasks are performed, the lower the error rate and the higher the user satisfaction and the usability the interface has. As considered in Ref. [59], usability is the ability of the software to allow the users to reach their goals of interaction with the system. The principles of good usability are: to be easy to learn, to allow efficient use, and to present few errors [59].

The first recommendation given by Pickering [62] is that the development of a technological product must be based on intuitive bases and it should not require prior knowledge. As per Ref. [59], it is recommended to keep a good contrast between the page background colors and the text.

Very bright backgrounds that completely obscure the dark letters should be avoided. When the background color of the web page is very bright, the elderly people find it difficult to perceive the text. A study in Ref. [59] suggests that in order to be more favorable for the elderly, web interfaces should appear with clear letters on a dark background with low brightness. It is convenient to avoid blue as the interface color and pay attention to the contrast indexes related with the text. The yellow, blue, and green tones should not be used nearby to each other.

The text view should have a font size compatible with the characteristic limitations of old age, being the most recommended a font up to 16 pixels that the user can adjust depending on the device and the viewing distance (National Institute on Aging and the National Library of Medicine, Making Your Web Site Senior Friendly, 2002 https://www.nlm.nih.gov/pubs/checklist.pdf). A sans serif font (Helvetica, Arial, Univers, or News Gothic) is a good choice (Making Your Web Site senior friendly). The text should be written in uppercase and lowercase letters, using only uppercase and italics in titles or headlines. A double spacing should be used in the body of the text, favoring rapid eye movements for the jumps between the end of one line and the beginning of the next.

The alignment of the text should be done by the left margin, as it favors reading by creating uniform spaces between words and by allowing jumps between the end of a line and the beginning of the next line [63].

With age, the elderly loses the ability to understand a text. Thus, the information should be clear and simple. To reduce the number of inferences in message comprehension, it is necessary to use positive statements using the active voice and avoid unnecessary punctuation marks. The information must be chained following an argument and logical order. Computer applications should use familiar words, phrases, and concepts, rather than technical terms. If the text includes technical terms, a glossary should be made available. The content of the information should be organized into shorter sections and segments, facilitating download time on older equipment. Elderlies usually have outdated equipment with less power.

The most important information should be placed in the upper left corner in the cases when the screen contains a lot of information. If the screen does not have much information, it can be placed in the central part.

Only relevant images should be used. Providing alternative text information with animation, video, and audio is generally well received by all users, including the elderly.

Study regarding contents for elders in Ref. [59] recommends avoiding the use of links in the middle of content that have associated the opening of other windows. Older people may get lost and disoriented by opening multiple links in new windows as it increases the set of actions to reach a goal or accomplish a task. The opening of new windows increases the perceptual and cognitive load of the elderlies. It is recommended that only one link can be opened from the primary page. This respects the perceptual, cognitive, and motor capacity of the elderly [59]. By decreasing the number of pages the user has to access, the workload and the probability of errors will be reduced.

The use of scroll bars to access longer text may be interesting, but this mechanism should be very visible and intuitive in its use.

Equipment with touch screen technology may be less user-friendly than equipment that uses buttons and keys. Thus, equipment should be simplified and tools such as fields and forms should be avoided. They should have a separation distance between interface elements of less than 2 mm [62]. Ref. [62] recommends that the buttons on the touch interfaces should be at least 9.6 mm diagonal (for example, 44 × 44 pixels on an iPad) for ages up to 70 and even larger for older people. Interface elements to be clicked with a mouse (such as forms and buttons) must be at least 11 mm diagonal.

When using icons in an interface, the number of elements and colors must be reduced in order to allow them to be identified and understood. Images must be enlarged and associated with textual labels. It is recommended to use large, legible, and significant icons that are easily discriminated and labeled.

The product must be tested on a screen reader and must provide captions whenever video or audio content is critical to the customer experience.

Sites must have a navigation map, allowing for greater understanding and guidance. The site map should clarify the organization of the site.

Security issues in accessing accounts that involve verification and validation procedures, reading difficult codes and letters are rarely recommended in the elderly. Also, validation issues that involve issues such as your preferred color, or a significant date may be confusing and demotivating for the older users. For those reasons, security processes must be streamlined and carefully considered.

In summary, we can conclude that there are a set of recommendations for the creation of applications, equipment, and websites for the elderlies that aim at their improved participation and social inclusion. A large proportion of elderly people present severe handicaps and changes in their functionality and they depend on third parties for a set of activities. These technologies can play an active and decisive role in the caring process. The previously described INTENT Care project (http://www.esenf.pt/pt/i-d/projetos-internacionais/intent-care/), is an example of this trend. The technologies associated with the care process should not replace professionals, but rather represent a resource that facilitates their approximation.

The emergence of technological products has come up at an accelerated pace creating an inability to keep abreast of all the proposals. Another problem that has recently appeared is related to the difficulty of articulating the different technological solutions due to the fact that they have different operating systems and present incompatibilities when used jointly. Therefore, it is desirable in the short term to develop criteria for the greater operability of technological products, in particular computer applications. The constitution of a set of free access technology repositories will be another relevant aspect for the creation of synergies in the field of active and participatory aging.

## Acknowledgements

This article was supported by FEDER through the operation POCI-01-0145-FEDER-007746 funded by the Programa Operacional Competitividade e Internacionalização – COMPETE2020 and by National Funds through FCT – Fundação para a Ciência e a Tecnologia within CINTESIS, R&D Unit (reference UID/IC/4255/2013).

## Author details

Maria José Lumini*, Fátima Araújo and Teresa Martins

*Address all correspondence to: lumini@esenf.pt

School of Nursing of Porto and Center for Health Technology and Services Research, Porto, Portugal

## References

[1] Portugal S. Famílias e Redes Sociais: Ligações fortes na produção de bem-estar. 1st ed. Coimbra: Almedina; 2014. 288 p. ISBN: 978-972-40-5471-1

[2] Silva J, Pereira M. Família e idoso. In: Silva J, Braga GC, editors. O envelhecimento no contexto interdisciplinar. 2nd ed. Curitiba: Prismas; 2016. pp. 253-270

[3] Figueiredo M. Modelo Dinâmico de Avaliação e Intervenção Familiar: Uma abordagem Colaborativa em Enfermagem de Família. 1st ed. Loures: Lusociência; 2012. 205 p. ISBN: 978-972-8930-83-7

[4] Pettengill M, Angelo M. Vulnerabilidade da família: Desenvolvimento do conceito. Revista Latino-americana de Enfermagem. 2005;**13**(6):982-988. Available from: http://www.scielo.br/pdf/rlae/v13n6/v13n6a10.pdf

[5] Brereton L, Nolan M. 'You do know he's had a stroke, don't you?' Preparation for family caregiving: The neglected dimension. Journal of Clinical Nursing. 2000;**9**:498-506

[6] Araújo I, Paúl C, Martins M. Cuidar das famílias com um idoso dependente por AVC: Do hospital à comunidade: um desafio. Revista Referência. 2008;**2**(7):43-53

[7] Shyu Y, Chen M, Wang H, Shao J. A family caregiver-oriented discharge planning program for older stroke patients and their family caregivers. Journal of Clinical Nursing. 2008;**17**:2497-2508. DOI: 10.1111/j.1365-2702.2008.02450.x

[8] Meleis A. Theoretical Nursing: Development and Progress. 4th ed. Philadelphia: Lippincott Williams & Wilkins; 2007. 807 p. ISBN: 0-7817-3673-0

[9] Revilla L, Corredor A, Quelc M, Quesada F. Tipolpgía psicosocial de las enfermedades crónicas en los mayors dependientes. Revista Atención Primaria. 2007;**39**(7):367-372

[10] Borges E, Franceschini J, Costa L, Fernandes A, Jamnik S, Santoro I. Sobrecarga do cuidador familiar: a sobrecarga de cuidar pacientes com câncer do pulmão, de acordo com o estágio do câncer e a qualidade de vida do paciente. Jornal Brasileiro de Pneumologia. 2007;**43**(1):18-23. DOI: doi.org/10.1590/S1806-37562016000000177

[11] Araújo F, Martins T. Avaliação dos cuidadores: Considerações e orientações para a prática. In: Martins T, Araújo F, Peixoto M, Machado P, editors. A pessoa dependente & o familiar cuidador. 1st ed. Porto: Enfermagem Porto; 2016 pp. 113-130. ISBN:978-989-20-7135-0

[12] Brito A. Reconstrução da autonomia: Uma teoria explicativa. In: Martins T, Araújo M, Peixoto M, Paulo Machado P, editors. A pessoa dependente & o familiar cuidador. Porto: Enfermagem Porto; 2016. pp. 113-130. ISBN: 978-989-20-7135-0

[13] Rezende G, Gomes C, Rugno F, Carvalho R, De Carlo M. Sobrecarga de cuidadores de pessoas em cuidados paliativos: revisão integrativa da literatura. Medicina (Ribeirão Preto). 2016;**49**(4):344-354. DOI: 10.11606/issn.2176-7262.v49i4p344-354

[14] Honea N, Brintnall R, Given B, Sherwood P, Colao D, Somers S, Northouse L. Putting evidence into Practice®: Nursing assessment and interventions to reduce family caregiver strain and burden. Clinical Journal of Oncology Nursing. 2008;**12**(3):507-516. DOI: 10.1188/08.CJON.507-516

[15] Hubbard A, McEvoy P, Smith L, Kane R. Brief group psychoeducation intervention for caregivers of individuals with bipolar disorder: A randomized controlled trial. Journal of Affective Disorders. 2016;**200**:31-36. DOI: 10.1016/j.jad.2016.04.013

[16] Arias C. El apoio social en la vejez: alternativas de acción frente a los desafíos del envejecimiento poblacional. Perspectivas en Psicología. 2008;**5**(2):54-61. Available from: http://www.mdp.edu.ar/psicologia/public/index.htm#vol5

[17] Vitor J, Moreira M, Lemes I. O cuidar do cuidador. In: Silva J, Cristiane C, editors. O envelhecimento no contexto interdisciplinar. 2nd ed. Curitiba: Prismas; 2016. pp. 561-571

[18] Belgacem B, Auclair C, Fedor M, Brugnon D, Blanquet M, Tournilhac O, Gerbaud L. A caregiver educational program improves quality of life and burden for cancer patients and their caregivers: A randomised clinical trial. European Journal of Oncology Nursing. 2013;**17**(6):870-876

[19] Gutierrez- madonado J, Caqueo-Urizar A. Effectiveness of a psycho-educational intervention for reducing burden in latin american families of patients with schizophrenia. Quality of Life Research. 2007;**16**(5):739-747. DOI: 10.1007/s11136-007-9173-9

[20] Stajduhar K. Burdens of family caregiving at the end of life. Clinical & Investigative Medicine. 2013;**36**(3):E121-E126. Available from: http://cahs-acss.ca/wp-content/uploads/2015/07/Burdens-of-Family-Caregiving-at-the-End-of-Life.pdf

[21] Brereton L, Carroll C, Barnston S. Interventions for adult family carers of people who have had a stroke: A systematic review. Clinical Rehabilitation. 2007;**21**(10):867-884

[22] Petronilho F. Preparação do regresso a casa. In: Martins T, Araújo F, Peixoto M, Machado P, editors. A pessoa dependente & o familiar cuidador. Porto: Enfermagem Porto; 2016. pp. 73-93. ISBN: 978-989-20-7135-0

[23] Chen M, Huang M, Yeh Y, Huang W, Chen C. Effectiveness of coping strategies intervention on caregiver burden among caregivers of elderly patients with dementia. Psychogeriatrics. 2015;**15**(1):20-25. DOI: 10.1111/psyg.12071

[24] Meleis A, Trangenstein P. Facilitating transitions: Redefinition of the nursing mission. Nursing Outlook.. 1994;**42**(6):255-259. DOI: http://dx.doi.org/10.1016/0029-6554(94)90045-0

[25] Chiang L, Chen W, Dai Y, Ho Y. The effectiveness of telehealth care on caregiver burden, mastery of stress, and family function among family caregivers of heart failure patients: A quasi-experimental study. International Journal of Nursing Studies. 2012;**49**(10):1230-1242. DOI: 10.1016/j.ijnurstu.2012.04.013

[26] OECD. Health at a Glance 2015: OECD Indicators. Paris: OECD Publishing. 2015. Available from: http://dx.doi.org/10.1787/health_glance-2015-en [Accessed: Sep 23, 2017]

[27] OECD. Focus on Health Spending: Health statistic 2015. Paris: OECD Publishing. 2015. Available from: https://www.oecd.org/health/health-systems/Focus-Health-Spending-2015.pdf [Accessed: Sep 23, 2017]

[28] Sousa F, Monteiro I. Colaborar para inovar – A inovação organizacional e social como resultado do processo de decisão. 1st ed. Lisboa: Sílabo; 2015. 343 p. ISBN: 978-972-618-790-5

[29] Resolução do Conselho de Ministros (RCM). No. 108/2017. Estratégia TIC 2020 – Estratégia para a Transformação Digital na Administração Pública. Diário da República, 1.a série-No. 143-26 de julho de 2017 [Internet]. Available from: https://tic.gov.pt/aprovados-a-estrategia-tic-2020-e-os-planos-setoriais-tic [Accessed: Sep 27, 2017]

[30] Varela M, Dias A. Introdução à Gestão – Gestão empresarial. Lisboa: Escolar Editora; 2015

[31] International Data Corporation (IDC). World Wild Internet of Things 2017-2021. [Internet] Available from: https://www.marketresearch.com/IDC-v2477/ [Accessed: Oct 3, 2017]

[32] Tao D, LeRouge C, Smith J, Fahima R, De Leo, G. Defining information quality into health websites: a conceptual framework of health website information quality for educated young adults. [Internet] JMIR Hum Factors. 2017;**4**(4):e25. DOI: 10.2196/humanfactors.6455

[33] Organização Mundial de Saúde (OMS). Relatório mundial de envelhecimento e saúde. Genebra: OMS. [Internet]. Available from: http://sbgg.org.br/wp-content/uploads/2015/10/OMS-ENVELHECIMENTO-2015-port.pdf [Accessed: Oct 3, 2017]

[34] Edquist C, Vonortas N, Zavala J, Edler J. Public Procurement for Innovation. Cheltenham: Edward Elgar Publishing Limited; 2015. 323 p

[35] Dantas J, Moreira A. O processo de Inovação. Como potenciar a criatividade organizacional visando uma competitividade sustentável. Lidel: Editora Lisboa; 2011. 284 p

[36] Organization for Economic Co-operation and Development, and Statistical Office of the European (OECD) Communities. The OECD Innovation Strategy. 2010. DOI: http://dx.doi.org/10.1787/9789264083479-en [Accessed: Sep 23, 2017]

[37] Organisation for Economic Co-operation and Development, and Statistical Office of the European Communities (OEDC). Demand-Side Innovation Policies. OECD Publishing. 2011. Available from: http://www.oecd.org/sti/inno/48081293.pdf [Accessed: Sep 23, 2017]

[38] Edquist C, Zabala J. Public procurement for innovation (PPI) as mission-oriented. Research Policy. 2012;**41**(10):1757-1769

[39] Edler J. Demand Policies for Innovation in EU CEE Countries. Manchester Business School Working Paper. 2009; 579 p. [Internet]. Available from: http://www.mbs.ac.uk/research/workingpapers/

[40] Georghiou L, Edler J, Uyarra E, Jillian Y. Policy instruments for public procurement of innovation: Choice, design and assessment. Technological Forecasting and Social Change. 2014;**86**:1-12

[41] Dias M. Contributo das tecnologias de informação na Gestão do Regime Terapêutico no Diabético [Tese]. Porto, Portugal: Instituto Superior das Tecnologias da Saúde; 2013

[42] Lopes P. A Web no apoio à gestão da Doença Pulmonar Obstrutiva Crónica (DPOC) [Tese]. Portugal: Universidade de Aveiro-Departamento de Educação e Arte; 2013

[43] Lumini M. Tecnologias educacionais interativas: contributo para o desenvolvimento de conhecimentos dos familiares cuidadores [Tese]. Biomédicas Abel Salazar-Universidade do Porto, Portugal; 2015. Available from: https://repositorio-aberto.up.pt/bitstream/10216/82527/2/113841.pdf

[44] Righi V. Re-thinking human-computer interaction research and design with a growing ageing population [Tese]. Universitat Pompeu Fabra, Barcelona, España; 2016. Available from: http://www.dtic.upf.edu/~jblat/material/tvr_2016.pdf

[45] World Health Organization (WHO). Active ageing: A policy framework. Geneva: WHO – Noncommunicable Disease Prevention and Health Promotion, Ageing and Life Course. 2002. Available from: http://apps.who.int/iris/bitstream/10665/67215/1/WHO_NMH_NPH_02.8.pdf [Accessed: Sep 20, 2017]

[46] European Commission (EC). Internet usage by individuals in 2014: Eurostat newsrelease. 2014. Available from: http://ec.europa.eu/eurostat/documents/2995521/6343581/4-16122014-BP-EN.pdf/b4f07b2a-5aee-4b91-b017-65bcb6d95daa [Accessed: Sep 10, 2017]

[47] European Commission (EC). A pocket guide on the innovation union. Luxemburgo: European Commission; 2014. Available from: http://ec.europa.eu/research/innovation-union/index_en.cfm [Accessed: Sep 10, 2017]

[48] European Commission (EC). European Commission. European Innovation Partnership on Active and Healthy Ageing [Internet]. [in press]. Available from: http://ec.europa.eu/research/innovation union/index_en.cfm?section=active-healthy-ageing&pg=about [Accessed: Sep 27, 2017]

[49] CE – Comissão Europeia (CE). Comunicação da Comissão ao Parlamento Europeu, ao Conselho, ao Comité Económico e Social Europeu e ao Comité das Regiões: Iniciativa emblemática no quadro da estratégia «Europa 2020» «União da Inovação» [Internet]. Bruxelas: Comissão Europeia; 2010. Available from: http://eur-lex.europa.eu/LexUriServ/LexUriServ.do?uri=COM:2010:0546:FIN:PT:PDF [Accessed: Sep 27, 2017]

[50] Malva J. Ageing@Coimbra, Região Europeia de Referência para o Envelhecimento Activo e Saudável "O Cluster de Envelhecimento Cerebral, Demência e Disfunções da Visão" [Internet]. 2013. Available from: https://www.fct.pt/apoios/cooptrans/jpi/docs/Ageing_Coimbra_JMalva.pdf [Accessed: Sep 27, 2017]

[51] Broek G, Cavallo F, Wehrmann C. AALIANCE ambient assisted living roadmap. In: Ambient Intelligence and Smart Environments. Amesterdão: IOS Press; 2010. ISBN: 978-1-60750-498-6

[52] Innovative ICT Solutions for Ageing – Ambient Assisted Living [Internet]. [in press]. Available from: www.aal-europe.eu/about us [Accessed: Oct 3, 2017]

[53] Lumini M, Peres H, Martins T. 2016. Evaluation of the educational technology "Caring for dependent people" by family caregivers in changes and transfers of patients and tube feeding. Revista Latino – Americana de Enfermagem. 2016;**24**:1-8. DOI: 10.1590/1518-8345.0846.2774

[54] European Commission (EC). How digital is your country? New figures reveal progress needed towards a digital Europe. Brussels: European Commission. 2015. Available from: http://ec.europa.eu/digital-agenda/en/news/how-digital-your-country-new-figures-reveal-progress-needed-towards-digital-europe [Accessed: Oct 1, 2017]

[55] Lumini M, Peres H, Martins T. Construction and evaluation of interactive educational technology for family members acting as caregivers on caring for dependent people. Revista Eletrônica de enfermagem. 2017;**19**(19):1-13. DOI: 10.5216/ree.v19.38115

[56] Girgis A, Durcinoska I, Levesque J, Gerges M, Sandell T, Arnold A, Delaney G, PROMPT-Care Program Group. eHealth system for collecting and utilizing patient reported outcome measures for personalized treatment and care (PROMPT-Care) among cancer patients: Mixed methods approach to evaluate feasibility and acceptability. Journal of Medical Internet Research. 2017;**19**(10):e330. DOI: 10.2196/jmir.8360

[57] Lumini M, Martins T, Peres H. Nurses' perception on the difficulties and information needs of family members caring for a dependent person. Texto & Contexto Enfermagem. 2016;**25**(1):1-9. DOI: 10.1590/0104-07072016000430015

[58] Leslie E, Marshall A, Owen N, Bauman A. Engagement and retention of participants in a physical activity website. Preventive Medicine. 2005;**40**:54-59. DOI: 10.1016/j.ypmed.2004.05.002

[59] Macedo M, Pereira A. Desenvolvimento de Recomendações de Acessibilidade e Usabilidade para Ambientes Virtuais de Aprendizagem Voltados para o Usuário Idoso. Revista Novas Tecnologias na Educação. 2009;**7**(1):E10. Available from: https://www.w3.org/WAI/older-users/developing.html

[60] Kachar V. A terceira idade e o computador: interação e produção no ambiente educacional interdisciplinar [Tese]. Currículo da PUC. São Paulo: PUC-SP; 2001

[61] Arch A, Abou-Zhara S. How Web Accessibility Guidelines Apply to Design for the Ageing Population. 2004. Available from: https://www.google.pt/search?q=Arch+%26+Abou-Zhara%2C+2004).&oq=Arch+%26+Abou-Zhara%2C+2004).&aqs=chrome..69i57.1238j0j1&sourceid=chrome&ie=UTF-8

[62] Pickering H. Inclusive design patterns. In: Magazine S, editor. Coding Accessibility into Web Design. 2016. 271 p

[63] Cybis W, Betiol A, Faust R. Ergonomia e Usabilidade: Conhecimentos, Métodos e Aplicações. 3rd ed. São Paulo: Novatec Editora Lta, 2007. 344 p

12

# Caregiving and the Family

Olawunmi Olagundoye and Morenike Alugo

**Abstract**

Caregiving is the routine rendering of care by a caregiver who has taken the sole responsibility for ensuring that the fundamental needs of the care recipient are met. With the population aging and the increasing trend of non-communicable diseases (NCDs), the need and the demand for home care will rise exponentially. Caregiving for most chronic illnesses has become a fastidious task requiring a combination of formal and informal caregivers to meet the needs of care recipients. The informal caregiving role falls squarely on the shoulders of the family, which remains the basic unit of every society connected biologically, legally or by choice, from which one expects a measure of physical, financial, and emotional support. This chapter discusses caregiving, home care, and the family against the backdrop of diverse world realities in beliefs and attitudes towards healthcare services and home care. It attests to the preferences for home care by some group of patients with chronic/terminal illnesses, especially the elderly, and it also expounds on reasons for this preference, the benefits to the patients and the family, including the family's need for support in dealing with the burden of caregiving for relatives with chronic illnesses.

**Keywords:** caregivers, healthcare financing, cross-cultural comparison, home care services, burden of care

## 1. Introduction

### 1.1. Caregiving: What, who, and why?

The term 'caregiving' as simply derived from the two separate words connotes the act of giving out care or extending care to an external body. The English Oxford Living dictionary describes it as the provision of the necessary and needful for the protection, welfare and total well being of an individual or a thing. Caregiving can simply be defined as the process or act of rendering care services to other people, who as a result of illness or disorder, have a deficit in or have lost the independent capabilities of carrying out certain fundamental activities on their own [1]. It encompasses the provision of assistance to another who needs help in the carrying out the activities of daily living [2]. Rendering of care, assistance, support, aid, all connote the term 'caregiving' to individuals unable to function independently due to some certain form of impairments/disability or the other, often involving two groups of individuals: the caregiver and the care recipient [3]. The caregiver is the active person who renders the care to the passive care recipient who is on the receiving end [1]. It is usually an ongoing process, which involves execution of duties and routines by somebody who has taken the sole responsibility of ensuring the fundamental activities of the individual in need of care [1]. According to the work and family research networks, caregiving is generally rendered in three dimensions, which are instrumental, informational and emotional caring [4]. Instrumental caring involves performing tasks as household chores, errands, cleaning. Emotional caring involves emotional support and companionship, counseling, listening, and attending to psychological needs. Informational caring involves learning about the ailment and how to provide favorable conditions for the patient [4]. This term caregiving is rarely used in reference to the form daily care rendered by parents to their children as this is often referred to as parenting [5]. Caregiving according to Sociologists is often discussed in the light of unpaid workers who are usually relatives and friends although, all forms of caregiving are also rendered by paid workers who are usually trained professionals [4]. Caregiving is of optimal importance as it is an inevitable way of ensuring that the ill and disabled can thrive.

### 1.2. Types of caregiving

The act of caregiving can be categorized into two major types based on the source of care being rendered:

#### *1.2.1. Informal caregiving*

Informal caregiving signifies a form of caregiving that is less structured and in which the caregivers are not paid for the services rendered. According to the Los Angeles public health publication, informal caregiving is the daily support and help rendered by family members and friends to their temporarily or permanently ill relatives who are unable to function independently [6]. Often, informal caregiving occurs in a family setting involving parents, grandparents, siblings, children, cousins, spouses, in-laws, and other relatives. In some cases, it could involve friends, neighbors, and good Samaritans [1]. It is usually based on some form of social relationship between the caregiver and the care recipient and often evolves partly out of societal expectations of a family, as well as the inherent obligation of one family member to the other [1]. According to a publication by the international federation on aging, informal caregivers are those caregivers who receive no payment or payment below the market value where the caregiver might refuse to perform the same task at the same wage if it were outside their social circle [7]. This simply signifies that a major factor in informal care revolves around the form of relationship and social responsibility the caregiver has to the care recipient. For example, a son who was brought up by his parents, an uncle, an aunt, stepparents or even a family friend would feel the obligation and responsibility to care for these people peradventure they became ill at any point in time. The role of informal caregivers is of paramount importance being an essential resource to the care recipient and to the healthcare system in general [8].

### 1.2.2. Formal caregiving

As the name implies, formal caregiving is a planned and structured form of caregiving where the caregivers are employed and get paid for the services they render. These caregivers are mostly professionals such as nurses, doctors and other professional health workers who are trained to carry out services. Due to this nature of formal caregiving, there exists the possibility of them rendering services that informal caregivers cannot render. Depending on the severity and specialty of the illness, formal caregivers are usually in demand alongside informal caregivers for home care services [9]. Formal caregiving is often times the last resort for families who face challenges in providing the necessary care for their ill relatives [7].

Informal caregiving can be categorized into primary caregiving and secondary caregiving.

In primary caregiving, the primary caregiver lives with the individual in need of the care and substitutes for the deficient activities or tasks such as bathing and feeding. They bear most of the recipient's burden of care in terms of emotional, financial and physical support [10].

In secondary caregiving, on the other hand, the secondary caregiver usually does not live with the care receiver but gives support and assistance in form of finances, visits, and transportation to and from the hospital [10]. In cases where family members are unable to provide the necessary attention and care needed by the ill relative, secondary caregiving is usually the form of care rendered by the family members in which they might, in turn, employ a formal caregiver who can be paid to render optimal care around the activities of daily living required for the subsistence of the ill relative.

A larger percentage of caregivers often fall under informal caregiving. According to the Utah coalition for caregiver support, there are more than 22.4 million persons who serve as informal caregivers rendering unpaid services to the elderly in the community [2]. Despite countering factors, family caregivers i.e. informal caregivers are the ones who produce up to 80-90% of both personal and medical related care of older relatives, and one in four American citizens' falls under the caregiver position [2].

## 2. Caregiving in diverse climes and at different times

The act of caregiving and the need for it are universal. However, caregiving varies in different contexts from the developing world to the developed world. The differing health systems, norms, values and beliefs in different parts of the world play significant roles in caregiving. A study carried out to explore the influence of culture on family caregiver experience revealed that among African American, Asian American, Hispanic American, and European American, there were commonalities in the experience of caregiving and the challenges that come with. However, significant distinctions appeared in the cultural norms, beliefs and values that shaped the caregiving experience of the people [11]. Cultural diversity across nations has resulted in the differences observed in the employment of informal caregiving or formal caregiving. Studies have revealed that minority caregivers are less likely to employ formal caregiving services in contrast with white caregivers who more often utilize formal support services [12]. There is consistency in the lower level of employment of formal caregiving services by minority groups and the findings, which show that minority caregivers provided more to their ill relatives in comparison to the whites [13]. The diversity in caregiving may also be assessed on the basis of the social orientation of the society. A society's orientation towards collectivism and individualism and the resulting values that guide their social behavior have been discovered to influence the caregiving role, in particular, the question of who takes the responsibility of rendering care [14, 15]. The informal form of caregiving predominates in most developing countries, which are collectivist in orientation. In these societies, family members play major roles in the care of their ill relatives. The role of caregivers in collectivist societies is usually culturally determined based on a set of hierarchy determining who is to render care and a traditional gender ideology that portrays care as a feminine role [14]. The national health systems are also a cogent factor that determines access to and uptake of health care services in general. Health infrastructure and the health care financing are influenced by the economic and political milieu. In many low and middle-income countries (LMIC), there appears to be poor access to health care services, which are grossly disproportionate to the population sizes. Access and equity are further impeded by the nature of health care financing where out-of-pocket payment still exceeds health insurance schemes. In the earlier century, there were few choices for family members who had ill relatives and care often fell on the family members, but in more recent times, there is easier access to information, more support and more resources available for both the caregivers and the care recipients [2]. The issue of health care financing has always posed a challenge, particularly in LMIC. Unlike the earlier times, health insurance schemes are evolving in LMIC, in addition to aids from nongovernmental organizations, welfare packages from local co-operative societies and other projects established to aid health financing. In Nigeria for instance, there is the National Health Insurance Scheme (NHIS), which was established to promote financial access to equitable health care for enrollees. Unfortunately, only about 10% of the population is currently covered by the NHIS [15]. The majority of the citizens finance their health care out-of-pocket.

Informal home caregiving may be the economically realistic alternative in these resource-constrained settings. In high-income countries, however, health insurance is a widely accepted practice. There are cross-cultural differences in the beliefs and attitude of the people towards healthcare and utilization of health insurance in the developing and developed worlds.

## 3. Home care: An inevitable part of chronic care

### 3.1. What is home care?

Home care is a form of caregiving rendered in the home of individuals in need of healthcare services. It includes a wide range of healthcare services that can be rendered within the home [16]. Rather than being present for healthcare services at the hospital, the individual receives care at home. An in-depth definition of home care was given in 2007 by the African Medical Research Foundation (AMREF) with respect to home and community-based care of people living with HIV/AIDs. Home care was defined as the form of care directed towards individuals with chronic/terminal illnesses, which is being extended from the hospital to the homes of the patients through a combination of both family and community involvement, within the available resources and in cooperation with other healthcare workers [17].

These health care services rendered in home care are usually as effective as hospital care, as the goal still remains to manage and treat the illness [18]. Literarily, with the term 'home care' it becomes apparent that the family plays a great role in this decision; it is either the home care is carried out by family members, by medical practitioners or by a combination of the two in the home. Often, home care involves four major components of care services, namely: clinical care, nursing care, counseling/psycho-spiritual care and social support [19]. With the inherent components of home care, it can be said to constitute a combination of formal and informal care carried out within the home. Depending on geographical, socio-cultural, and economic factors, one of the two, i.e., formal or informal care may predominate in the rendering of home care services. Informal home care services can be explained as the services rendered by the family members and other community members within the confines of the home whilst formal home care services are rendered by medical practitioners and experts who receive payment for their services.

### 3.2. Why home care?

Home care often times appears to be an inevitable part of chronic care. In cases where people are faced with a range of chronic illnesses, which are usually long lasting and demanding of effective treatment/management to avoid further disability, home care becomes a necessity as it ensures that patients do not have to be kept within the confines of the hospital before healthcare can be accessed [19]. Patients with chronic diseases are often recommended for home care as they cannot be restricted to the hospital for as long as the illness lasts. Home care allows for more flexibility because it allows for patients to go on with their lives without having to be limited by hospital time schedules [20]. Home care is a major form of care for the elderly who have become too frail and weak to function and live independently. Also, in cases of mental illnesses, treatment, and monitoring often result in the demand for effective home care services so as to improve function and prevent relapse [20].

### 3.3. Benefits of home care

Home care has numerous benefits. Studies have revealed the positive impacts of home care in the physical, psychological, social, and economic well-being of the patients, the family, community, and the healthcare system [19]. One is the fact that patients do not have to be kept in the hospital environment indefinitely. This reduces the risk of hospital-acquired infection in individuals who were on admission for other non-communicable diseases (NCDs). Being nursed at home provides an increased sense of recovery. Although home care might initially be perceived to be less efficient in comparison to care in the hospital where the facilities are at the beck and call of the physicians, the truth remains that it is as effective as the care received in the hospital. Home care comes with numerous benefits for the patients, the family, and the community. Starting with the patient, home care provides a sense of comfort and belonging as they receive treatment at the home, which is a familiar environment where other supportive family members may be present [21]. It helps to maintain independence [22], allowing the patients to go on with their normal lives and remain in contact with family members. For example, patients who are head of their homes continue doing so and are able to fully getting in family matters and decision making [19]. In most cases, home care appears to be more affordable as it costs less than hospitalizing patients especially in cases of chronic and palliative care. Generally, for the patient, home care allows for a more stable emotional health, being surrounded by loved ones in the comfort of the home makes a lot of difference, being in a familiar environment makes the illness more tolerable [19]. The patients are able to get assistance in carrying out their daily activities. Home care is also very advantageous for one-on-one focus on the patient, it allows for the rendering of individualized services, which focuses on the recipient's health needs [23]. It has been reported that a patient who is being attended to by a clinician or medical personnel in the comfort of their home often displays levels of trust that the Physician places their needs first [24]. For the family and community, home care allows for a steady relationship between the family members and their ill loved ones [25]. It maintains the family bond without any form of separation due to illness [19]. It also alleviates stress for the family member as constant visits to the hospital to monitor the progress in the health of a sick relative might result in some degree of stress and increased financial cost. The additional expenses that might be incurred from bed charges, food items and the likes if the patients were in the hospital are eliminated through home care. It also enables the family members to be present during the time of death [19]. For the community, home care permits a more affordable provision of support for the ill and also ensures that there is existent cohesiveness in the community with regards to caring for others in need [26].

To the healthcare system, home care helps to reduce the exasperating demand of health care on the health system by eliminating overcrowding of in-patient facilities, and ensuring effectiveness. Healthcare practitioners' workload is also reduced and where structural resources are limited, the demand on the health facility is reduced [19].

### 3.4. Major role players in home care

Home care basically involves two key players without whom no form of care will take place. The caregivers themselves are the active players who render care to the passive players who are at the receiving end. The active players in relation to home care can vary depending on several factors, such as the nature of the illness and the demands of care, epidemiological, socio-cultural and socio-economic factors. They can either be informal caregivers or formal caregivers depending on these factors. According to the African medical research foundation, the key providers of home care were classified as the patient, the family, the health workers, the community, and the government [19]. This list presents a combination of both formal and informal caregivers. Formal caregivers involved in the provision of home care services are practitioners as doctors, Family Doctors, Community Nurses, Social workers, also specialized practitioners such as Oncologists, Pediatricians, Gynecologists, Palliative care providers, Psychologists, and others. The nature of the illness usually determines the type of healthcare practitioner to be involved. Friends, nuclear, and extended family members are involved in home care in an informal capacity. The structure and functionality of the home is also a cogent factor as the state/condition of the facilities in the home may influence the nature and the extent of caring that can be done.

There are volunteer workers who offer home care services, and they may be retired professionals or others with interest in healthcare or healthcare charity organization workers [7]. Community service in the form of home care services may be meted out to public offenders through the legal system in some developed countries. The community and government cannot be left out of the equation as they also exert great influence on the wellbeing of the ill in the community. The government plays a significant role in creating a supportive environment by establishing policies, setting and maintaining standards to support caregiving [19].

### 3.5. Elderly patients with terminal/chronic illnesses and their care preferences

Terminal and chronic illnesses are medical situations that require constant medical attention. Chronic illnesses are long-lasting illnesses that progress gradually with time; these illnesses often affect the quality of life of the patients if they are not properly managed [19]. They include hypertension, bronchial asthma, diabetes mellitus, Parkinson's disease, and neurocognitive disorders/dementia, which majorly affect the elderly. These conditions often require continuous medical care so as to sustain functioning and prevent deterioration. The preference of patients with these chronic illnesses usually falls within home care, the case being that these patients cannot remain within the confines of the hospital for as long as their illness lasts. Once the major treatment has been received where the doctor does the necessary medical treatment, prescribes drugs, and does the necessary therapy and counseling, the patients and their relatives can make decisions to continue with home care. Some patients and their families favor home care services carried out by family members, in addition to home visits by medical practitioners as the situation demands [19]. Home care allows for more emotional support and a quick sense of recovery for these patients ensuring they go on with their daily lives [22]. Although there are several factors that may affect the decisions of these patients regarding home care; factors such as the availability of family members to take up the responsibility of acting as primary caregivers, providing support, and constant care. In the absence of these informal primary caregivers or in situations where the family desires to ease members of the physical burden of care, the tasks may be shifted to nursing homes. In the case of terminal illnesses where death is inevitable, the goal is to improve the quality of life, by relieving pain, discomfort and ensuring more emotional balance, support, and happiness for the patients. Palliative care is the form of care rendered to terminally ill patients to make pain and sorrow easier to bear though curing is unattainable and death inevitable [27]. Home care is usually more preferable for terminal illnesses as these patients need to feel more accepted and loved in their remaining days [19]. Although home care is a more preferred option for elderly and terminally ill patients, the society, and cultural beliefs also determines the choice of home care for terminally ill patients. In countries ruled by the idea of collectivism, the act of family members caring for their older relatives, their chronically/terminally ill relatives are common [11]. On the other hand, in individualistic societies, there is usually a shift away from informal care in the home for chronically/terminally ill relatives to a more formalized form of care [11]. Thus, a form of care, which is designed basically for patients nearing the end of life, i.e. the terminally ill, becomes more popular [25]. This care was designed to provide professional care to maximize comfort for terminally ill patients by looking into the psychological, physical, spiritual and physical needs of the patients. Hospice care is often the resort for terminally ill patients in most developed countries to ease relatives of some of the burden of care, and to prepare the patients and their families for the end [25]. In most African countries, family relatives hold the belief that their elderly relatives who are ill should preferably die at home. It is a custom in some African societies for older relatives to return home once they are approaching death. The employment of hospice care is still at the evolutionary stage in most developing countries and where they currently exist; they may be elitist and out of the reach of the common man.

## 4. Family and care giving

The family is the basic unit of every society; it is defined as a social and intimate nurturing group of individuals connected biologically, legally or by choice from whom one expects a measure of support in form of food, shelter, clothing, finance, emotion and natural nurturing as well as sharing a past, present and future together [28]. The family forms the basic unit of care for every individual; it is in the family setting that every individual receives first-hand attention whenever an ailment is discovered. In cases of less severe illnesses, family members are mostly capable of bringing about recovery without the ill relative having to visit the hospital [8]. This makes the act of caregiving to fall majorly within the family. Informal caregiving appears to be the more predominating form of care. Consequently, the members of the family are regarded as critical partners in the care of the patients, and family functioning becomes a significant factor in determining the quality of care rendered by informal caregivers. Families play very significant roles in the treatment of their ill relatives [7]. The existence of an emotional bond and a sense of belonging explains the clear differences in the approach to care by families in comparison with the professional and mostly formal relationship that patients have with their healthcare providers.

Most patients find it very rewarding to have their loved ones around to care for them, and to accompany them through their healing process. However, this does not imply that family caregivers are adequately equipped to provide most of the care needs to hasten recovery. They are not professional caregivers, and they often have multiple roles and tasks to attend to [9]. These constitute some form of stress, both physical and emotional as they try to meet up with several demands [29]. Family members as caregivers are also not trained and are usually less skilled in rendering care for particular illnesses [9]. In view of the foregoing, it becomes expedient to combine both formal and informal caregiving services to guarantee effective outcomes.

## 5. Burden of care on informal (family) caregivers

The burden of care is a complex, multifactorial construct, which includes emotional, psychological, physical and economic impact as well as related distressing feelings such as shame, embarrassment, anger, feeling of guilt, and self-blame [29]. It is customary to describe burden as for either objective or subjective. A researcher differentiated between objective and subjective burden [30]. Objective burden is a disruption to family/household life, which is potentially verifiable and observable. It refers to changes in household routine, family or social relations, work, leisure, and physical health. Subjective burden consists of subjective distress among relatives including the impact on mental health, personal feelings of carrying a burden, being unhappy or upset [30, 31]. It was also pointed out that one aspect of the objective burden is in fact based on a subjective experience {distress} whose presence or absence is logically assumed by the investigator [30]. Thus, the investigator is consistently considered a better judge of caregivers' feelings than the caregivers themselves. Family caregivers have been described as forgotten or hidden patients and it was suggested that caregivers' symptoms such as mood swings, headache, joint and muscle pain, marital and family conflicts, and financial problems may be a reflection of caregivers' stress in looking after a sick relative [32]. Most studies of family burden in severe mental illness have taken place in developed countries and they reported that family caregivers experience high levels of burden [33, 34]. There has been an emergence of self-help and advocacy groups of affected families and also a rising pressure towards involving consumer groups in service planning during the last two decades, which has helped in bringing the needs of the informal caregivers into increasing focus [35]. From the result of a study conducted in 2009, it was revealed that providing support that enhances the quality of life of patients with mental illness may indirectly help reduce the sense of burden felt by family members caring for them [36]. Caregivers have been described as hidden patients who also need attention so as to be protected from both physical and emotional harm. Interventions to reduce burden are important in directly curtailing caregiver distress and promoting overall well being whilst the care recipient also benefits secondarily from such interventions [27]. Intervention for caregivers can come in different forms to help increase the confidence and competence of caregivers in providing effective care for the care recipients which in turn help in eliminating the feelings of distress among caregivers [37]. Healthcare professionals have significant roles to play in alleviating the burden on informal caregivers. More involvement by health practitioners in the duties carried out by informal caregivers often proves effective. Counseling sessions carried out by healthcare practitioners to enlighten and educate caregivers often results in a significant reduction in burden [38].

The significance of support for informal caregivers cannot be overemphasized as it has also been suggested that burden of care indirectly affects medication adherence and by extension the course of illness [39]. This gives credence to the fact that family intervention is needful as part of the holistic care of the patient with a chronic illness. Gender, socio-economic, and cultural factors also influence the experience of caregiver burden by the family members. Most often, mothers take up the most of the physical responsibilities for caring for the patients, and women have been found to report poorer states of perceived health [40]. Fathers, on the other hand, take up the financial responsibilities and are more likely to experience burden in relation to their finances. A number of socio-demographic characteristics of the caregivers exert great influence on the levels of burden. A study in the province of Arica, Chile involving 41 relatives of patients with schizophrenia who were attending a public mental health outpatient service showed a very high degree of a burden especially in mothers, older relatives with low educational level, unemployed caregivers and those taking care of young patients and caregivers of patients with more hospitalization in the previous 3 years. Similar findings were made in an African context, where it was observed that those who cared for patients in the age range 21–45 years were the most burdened [40]. A more recent study in a similar context revealed a significant relationship between gender and the experience of caregiver burden, with females accounting for 67.3% of those with a high burden [3]. A high level of burden was also found among mothers (35.1%) and spouses (33.9%). It was also revealed that level of income played a significant role as the majority of the participants who experienced low burden earned above $125 whilst those with high burden earned less than $62.50 [3]. Furthermore, living in rural areas, large family size, the severity of patients' illness, and caregivers' low level of education were associated with a high level of burden in Nigeria [41–43].

It has been shown that the incidence of depression in caregivers is high, ranging from 18 to 47% and caregivers who are depressed experience higher degrees of burden [44]. A landmark study of caregivers' health revealed that elderly spousal caregivers who experienced caregiver strain had a mortality risk that was 63% higher than that in control subjects [45]. The implications of this study make early identification of caregiver burden and appropriate intervention even more critical. The caregiver burden experience can be controlled by a process of family intervention. This is an essential plan for assessing the family functioning and establishing ways of managing the experience of burden. Emotional burden experienced by primary caregivers is a pressing factor that cannot be overlooked. This factor spells out the need to care for caregivers through therapy sessions and enlightenment on how they can manage their emotional health and wellbeing. Counseling and educating caregivers on how they can adopt coping strategies and deal with stress will go a long way. Adjustments in Government policies regarding health financing and insurance are also ways of improving access to healthcare and reducing the financial burden on middle and low-income families.

## Author details

Olawunmi Olagundoye[1*] and Morenike Alugo[2]

*Address all correspondence to: olabima@yahoo.com

1 Department of Family Medicine, General Hospital Lagos, Lagos, Nigeria

2 Department of Psychology, Faculty of Social Sciences, University of Lagos, Lagos, Nigeria

## References

[1] Schulz R, Patterson TL. Caregiving in geriatric psychiatry. The American Journal of Geriatric Psychiatry. 2004;**12**(3):234-237

[2] Utah Coalition for Caregiver Support. What is caregiving? Available from: http://utahcares.org/caregiving-2/ [Accessed: September 16, 2016]

[3] Olagundoye O, Akhuemokhan V, Alugo M. Towards caring for caregivers: Assessing the burden of care and experience of associative stigma among caregivers of patients with 17 chronic mental illnesses at a mental health care facility in Lagos Metropolis, Nigeria. Family Medicine & Primary Care Review. 2017;**19**(2):149-155

[4] Care Giving Definitions. Work and Family Researcher's Network. Available from: https://workfamily.sas.upenn.edu/glossery/c/caregiving-definations [Accessed: October 2, 2017]

[5] Drentea P. Caregiving. In: Ritzer G, editor. Blackwell Encyclopedia of Sociology. New Jersey: Blackwell Publishing; 2006. Blackwell Reference Online. Available from: http://www.blackwellreference.com/ [Accessed: June 23, 2007]

[6] Los Angeles County Department of Public Health, Office of Health Assessment and Epidemiology. Informal Caregiving: Implications for Public Health, LA Health. Available from: www.publichealth.lacounty.gov/ha/reports/habriefs/2007/Caregiving_Final [Accessed: February 2010]

[7] Connecting the Dots: Formal and Informal Care. International Federation on Aging. 2014. Available from: www.IFA-FIV.ORG [Accessed: June 10, 2014]

[8] Schulz Rand Tompkins CA. Informal Caregivers in the United States: Prevalence, Caregiver Characteristics, and Ability to Provide Care. The Role of Human Factors in Home Health Care: Workshop Summary. National Academy of Sciences. 2010. Available from: https://www.ncbi.nlm.nih.gov/books/NBK210048/

[9] There is No Place Like Your Home. Understanding the Roles of Formal and Informal Caregivers. Community Care. 2010. Available from: http://www.communitycarehhs.com/formal-informal-caregivers.html

[10] Thomas D. About Caregiving: Community Health Services. Available from: www.about-caregiving.com [Accessed: March 20, 2006]

[11] Pharr JR, Francis CD, Terry C, Clark MC. Culture, Caregiving, and Health: Exploring the Influence of Culture on Family Caregiver Experiences. ISRN Public Health, 2014. Retrieved from: http://dx.doi.org/10.1155/2014/689826

[12] Napoles AM, Chadiha L, Eversley R, Moreno-John G. Reviews: Developing culturally sensitive dementia caregiver interventions: Are we there yet? American Journal of Alzheimer's Disease and Other Dementias. 2010;**25**(5):389-406

[13] McCann JJ, Hebert LE, Beckett LA, Morris MC, Scherr PA, Evans DA. Comparison of informal caregiving by black and white older adults in a community population. Journal of the American Geriatrics Society. 2000;**48**(12):1612-1617

[14] Lee KS. Gender, care work, and the complexity of family membership in Japan. Gender and Society. 2010;**24**(5):647-671

[15] Nigeria's Health Insurance Scheme. Insurance. Available from: www.einsurance.com.ng/nigerias-national-health-insurance-scheme-nhis/ [Accessed: September, 2017]

[16] Wallhagen MI, Yamamoto-Mitani N. The meaning of family caregiving in Japan and the United States: A qualitative comparative study. Journal of Transcultural Nursing. 2006;**17**(1):65-73

[17] What's Home Healthcare? Medicare.gov. Available from: www.medicare.gov/what-medicare-covers/home-health-care/home-health-care-what-is-it-what-to-expect [Accessed: November 15, 2017]

[18] What is Medicare? medicare.gov Available from: https://www.medicare.gov/what-medicare-covers/home-health-care/home-health-care-what-is-it-what-to-expect.html [Accessed: September 17, 2017]

[19] Van Acker IN. Home and Community Based Care of PLWHA. Integrated HIV/AIDS Prevention, Treatment and Care. A distance learning course of the Directorate of Learning Systems (AMREF) 2007. Available from: www.colfinder.net/materials/HIV_Course/HIV_Unit_11_SG.odt [Accessed February 4, 2015]

[20] Effiong A. Palliative care for the management of chronic illness: A systematic review study protocol. BMJ Open. Available from: www.bmjopen.bmj.com/content/2/3/e000899 [Accessed: November 15, 2017]

[21] Benefits of Home Care for the Elderly. Precision Home HealthCare, Inc. Available From: www.precision-hhc.com/benefits-of-home-care-for-the-elderly/ [Accessed: September 18, 2017]

[22] Home Healthcare Advantages & Disadvantages. Livestrong.com. Available from: www.livestrong.com/article/79680-home-health-care-advantages-/ [Accessed: September 17, 2017]

[23] Advantages of Home Care. Rhode Island Partnership for Home Care. Available from: www.riphc.org/advantages-of-home-care [Accessed: October 4, 2017]

[24] 10 Benefits of Home Health Care. Bayada Home Health Care 2017. Available from: Blog.bayada.com/cares/bid/344508/24.-benefits-of-home-health-care [Accessed: September 18, 2017]

[25] Hospice Care: Comforting the Terminally Ill. Mayo Clinic. Available from: www.mayo-clinic.org/healthy-lifestyle/end-of-life-/in-depth/hospice-care/art-20048050 [Accessed: September 15, 2017]

[26] WHO. AIDS Home Care Handbook. Geneva: World Health Organization; 1993

[27] Lynch T, Connor S, Clark D. Mapping levels of palliative care development: A global update. Journal of Pain and Symptom Management. 2013;**45**(6):1094-1106

[28] Sloane PD, Slatt LM, Ebell MH, et al., eds. Essentials of Family Medicine. 4th ed. Philadelphia: Lippincott Williams & Wilkins; 2002

[29] Alejandra C, Maldonado JG. Burden of care in families of patients with schizophrenia. Quality of Life Research. 2000;**15**(4):719-724

[30] Platt S. Measuring the burden of psychiatric illness in the family: An evaluation of some rating scales. Psychological Medicine. 1985;**15**:383-393

[31] Rein G, Lancon C, Simeon M, Duplin S. Caregiver burden in relatives of persons with schizophrenia: An overview of measure instruments. Encephale. 2003;**29**(2):137-147

[32] Medalie J. The caregiver as hidden patient; theory and research on healthcare triads. Journal of Health and Social Behavior. 1994;**35**:1-12

[33] Awad G, Vonugant L. The burden of schizophrenia on caregivers: A review. Pharmaco-Economics. 2008;**26**(2):149-162

[34] Harish K, Anil N. Extent and determinants of burden of care in Indian families: A comparison between organic brain disorders (OBD) and Schiz. International Journal of Social Psychiatry. 2009;**55**(1):28-38

[35] Kreisman D, Joy V. Family response to the illness of a relative: A preview of the literature. Schizophrenia Bulletin. 2001;**1**:34-57

[36] Fujino N, Okamura H. Factors affecting the severity of burden felt by family members caring for patients with mental illness. Archives of Psychiatric Nursing. 2009;**23**:128-137

[37] Reinhard SC, Given B, Petlick NH, Bemis A. Supporting family caregivers in providing care. Patient Safety and Quality: An Evidence-Based Handbook for Nurses. Available from: https://www.ncbi.nlm.nih.gov/books/NBK2665/ Accessed: October 4, 2017

[38] Acton GJ, Kang J. Interventions to reduce the burden of caregiving for an adult with dementia: A meta-analysis. Research in Nursing & Health. 2001;**24**:349-360

[39] Perlick DA. Impact of family burden & affective response on clinical outcome among patients with bipolar affective disorder. American Psychiatric Association, Psychiatric Services. 2004;**55**:1029-1035

[40] Martyns Yellowe IS. The burden of schizophrenia on the family: A study from Nigeria. British Journal of Psychiatry. 1992;**161**:779-782

[41] Owoeye O. The Mentally Ill and the Nigerian Society. Available from: http//neuropsychiatrichospitalyaba.org [Accessed: October 10, 2010]

[42] Olukayode JR, William AO, Sijuwola AO. Recent developments in the care, treatment and rehabilitation of the chronic mentally ill in Nigeria. Hospital & Community Psychiatry. 1985;**36**:658-661

[43] Akinbiyi A. The psychosocial burden of caring for some Nigerians with dementia. National Postgraduate Medical College of Nigeria Part II Dissertation in Psychiatry. October 2001

[44] Ostman M, Kjellin L. Psychological factors in relatives of people with mental illness. The British Journal of Psychiatry. 2002;**181**:494-498

[45] World Health Organisation. Mental Health Atlas. Geneva: World Health Organisation; www.globalatlast.who.int/globalatlast/default.asp [Accessed: December 20, 2008]

# Permissions

All chapters in this book were first published in CHC, by InTech Open; hereby published with permission under the Creative Commons Attribution License or equivalent. Every chapter published in this book has been scrutinized by our experts. Their significance has been extensively debated. The topics covered herein carry significant findings which will fuel the growth of the discipline. They may even be implemented as practical applications or may be referred to as a beginning point for another development.

The contributors of this book come from diverse backgrounds, making this book a truly international effort. This book will bring forth new frontiers with its revolutionizing research information and detailed analysis of the nascent developments around the world.

We would like to thank all the contributing authors for lending their expertise to make the book truly unique. They have played a crucial role in the development of this book. Without their invaluable contributions this book wouldn't have been possible. They have made vital efforts to compile up to date information on the varied aspects of this subject to make this book a valuable addition to the collection of many professionals and students.

This book was conceptualized with the vision of imparting up-to-date information and advanced data in this field. To ensure the same, a matchless editorial board was set up. Every individual on the board went through rigorous rounds of assessment to prove their worth. After which they invested a large part of their time researching and compiling the most relevant data for our readers.

The editorial board has been involved in producing this book since its inception. They have spent rigorous hours researching and exploring the diverse topics which have resulted in the successful publishing of this book. They have passed on their knowledge of decades through this book. To expedite this challenging task, the publisher supported the team at every step. A small team of assistant editors was also appointed to further simplify the editing procedure and attain best results for the readers.

Apart from the editorial board, the designing team has also invested a significant amount of their time in understanding the subject and creating the most relevant covers. They scrutinized every image to scout for the most suitable representation of the subject and create an appropriate cover for the book.

The publishing team has been an ardent support to the editorial, designing and production team. Their endless efforts to recruit the best for this project, has resulted in the accomplishment of this book. They are a veteran in the field of academics and their pool of knowledge is as vast as their experience in printing. Their expertise and guidance has proved useful at every step. Their uncompromising quality standards have made this book an exceptional effort. Their encouragement from time to time has been an inspiration for everyone.

The publisher and the editorial board hope that this book will prove to be a valuable piece of knowledge for researchers, students, practitioners and scholars across the globe.

# List of Contributors


**Kendra Ray**
MJHS, Menorah Center for Nursing and Rehabilitation, Brooklyn, NY, USA Drexel University, Philadelphia, PA, USA

**Ayelet Dassa**
Bar-llan University, Ramat Gan, Israel Alzheimer's Medical Center, Ramat Gan, Israel

**Jan Maier**
Jemsong, LLC, Waltham, MA, USA

**Renita Davis**
Troy University at Phenix City, AL, USA

**Olayinka Ogunlade**
Gemma Regis Center for Music Therapy, Lagos, Nigeria

**Assol Cortés-Moreno**
National Autonomous University of Mexico, Faculty of Higher Education Iztacala, Mexico

**Natalia López Celani**
Gabinete de Tecnología Médica, Universidad Nacional de San Juan - Consejo Nacional de Investigaciones Científicas y Técnicas, Argentina GADIB, Facultad Regional San Nicolás, Universidad Tecnológica Nacional, Buenos Aires, Argentina

**Sergio Ponce**
Gabinete de Tecnología Médica, Universidad Nacional de San Juan - Consejo Nacional de Investigaciones Científicas y Técnicas, Argentina

**Olga Lucía Quintero**
Mathematical Modeling Research Group, Universidad EAFIT, Medellín, Colombia

**Francisco Vargas-Bonilla**
SISTEMIC Research Group, Universidad de Antioquia, Medellín, Colombia

**Birgül Özkan**
Ankara Yildirim Beyazit University, Faculty of Health of Sciences, Turkey

**Selahattin Menteş**
Adana Numune Education and Research Hospital, Department of Radiation Oncology, Turkey

**Gökmen Zarasız**
Department of Biostatistics, Faculty of Medicine, Erciyes University, Kayseri, Turkey

**Ulrika Ferm**
DART Centre for Augmentative and Alternative Communication and Assistive Technology, Sahlgrenska University Hospital, Göteborg, Sweden

**Stefan Nilsson and Margaretha Jenholt Nolbris**
Institute of Health and Care Sciences, Sahlgrenska Academy, University of Gothenburg, Göteborg, Sweden

**Petra Linnsand**
Dalheimers hus, Social Resursförvaltning, Göteborg, Sweden

**Annikki Jonsson**
Faculty of Caring Science, Work Life and Social Welfare, University of Borås, Borås, Sweden

**Boštjan Kerbler**
Social Geography, Urban Planning Institute of the Republic of Slovenia Ljubljana, Slovenia

**Birsel Canan Demirbağ**
Public Health Department, Faculty of Health Sciences, School of Nursing, Karadeniz Technical University, Trabzon, Turkey

**Çiğdem Gamze Özkan, Betül Bayrak and Yeter Kurt**
Fundamentals of Nursing Departmant, Faculty of Health Sciences, School of Nursing, Karadeniz Technical University, Trabzon, Turkey

**Fernando L. Vázquez, Vanessa Blanco, Lara López and Ángela Torres**
University of Santiago de Compostela, Santiago de Compostela, Spain

**Patricia Otero**
University of A Coruña, A Coruña, Spain

**María del Carmen Pérez-Fuentes, María del Mar Molero Jurado and José Jesús Gázquez Linares**
University of Almeria, Almeria, Spain

**Antonio G. Lentoor**
UCT Department of Psychiatry and Mental Health, Valkenberg Hospital, Cape Town, South Africa

**Maria José Lumini, Fátima Araújo and Teresa Martins**
School of Nursing of Porto and Center for Health Technology and Services Research, Porto, Portugal

**Olawunmi Olagundoye**
Department of Family Medicine, General Hospital Lagos, Lagos, Nigeria

**Morenike Alugo**
Department of Psychology, Faculty of Social Sciences, University of Lagos, Lagos, Nigeria

# Index

www.ingramcontent.com/pod-product-compliance
Lightning Source LLC
LaVergne TN
LVHW060522210926
848485LV00005B/1128
* 9 7 8 1 6 3 9 8 7 3 9 4 4 *